RADIOGRAPHIC EXPOSURE

Principles & Practice

RADIOGRAPHIC EXPOSURE
Principles & Practice

Jerry Ellen Wallace, MEd, RT(R)
Program Director
School of Radiologic Technology
Mercy Hospital Hamilton
Hamilton, Ohio

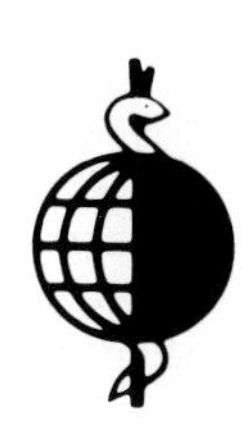

F.A. DAVIS COMPANY • PHILADELPHIA

F. A. Davis Company
1915 Arch Street
Philadelphia, PA 19103

Printed in the United States of America

Last digit indicates print number: 19 18 17 16 15 14 13 12

Publisher, Allied Health: Jean-François Vilain
Allied Health Editor: Lynn Borders Caldwell
Production Editor: Glenn L. Fechner
Cover Designer: Louis J. Forgione
Art Assistant: Jack Kiefer

Library of Congress Cataloging in Publication Data

Wallace, Jerry Ellen, 1945-
Radiographic exposure: principles & practice / Jerry Ellen Wallace.
p. cm.
Includes index.
ISBN 10: 0-8036-0051-8 (pbk. : alk. paper) ISBN 13: 978-0-8036-0051-5
1. Radiography, Medical—Exposure. I. Title.
[DNLM: 1. Radiography 2. Technology, Radiologic. 3. Radiography—problems. 4. Technology, Radiologic—problems. WN 180 W191r 1995]
RC78. W27 1995
616.07'572 — dc20
DNLM/DLC
for Library of Congress 95-741
CIP

To

my husband, Ron and my parents, Ann and Sonny.

Acknowledgments

Many people have helped with the production of this book. I would like to thank my editor, Lynn Borders Caldwell, for her encouragement. I valued the ideas and critiques of all the reviewers of the manuscript, and I am grateful for the many hours they spent on the various drafts. The reviewers included:

Sandsha Abuschinow, BS, RT, Holy Family College, Philadelphia

Joseph R. Bittengle, MEd, RT(R), University of Arkansas Medical Center, Little Rock

Mary Cullen, BS, RT(R), Elkins Park Radiology, Ltd., Elkins Park, Pennsylvania

Eugene D. Frank, BS, RT(R), FASRT, Mayo Clinic Foundation, Rochester, Minnesota

Diane Mayfield, RT(R), Indian Hills Community College, Ottumwa, Iowa

MaryLou Walsh Phillips, MBA, RT(R), Holy Family College, Philadelphia

Elizabeth W. Price, AAS, RT(R), Community General Hospital, Reading, Pennsylvania

Wanda E. Wesolowski, MAEd, RT(R), Community College of Philadelphia.

The following people graciously provided some of the illustrations in the book: Martin Ratner of Nuclear Associates, Tom Colucchi and Pam McCormack of AGFA Corporation, and Ike Pipkin of Fuji Medical Systems.

I appreciate the interest and encouragement of the staff of Mercy Hospital Hamilton and Fairfield. I am especially grateful to my colleagues, Cindy Hale and Susan Michael, for their critiques. I thank all of my students who taught me as much as I taught them, especially the class of 1994 and 1995 for being "guinea pigs."

My children and family encouraged me through the whole long process. My niece, Mary Jo Petrocelli, helped by reviewing the math appendix. Thank you to my parents, Sonny and Ann, who provided my education. Most of all, a special thank you goes to my husband, Ron, for his support and encouragement and for being my best friend.

Contents

Introduction

THE RADIOGRAPHIC BALANCING ACT

In the movie *The Karate Kid*, Mr. Miage tells the hero of the importance of seeking balance in his life. If you get a chance, rent the movie. It's great! Balance is very important in radiography also. In this book you are going to learn about all the factors that work together to produce a radiographic image, which is the picture of the patient's body on a film. Then you must learn to balance these factors, so the radiograph shows the image of the patient that you are trying to see, appears pleasant to look at, and enables the radiologist to make the diagnosis of what might be wrong with the patient.

The quality of the image is an important aspect of radiography. (Isn't it interesting that the words Miage and image are anagrams? There is probably some significant philosophical point here. If you figure it out let me know.)

Learning about all the technical things that make up a radiographic image is difficult work. Each factor must be examined separately and in depth. Students often get bogged down in this process and forget that the main goal is to seek balance in the finished product. When that goal is achieved, you will be proud to put a marker with your initials on the radiograph. It's just like an artist's signature on a painting.

Radiographic exposure is one of the most difficult subjects for students to learn. Many of the textbooks are written in highly technical language, and they are hard to read and understand. This book is written for students who want a complete book on the principles of radiographic exposure, but one that is understandable.

The text includes activities. Reading is nice for learning, but reading and doing is better. When it is time for you to perform an activity the text will say "Perform activity XX. (The activity will be identified by chapter number and letter, for instance, 3-A, 3-B, and so on.) The activities are numbered to coincide with the chapters in the text.

Many of the activities involve mathematical calculations. If you need to review your math skills, there is a math review in Appendix A.

In this book you first will learn about the balance of four important qualities in a good radiographic image. You will also learn how radiation is produced, and how the radiation produces an image of the patient on a film.

After these introductory chapters, you will investigate in depth each factor that influences the quality of the finished radiograph. There are many of these, and which one to investigate first is not easy to decide. This book is written in sections, and each section can be investigated separately. It is all right if your instructor starts with a different section than the book does.

The book begins with the radiographic qualities that are easiest for students to understand and then moves to the more difficult ones. By then you may have seen some of these things in your clinical education, which will make it easier to relate to the information in the book. At the end of the book, you will understand the balancing act of putting all the factors and qualities together to make a good radiographic image.

New students often watch experienced technologists stand at the control panel and push the buttons and flip the dials around for a few seconds. Then they make the exposure and the radiograph turns out fine most of the time. Students think they'll never be able to do that.

Pushing the buttons and flipping the dials is easy. Knowing which button to push and where to flip the dials and why is the difficult part. But never think of yourself as a button pusher. You are an artist and the good part is that it only takes about ninety seconds to see your art work.

Jerry Ellen Wallace

SECTION I

IMAGE QUALITIES AND IMAGE PRODUCTION

CHAPTER 1

THE FOUR RADIOGRAPHIC QUALITIES

CHAPTER OUTLINE

OBJECTIVES

At the end of this chapter you should be able to:

- List the four radiographic qualities that are used together to produce a radiographic image.
- Define each of the four radiographic qualities.
- Begin to recognize the four radiographic qualities on a radiograph.
- Identify the radiographic qualities that are considered photographic properties and those that are considered geometric properties.
- Identify the radiographic qualities that influence the sharpness of the image and those that influence the visibility of the image.
- List some of the factors that control or influence each radiographic quality.
- Explain how the sharpness and visibility of the image can be separate entities.

The balancing act of radiography is difficult to understand at first. There are four individual qualities that must blend to produce a radiographic image with good overall quality. On one end of the scale are the *photographic* qualities, which allow us to see the image, and on the other end of the scale are the *geometric* qualities, which produce a sharp image. Radiographers have to be careful not to tip the scale in favor of one quality over another or they will not have a good radiograph.

PHOTOGRAPHIC VERSUS GEOMETRIC PROPERTIES

Photographic Properties

The qualities on one end of the image scale are those that affect the visibility of the image. These qualities are **density** and **contrast**. There are many factors that affect

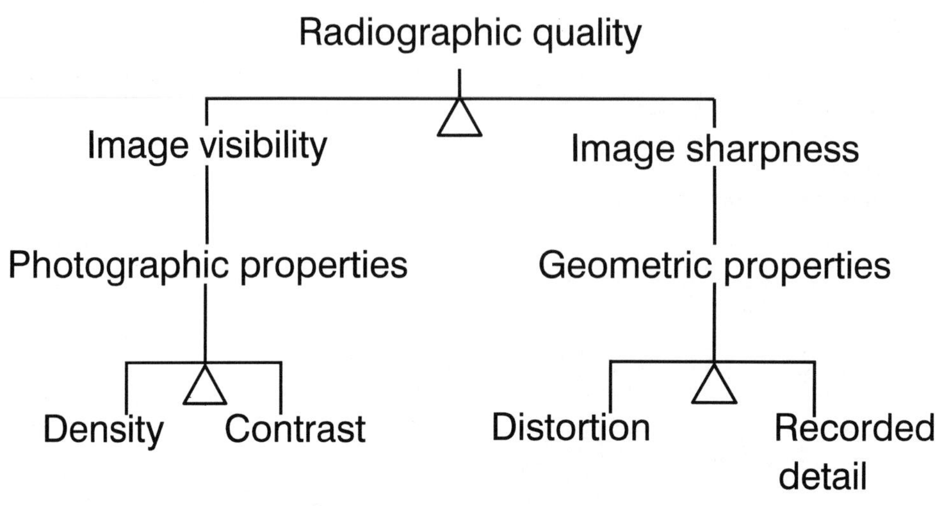

FIGURE 1–1. Radiographic properties and qualities.

these two qualities and this book will investigate each one of these in depth. The qualities on this end of the scale are referred to as **photographic properties**.

Geometric Properties

The qualities on the other end of the image scale are those that affect the sharpness of the image. These qualities are **recorded detail** and **distortion**. There are many factors that affect these two qualities, and this book will investigate each one in depth also. The qualities on this end of the scale are referred to as **geometric properties**.

Figure 1–1 is a chart of these primary qualities and properties.

PERFORM ACTIVITY 1.A

THE FOUR RADIOGRAPHIC QUALITIES

The four radiographic qualities are very important, and it is necessary to understand each before investigating the factors that influence them.

Density

Density is the overall blackness of a radiograph. This is controlled by the quantity of x-rays produced and used to form the image. If a radiograph is too dark or black, it has too much density. If a radiograph is too light or white, it does not have enough density.

Density is the overall blackness of a radiograph.

Contrast

Contrast is the difference between adjacent densities on a radiograph and refers to the number of black, white, and gray tones that appear on the radiograph. Contrast is controlled by the energy of the x-rays in the x-ray beam. A radiograph that has very high contrast will appear too black and white. A radiograph that has very low contrast will appear too gray.

Contrast is the difference between adjacent densities on a radiograph.

Recorded Detail

Recorded detail is the sharpness of the lines of the image. This is controlled by the distances between the x-ray tube, patient, and film. It is also controlled by the devices used to produce the radiograph, which are the film and intensifying screens. A radiograph that appears very sharp or clear has good recorded detail. A radiograph that appears blurry has poor recorded detail.

Recorded detail is the sharpness of the lines of the image.

Distortion

Distortion is the misrepresentation of the true size or shape of the image as compared to the object. The object is the part of the patient's body that is being examined with x-rays. Distortion is controlled by the distance between the x-ray tube, patient, and film, and the alignment of the x-ray tube, patient, and film. When the image of the object on the radiograph looks much bigger than the real object, the image is distorted. This type of distortion is called **magnification** or **size distortion**. When the image of the object on the radiograph looks out of shape compared with the actual object, the image is also distorted. The image may appear to be stretched out of shape as when you pull on a piece of taffy, or it may appear squashed together as when you look at yourself in a funny mirror at an amusement park. This type of distortion is called **shape distortion**.

Distortion is the misrepresentation of the true size or shape of the image as compared to the object.

FACTORS THAT CONTROL AND INFLUENCE RADIOGRAPHIC QUALITY

Each of the four radiographic qualities has factors that control it and factors that influence it. The factors that *control* are considered primary factors, which means the primary factor should be used to change a specific radiographic quality. The factors that *influence* or affect are considered secondary factors, which means they usually play a more minor role in changing the radiographic quality. Some of the factors can affect more than one of the four qualities.

Table 1–1. Factors Affecting the Four Radiographic Qualities

Density	Distortion
mAs* (milliampere-seconds)	OID (object-image distance)
kVp (kilovolts peak)	SID (source-image distance)
SID	Object alignment
Film	Film alignment
Screen	Central ray alignment
Grid	
Beam restriction	
Processing	
Filtration	
Pathology	
OID (used in air gap)	
Patient	
Contrast	**Recorded Detail**
kVp*	SID
Beam restriction	OID
Grid	Focal spot
Processing	Screen
Filtration	Film
OID (used in air gap)	Contact
Patient	Motion
Film	

*These are controlling factors. All the others listed are affecting factors.

Table 1–1 shows a chart of the most important factors that control or influence each of the four primary qualities. A lot of these terms will be new to you. Don't be discouraged that you don't understand them yet. Keep referring to this important chart as you learn about the factors later on in this book. It's good to get an overall picture first and then be able to refer back to the chart if you lose perspective. Table 1–2 gives a brief definition of each term listed in Table 1–1.

PERFORM ACTIVITY 1.B

Table 1–2. Definitions of the Terms Used in Table 1–1.

mAs—Milliampere-seconds. The milliamperage (current in the x-ray tube) multiplied by the exposure time; mAs determines the quantity of x-rays produced and the amount of density on the film.
kVp—Kilovolts peak; determines the energy of the x-ray beam.
SID—The source-image distance; the distance from the x-ray tube to the film.
Processing—Development of the film; makes the image visible.
Film—A sheet of plastic coated with a photographic emulsion; the image is formed on the film, which is placed in a cassette.
Screen—A piece of plastic coated with phosphors; the phosphors light up when struck by x-rays; the light forms the image on the film; the screen is located in the cassette (film holder) along with the film.
Grid—A device that absorbs x-rays and improves contrast; it is made of a layer of lead strips covered with aluminum.
Beam restriction—The collimator; adjusts the size of the area of radiation.
Filtration—Used with the x-ray tube; absorbs low energy x-rays.
Pathology—Disease conditions.
OID—The object-image distance; the distance between the film and the part inside the patient that is being examined.
Central ray—The x-ray that is in the exact center of the x-ray beam.
Focal spot—The place on the anode of the x-ray tube where x-rays are produced.
Contact—The place inside the cassette where the intensifying screen and film meet.
Motion—Movement of the patient during the exposure; this blurs the image.

SHARPNESS VERSUS VISIBILITY

The balance of sharpness and visibility can seem confusing at first. It's difficult to understand how a very sharp image can be produced but we might not be able to see well. It's also difficult to understand how we can see the image well, but at the same time it might not appear sharp or even look like the object we are trying to make an image of. A radiographic image may be sharp but not visible, and it may be visible but not sharp.

Imagine this. Think of driving to the hospital on a foggy day. You always drive past a very pretty house that sits back from the road on a rise. Only today you can't see the house because of the fog. You know the house is still there, and when the fog lifts you will be able to see it again. On a radiograph, the image like the house can be recorded on the film, but it may not be visible due to various conditions like too much density.

Now imagine riding past the same house, but this time you are on your way home after an appointment with an eye doctor. The doctor put drops in your eyes, and your vision is still slightly blurred. When you look at the house it appears blurry. You know that it really isn't blurry, and that tomorrow you will be able to see it clearly again. On a radiograph, the image may not be recorded sharply, but it is still visible.

GOOD IMAGES AND BAD IMAGES

When a radiograph is produced with too much density, it appears too dark or black and the body parts in the image are not visible. The image of the body is still there under the darkness, and if some of the darkness is removed, the image of the body parts will be visible again. If too much of the darkness is removed, the image will become too light or white to see the patient's anatomy. Figure 1 – 2 shows a radiograph with good density, one that is too light, and one that is too dark.

When a radiograph is produced with a **contrast** that is too high or too low, certain parts of the image are emphasized and other parts are de-emphasized. All the parts are still there, but it is impossible to see them all at the same time on the image. Figure 1 – 3 shows a radiograph with good contrast, one with a contrast that is too high, and one with a contrast that is too low.

If a radiograph is produced with poor recorded detail, the image will appear blurry. The image is still there, and if it is cleared up it will be easier to see. Figure 1 – 4 shows a radiograph with good recorded detail and one that appears blurred because of motion of the patient during the exposure.

If a radiograph is produced that is distorted, the image will appear different from the actual object. The image may appear larger than the actual object or not the same shape as the actual object. This can be very confusing to the radiologist and to anybody else who looks only at the image and hasn't seen what the real object looks like. It is the radiographer's job to make the image look as much like the real object as possible. Figure 1 – 5 shows a radiograph without distortion, one with magnification distortion, and one with shape distortion.

PERFORM ACTIVITY 1.C

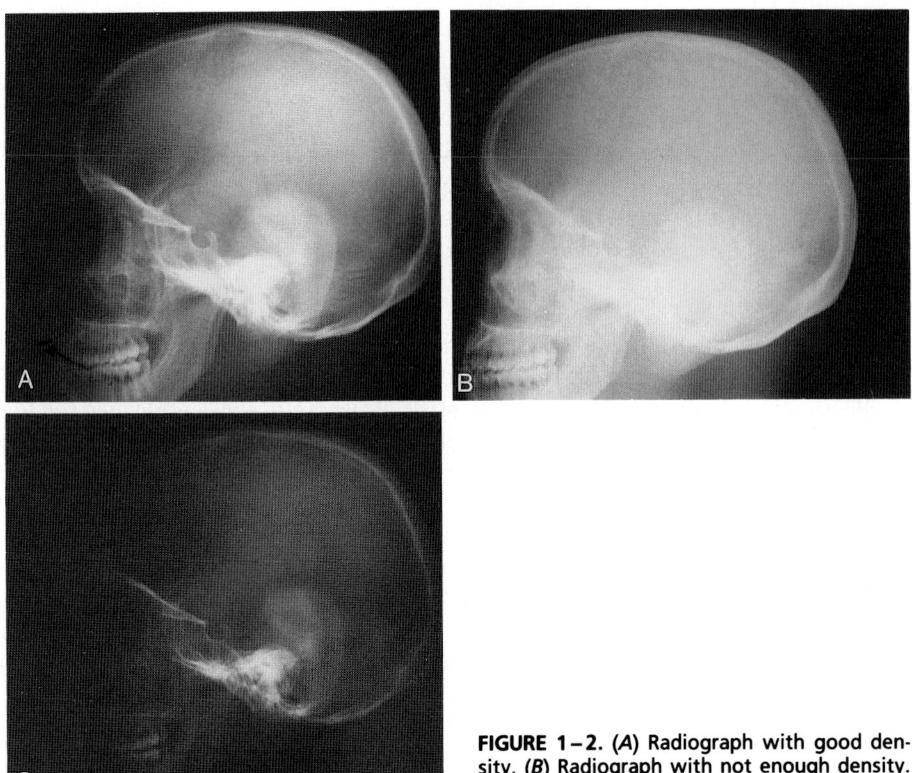

FIGURE 1–2. (*A*) Radiograph with good density. (*B*) Radiograph with not enough density. (*C*) Radiograph with too much density.

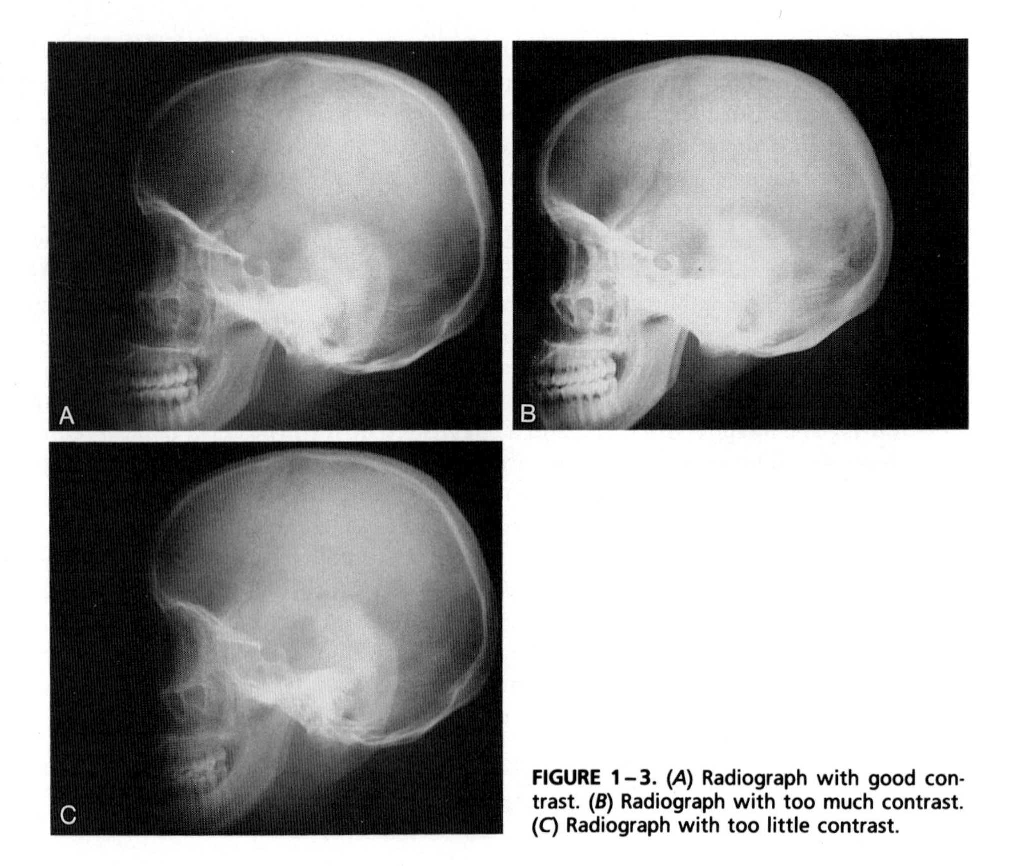

FIGURE 1–3. (*A*) Radiograph with good contrast. (*B*) Radiograph with too much contrast. (*C*) Radiograph with too little contrast.

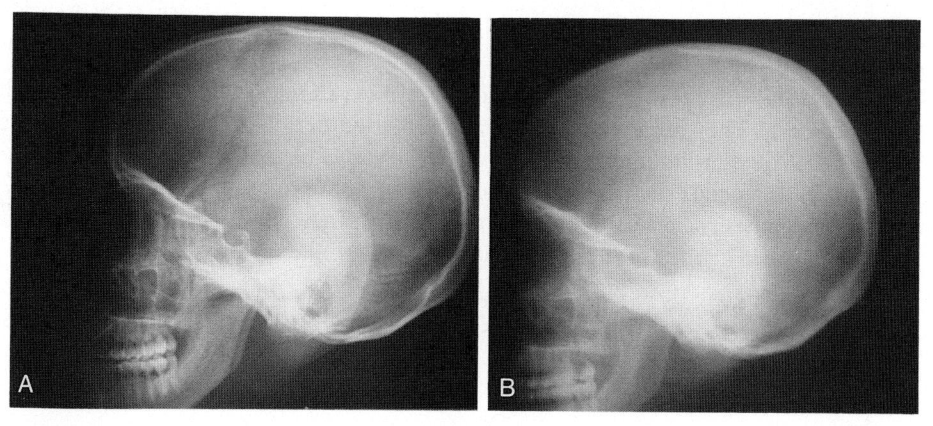

FIGURE 1-4. (*A*) Radiograph with good recorded detail. (*B*) Radiograph with poor recorded detail due to motion.

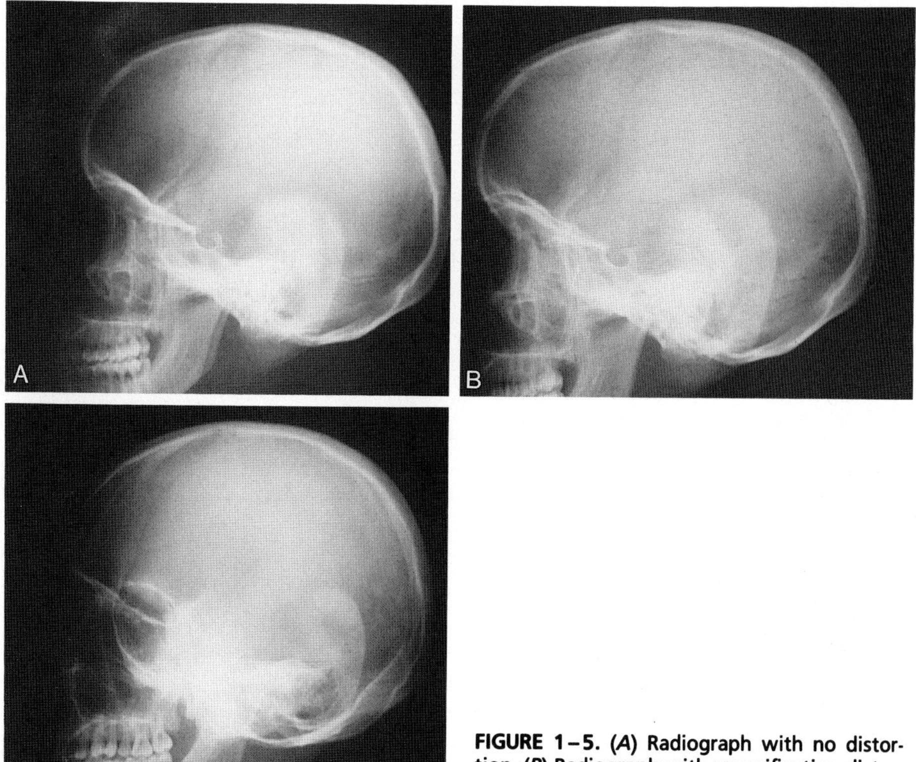

FIGURE 1-5. (*A*) Radiograph with no distortion. (*B*) Radiograph with magnification distortion. (*C*) Radiograph with shape distortion.

SUMMARY

There are four radiographic qualities that affect the overall quality of the finished radiograph. They are density, contrast, recorded detail, and distortion. Density and contrast are called photographic properties, and recorded detail and distortion are called geometric properties. A good radiographic image will have a balance of the four qualities. There are many factors that influence these qualities, and a good radiographer can manipulate the factors to produce an excellent radiograph.

PERFORM ACTIVITY 1.D

CHAPTER 2

The Production and Properties of X-Rays

CHAPTER OUTLINE

OBJECTIVES

At the end of this chapter you should be able to:

- Name and describe the two parts of the cathode.
- Describe the appearance of the anode.
- Explain the purpose of the two x-ray tube housings.
- Draw a diagram of an x-ray tube and label the parts.
- Explain how the parts of the x-ray tube function to produce x-rays.
- Place the events involving the production of x-rays in chronological order.
- Differentiate between the terms anode, target, and focal spot.
- Explain these properties of x-rays: divergent rays, photon energy, visibility, speed, ability to produce scatter, effect on film, effect on phosphors, and the ability to cause biological damage.

In this chapter you will learn about the construction and function of the x-ray tube. X-rays are produced in the x-ray tube, and it is necessary to understand how this occurs before learning how to determine the exposure factors to set on the x-ray control panel.

You will also learn about the properties of x-rays and how x-rays act to produce a radiographic image. This is important to know before you learn to evaluate the quality of the image.

X-RAY TUBE CONSTRUCTION

The inside of the x-ray tube consists of two main parts: the cathode and the anode. These two parts work together to produce x-rays. Electrons are released from the cathode, they zoom over to the anode, and when they collide with the anode, x-rays are produced.

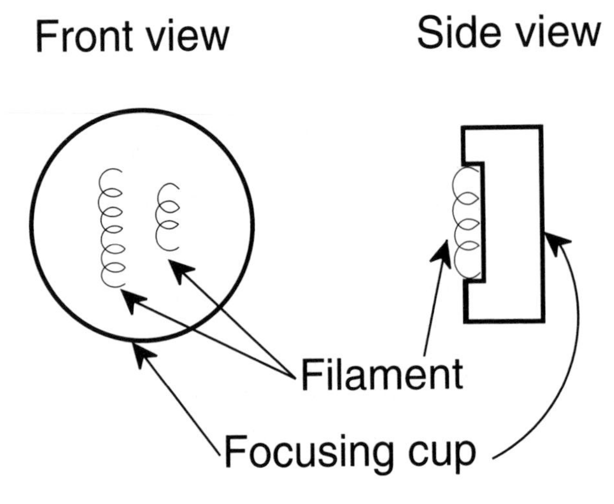

FIGURE 2–1. The cathode of the x-ray tube.

The Cathode

The x-ray tube has two electrodes, the cathode and the anode. When x-rays are produced, current passes between these two electrodes that have opposite charges. The cathode (Fig. 2–1) is the negatively charged electrode. It consists of a focusing cup and two filaments.

The **filament** is a tiny wire made of tungsten and shaped into a coil. It looks a little bit like the spring inside a ballpoint pen. There are usually two filaments, and this type of tube is called a dual-focus x-ray tube. The two filaments are positioned next to each other and are parallel to each other. The large filament is longer than the small filament.

The **focusing cup** surrounds the filament on three sides. The cup is made of molybdenum and it is negatively charged.

The Anode

The anode (Fig. 2–2), which is the positively charged electrode, is a disc made of molybdenum and coated with tungsten, which has a little rhenium added to it. The anode is shaped like a saucer. When visualizing how the anode sits in the x-ray tube, think of a saucer standing on end with its bottom facing the filament wires.

The edge of the anode that tilts back is where the x-rays are produced. The anode rotates while the x-rays are being produced so that the production of x-rays takes place all around the edge of the anode in an area called the **focal track**.

The Glass Envelope

The inside parts of the x-ray tube (the cathode, consisting of the filament and focusing cup, and the anode) are surrounded by a glass housing made of Pyrex (Figure 2–3). This Pyrex glass has lead added to it. While the x-ray tube is being manufactured it is baked, and this removes the air inside the glass housing, creating a vacuum. If the glass envelope cracks, the vacuum is destroyed and it's time to buy a new x-ray tube.

The glass housing has a thin spot in it called the **window**. The x-ray beam is produced at the anode and first exits from the tube through this window before it travels toward the patient's body.

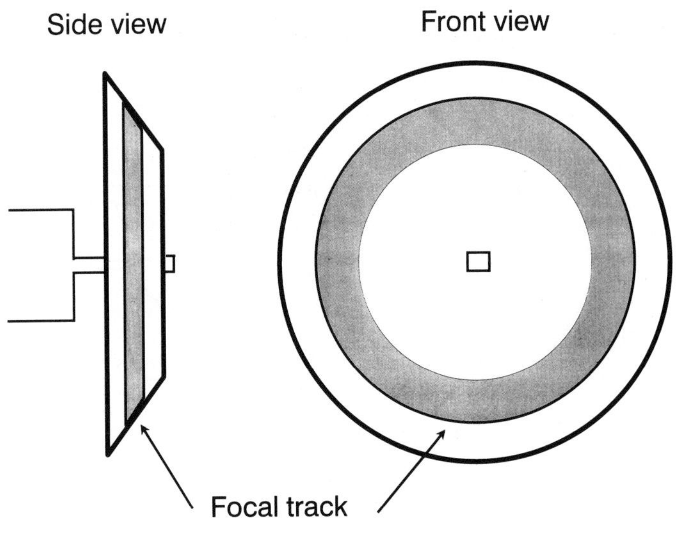

FIGURE 2–2. The anode of the x-ray tube.

The Metal Housing

A metal housing is built on the outside of the glass envelope. One of its purposes is to protect the glass housing. The metal housing is what the radiographer sees when looking at the x-ray tube. The insides of the tube and the glass envelope are hidden by the metal housing. At first students often confuse the collimator box with the tube. The x-ray tube sits above the collimator box (Fig. 2–4).

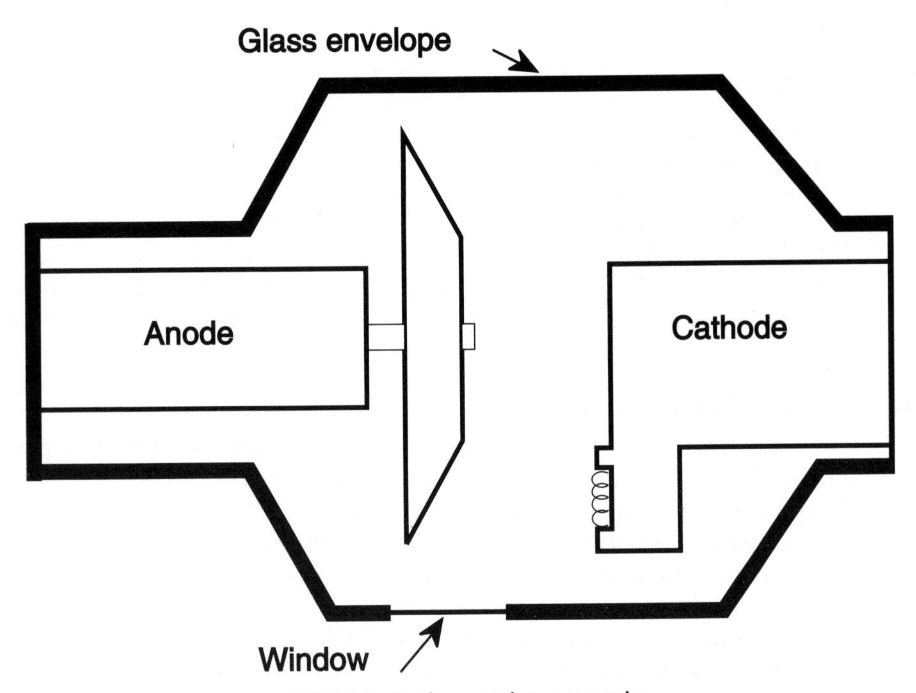

FIGURE 2–3. The complete x-ray tube.

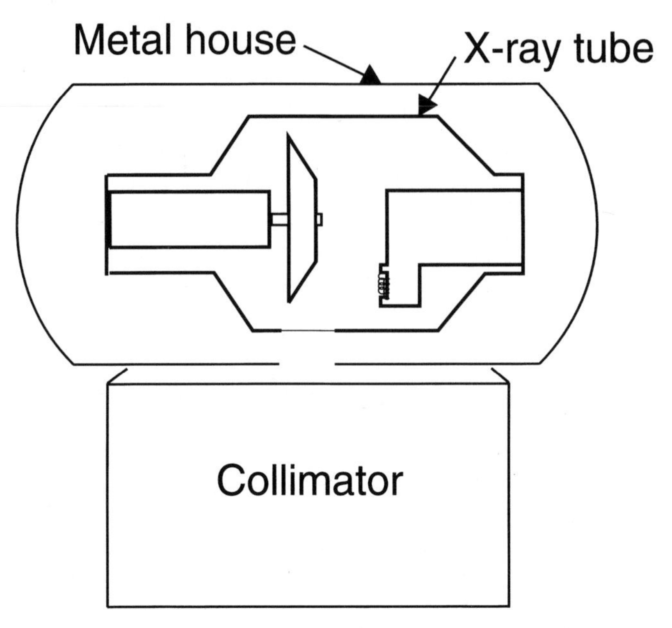

FIGURE 2–4. The x-ray tube with metal house and collimator.

PERFORM ACTIVITY 2.A

PRODUCTION OF THE X-RAY BEAM

X-rays are produced inside the x-ray tube after a chain of events involving the filament, focusing cup, and anode. The chain of events involves releasing electrons from atoms at the filament, giving the released electrons a high speed, focusing these electrons, and then stopping them suddenly at the anode where the x-rays are produced.

Releasing the Electrons

The first event is the removal of electrons from the atoms contained in the filament wire. The filament is the source of the electrons. The filament wires are connected in a circuit, which is a group of wires that can conduct electricity. The circuit containing the filament wires is called the filament circuit. When current is sent through this circuit, one of the two filament wires gets hot.

The filament wires are made of tungsten, which has a high melting point. The high melting point is important because the current causes the wire to get hot enough to actually glow. This glowing is called **incandescence**. When the filament gets this hot, electrons are "boiled off" or freed from the atoms of the filament. This process of releasing electrons is called **thermionic emission**.

For a fraction of a second these electrons sit right beyond the filament in a group called the **space charge** (Fig. 2–5). All electrons are negatively charged, and since charges that are the same repel each other, the electrons in this group want to escape from each other. So the focusing cup is used to hold the group of electrons together.

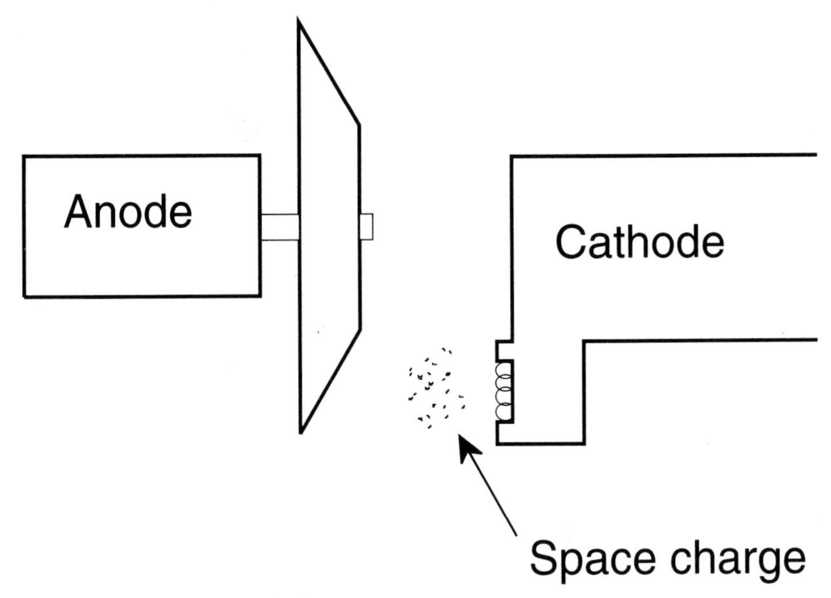

FIGURE 2–5. The space charge.

Producing High Speed Electrons

The electrons must travel from the cathode to the anode at great speed to produce x-rays. Two forces work together to produce this high speed. During the exposure, the focusing cup gets a strong negative charge and the anode gets a strong positive charge. The negatively charged electrons sitting in their group (the space charge) just beyond the filament are repelled by the negative focusing cup. This causes the electrons to leave the filament as a group and shoot over to the anode.

Since the anode is positively charged, and opposite charges attract, the positive anode pulls the negative electrons from the filament at the same time that they are being repelled from the focusing cup. This combination of push and pull forces the electrons to travel at high speed between the filament and the anode. The high speed gives the electrons a large amount of kinetic energy, which is the energy of motion.

Focusing the Electrons

The focusing cup helps the electrons hit the anode in a small area. The actual place that the electrons hit on the surface of the anode is called the **target**. The anode disc is made of molybdenum, which is coated with tungsten so the anode surface or the target area is made of tungsten. The size of the area that the electrons hit is called the **focal spot** (Fig. 2–6). The anode disc, the target, and the focal spot are all physically located in the same place (at the anode), but the terms should not be interchanged since they each mean something different.

The size of the focal spot helps control the radiographic quality of recorded detail. A small focal spot will produce better recorded detail on the radiograph than a large focal spot.

In a dual-focus x-ray tube either the small filament or the large filament could be heated. If the large filament is heated, the electrons released from it would create a large space charge, and thus hit a large area on the anode. This would produce a large focal spot. If the electrons are released from the small filament, they would create a

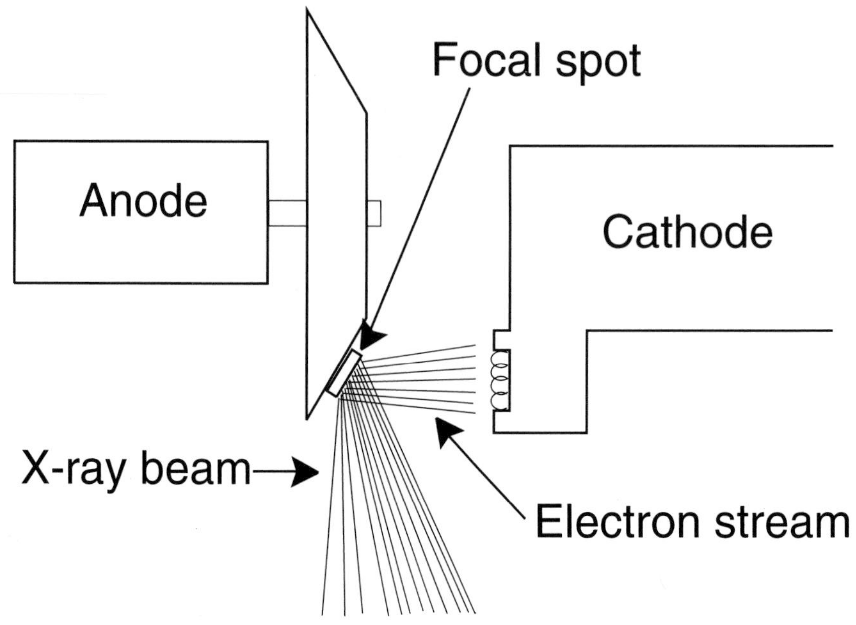

FIGURE 2–6. The focal spot.

small space charge, thus hit a small area on the anode. This would produce a small focal spot.

When the x-rays are produced at the focal spot, they fly off in all directions, like the sparks from a Fourth of July sparkler. This spherical pattern is called **isotropic emission** (Fig. 2–7). Only the x-rays that are aimed at the patient are useful to us. The rest of the x-rays could fly out of the tube and hit people other than the patient. This is why a lead glass and metal housing are put around the cathode and anode. These housings and the anode disc absorb this unnecessary radiation. A tiny bit of radiation still might get through, and this is called **leakage radiation**.

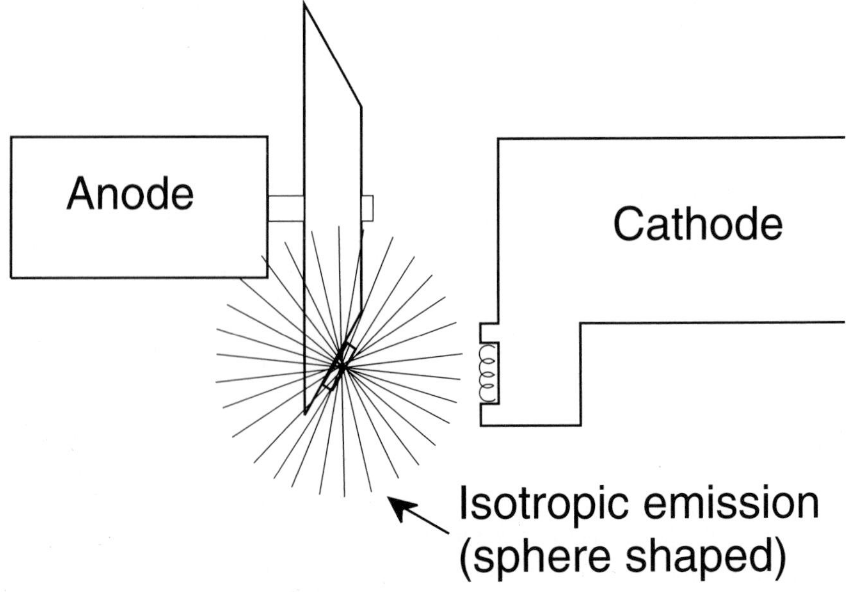

FIGURE 2–7. Isotropic emission of x-rays.

Stopping the Electrons

When the electrons slam into the anode at high speed, they lose their kinetic energy. This lost energy is transformed into a great amount of heat, a little light, and less than 1% x-ray. It seems like this whole process is inefficient, since very little of the lost energy is converted to x-rays, but nobody has been able to improve on the process.

PERFORM ACTIVITY 2.B

PERFORM ACTIVITY 2.C

PROPERTIES OF X-RAYS

After the x-rays are produced they have some properties that are important to understand because the properties affect the quality of the radiograph. The properties also help determine what technical factors the radiographer should use to produce a good radiograph. The properties that are listed in this book are not all the x-ray properties, but they are the ones that pertain to radiographic quality.

X-RAY PROPERTY. X-rays travel in straight lines and diverge from their point of origin at the focal spot.

The part of the x-ray beam that is directed at the patient is only a section of the x-rays produced at the anode (Fig. 2–8). Since the remainder of the x-rays are absorbed by the anode and the glass and metal housings, they are virtually eliminated. The x-rays that are aimed at the patient are still moving away from the focal spot. They all keep traveling in straight lines, but because they are still moving isotropically, they diverge or move away from each other, creating a **cone-shaped beam**.

X-RAY PROPERTY. X-ray photons have many different energies.

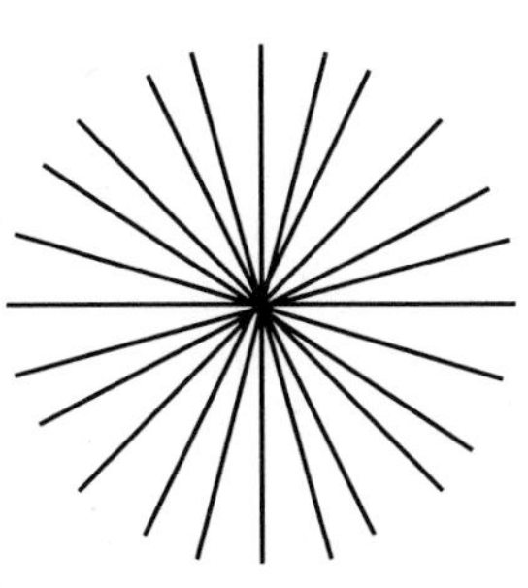

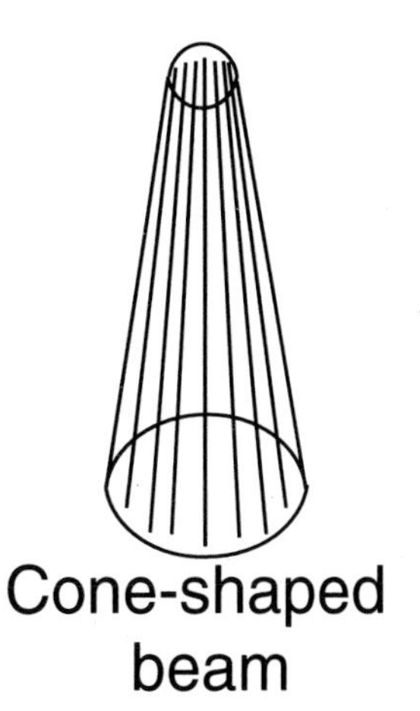

FIGURE 2–8. The cone-shaped x-ray beam directed at the patient.

The x-ray beam that is directed at the patient consists of millions of x-rays or what are better called x-ray photons. A **photon** is a tiny particle of energy. The energy of each of the photons in the x-ray beam can be different. The technical terms for this are **heterogeneous** or **polyenergetic**.

X-RAY PROPERTY. X-rays are highly penetrating.

Photons with less energy are absorbed more easily by the patient's body parts, whereas photons with more energy will penetrate right through the patient's body. The photons that get through the patient's body will hit the x-ray film and eventually produce an image of the patient's body on the film.

X-rays are a form of electromagnetic radiation. There are many different kinds of electromagnetic radiation, such as radio waves and light waves, but x-rays are a type that are able to penetrate through matter such as the patient's body.

X-RAY PROPERTY. X-rays are invisible.

Since x-rays are invisible, they often seem mysterious, and this is why many people are afraid of them. X-rays cannot be seen as they are produced, as they leave the x-ray tube, or as they enter the patient's body. It's obvious that they were there, though, when the film is developed and the image of the patient's body is on the radiograph.

X-RAY PROPERTY. X-rays travel at the speed of light.

The speed of light is approximately 186,000 miles per second, and x-rays travel at the same speed as light. The walls in an x-ray room are lined with lead, which is good at absorbing x-rays. The radiographer stands in a lead-shielded area when making the exposure, and since x-rays travel so fast, they will already be absorbed by the lead in the walls by the time the radiographer lets go of the exposure button and gets back inside the x-ray room.

X-RAY PROPERTY. X-rays produce scattered radiation.

Scattered radiation is produced when x-rays enter the patient's body. The x-ray beam that is directed at the patient's body is called the **primary beam** (Fig. 2–9). When the primary beam enters the patient's body, three things could happen to the photons:

1. Photons could be absorbed by the patient's body parts.
2. Photons could pass right through the patient's body and enter the film, putting density on the film. These photons are called **exit radiation** or remnant radiation.
3. Photons could hit something in the patient's body, bounce off, and fly out in a new direction. This last event produces **scattered radiation**.

Scattered radiation that hits the film creates several significant problems for the quality of the radiographic image. Scatter reduces radiographic **contrast.** Loss of

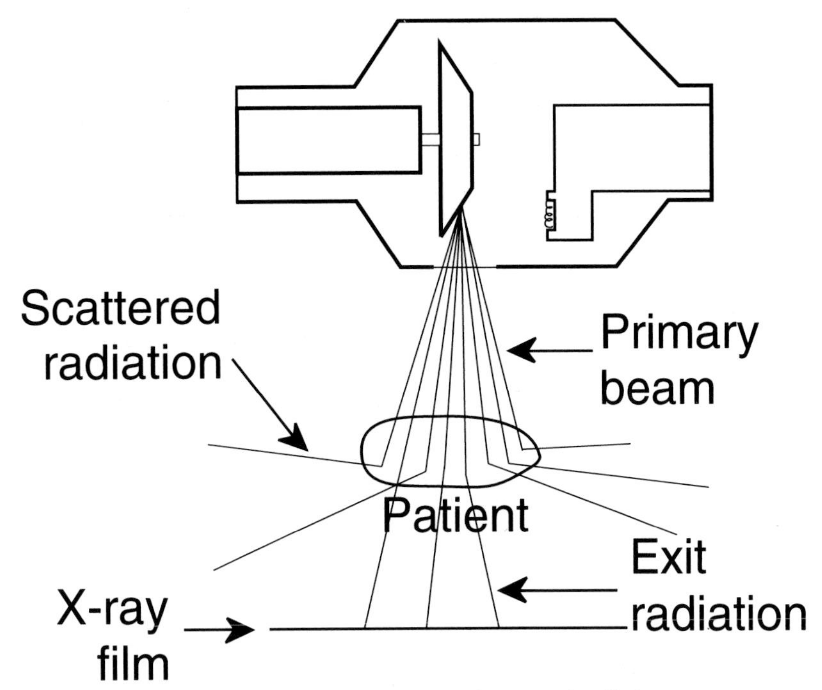

FIGURE 2–9. Primary, exit, and scattered radiation.

contrast is not good, and there are a variety of things the radiographer can do to avoid the problems associated with scatter. Chapters 9 and 10 of this book are devoted to the problem of scatter.

X-RAY PROPERTY. X-rays affect radiographic film.

X-rays produce an image of the patient's body by affecting radiographic film. When x-ray photons hit the film, they interact with the atoms in the film and cause changes in the atoms. This exposes the film. When this exposed film is put into the radiographic processor, the processing chemicals that develop the film are able to act on these changed atoms. This action is what produces the image on the film.

In areas where the film received a lot of radiation, a great many atoms will be changed and the action of the developing chemicals will be stronger in these areas. These areas of the film will be very black when developed. These areas on the radiograph would be referred to as having a lot of **density**. Areas which receive less radiation or no radiation will be gray or white when developed and would show varying degrees of density on the radiograph. The variation in densities on a radiograph is called **contrast**.

X-RAY PROPERTY. X-rays cause some materials to fluoresce.

X-rays can cause certain materials called **phosphors** to glow or light up. This glowing is called **fluorescence**. The phosphors light up in proportion to the amount of radiation that hits them. If a large quantity of radiation hits a phosphor, that

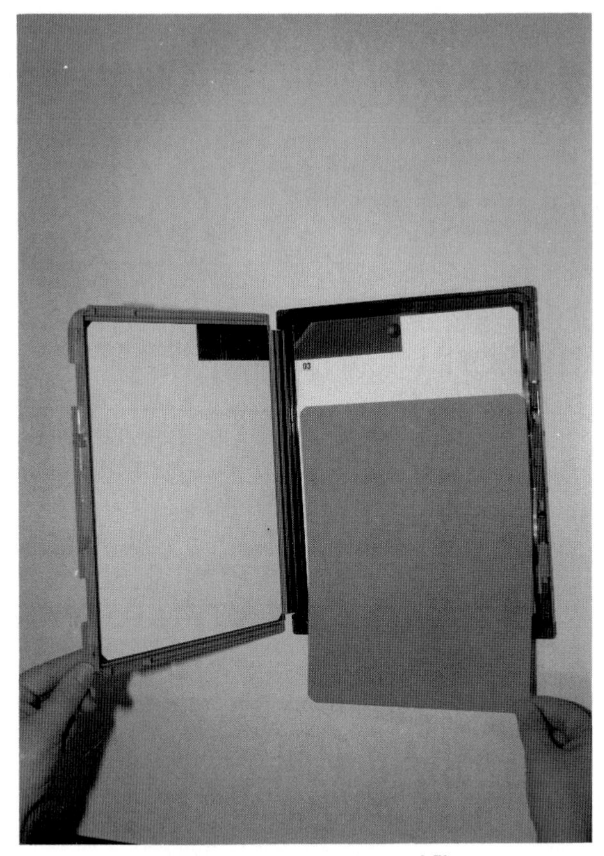

FIGURE 2–10. A cassette and film.

phosphor lights up very bright. If only a little radiation hits the phosphor, the phosphor gives off only a little light.

A radiographer getting ready to make a radiograph first puts a piece of radiographic film into a device called a **cassette** (Fig. 2–10). The cassette contains **intensifying screens** that touch both sides of the film when the cassette is closed. The intensifying screens are coated with phosphors.

When exit radiation comes into the cassette, the phosphors on the intensifying screens glow, producing a fluorescent light. The fluorescent light from the phosphors hits the film and exposes it. Exposure of the film to light causes changes in the atoms of the film in the same way that x-rays can expose the film. When the film is developed, it will have areas of black where a large amount of radiation got through the patient's body and into the cassette, producing a large amount of fluorescent light. The film will be different shades of gray where moderate amounts of radiation got through, and white where no radiation got through the patient's body and into the cassette.

X-RAY PROPERTY. X-rays cause biological damage.

The x-ray properties we have been discussing so far are all fascinating and exciting. This last one isn't so great for us or our patients. X-rays can damage biological or

Table 2–1. Properties of X-rays that Affect Radiographic Quality

1. X-rays travel in straight lines and diverge from their point of origin at the focal spot.
2. X-ray photons have many different energies.
3. X-rays are highly penetrating.
4. X-rays are invisible.
5. X-rays travel at the speed of light.
6. X-rays produce scattered radiation.
7. X-rays affect radiographic film.
8. X-rays cause fluorescence of some materials.
9. X-rays cause biological damage.

living matter. X-ray photons can change the atoms in a living body by causing electrons to leave some of the atoms in the body. This process of removing an electron from an atom is called **ionization**. If many atoms are disrupted in this way, the DNA in the cells of the living body can be damaged. This can cause the cell to either die or malfunction. If DNA damage occurs in sperm or ova that are then used to produce a baby, the damage can be transferred to the baby's body. This is why radiographers must be so careful about protecting themselves, their patients, and others from unnecessary radiation.

PERFORM ACTIVITY 2.D

SUMMARY

The inside parts of the x-ray tube are the anode and the cathode. The cathode consists of the focusing cup and filament. When x-rays are produced, electrons are released from the filament, given a high speed, and focused into a small group by the focusing cup. When they zoom over to the anode, they are stopped suddenly. The kinetic energy of the electrons is converted to x-rays.

X-rays have certain properties. These properties are summarized in Table 2–1.

PERFORM ACTIVITY 2.E

SECTION II

DISTORTION

CHAPTER 3

SIZE DISTORTION

CHAPTER OUTLINE

OBJECTIVES

At the end of this chapter you should be able to:

- Define these terms: source-image distance, focus-film distance, object-image distance, object-film distance, source-object distance, and focus-object distance.
- Given two of the three distance measurements, calculate the third unknown distance.
- Define size distortion.
- Explain how the object-image distance is used to control magnification.
- Explain how the source-image distance is used to control magnification.
- Describe the clinical applications of the most common source-image distances.
- Recognize obvious magnification on a radiograph.
- Calculate the image size, object size, magnification factor, and percent of magnification.

Size distortion causes the image to appear larger than the object being radiographed. Size distortion is also called magnification. All radiographs have some magnification, but with good clinical practices, the problem is kept at an acceptable level. The radiographer can avoid most size distortion by paying attention to proper positioning principles.

In this chapter you will first learn about the distances that affect size distortion. Then the ideal distances that will help avoid size distortion are discussed. You will also learn to calculate factors concerning the size of the image and object.

DISTANCES

Before learning about size distortion and how to avoid it, students must learn some basic terminology associated with distances. This sounds simple, but in clinical practice radiographers, instructors, and physicians can all use different terms that mean the same thing. This can be confusing, so students must become familiar with all the synonyms.

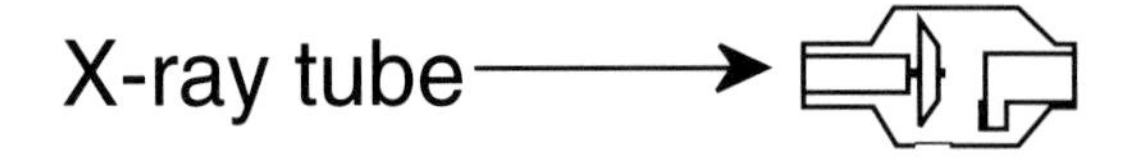

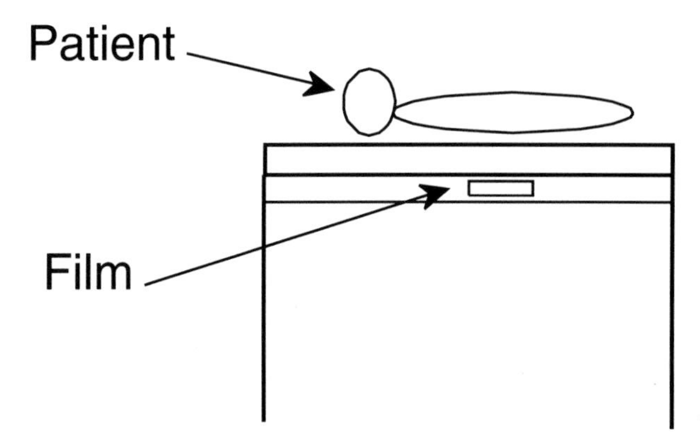

FIGURE 3–1. The arrangement for a basic x-ray exposure.

Figure 3–1 shows the basic arrangement used for many radiographs. The patient lies flat on the x-ray table, the x-ray tube is positioned above the patient, and the film inside the cassette is placed in the Bucky tray. The Bucky tray can be stationary or it can slide back and forth in a slot right under the table.

The distance between the x-ray tube and the patient can be measured, as can the distance between the patient and the film. Also, the distance between the x-ray tube and the film can be measured. These distances are important and have specific names and several synonyms.

Source-Image Distance (SID)

The distance between the x-ray tube and film is called the **source-image distance (SID)**, or the **focus- (or focal-) film distance (FFD)**. This distance is called the source-image distance because it is the distance from the source of the x-ray beam, which is in the x-ray tube, to the spot where the image is formed, which is usually at the film for radiography. This term can also be called the source-to-image receptor distance.

The "focus" part of the term focus-film distance originates from a component of the x-ray tube. The anode, one of the major parts of the x-ray tube, is where x-rays are formed. X-rays are formed after electrons hit the anode. The size of the area where the electrons hit the anode is called the focal spot, and this is where the "focus" in focus-film distance comes from.

The distance between the x-ray tube and film:
Source-image distance (SID)
Focus-film distance (FFD)

The distance between the x-ray tube and film has also been called the anode-film distance and target-film distance, but these are older terms. This book will use the term source-image distance (SID).

Object-Image Distance (OID)

The patient is inelegantly referred to as the object in these distance terms. However, referring to the patient as the object is not always precise. The patient's body is a three-dimensional structure. If the radiographer is interested in producing a radiograph of just one part inside of the patient, then that part becomes the object.

The distance between the part inside the patient's body that is being radiographed and the place where the image is formed, which is usually at the film, is called the **object-image distance (OID)**. Another term that means the same thing is the **object-film distance (OFD)**, the distance between the object and the film.

The distance between the object and film:
Object-image distance (OID)
Object-film distance (OFD)

This book will use the term object-image distance (OID).

Source-Object Distance (SOD)

The last distance is the distance from the x-ray tube to the object. This distance is called the **source-object distance (SOD)**, or the **focus-object distance (FOD)**. This term is used less frequently in clinical situations than SID and OID, but it is used in several calculations.

The distance between the x-ray tube and object
Source-object distance (SOD)
Focus-object distance (FOD)

Calculating the Distances

If two of these three distances are known, the other one can be calculated. Refer to Figure 3–2. If the source-image distance (SID) is 40 inches and the object-image distance (OID) is 4 inches, the source-object distance (SOD) can be calculated by subtracting the OID from the SID. The SOD is 36 inches. Adding the OID of 4 and the SOD of 36 gets the SID of 40. And subtracting the SOD of 36 from the SID of 40 gets the OID of 4.

Here are the formulas:

$$\text{SID} = \text{OID} + \text{SOD}$$
$$\text{OID} = \text{SID} - \text{SOD}$$
$$\text{SOD} = \text{SID} - \text{OID}$$

PERFORM ACTIVITY 3.A

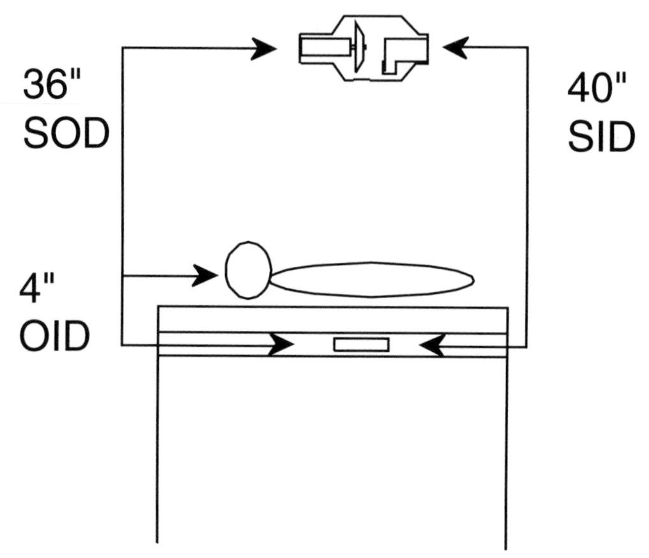

FIGURE 3–2. Source-image distance (SID), source-object distance (SOD), object image distance (OID).

SIZE DISTORTION

Size distortion is defined as the misrepresentation of the true size of the image as compared to the object. Size distortion, or magnification distortion, occurs when the image of the object on the radiograph appears larger than the actual size of the object. When this occurs, the image is magnified. The job of the radiographer is to make the image appear as close to the true size of the actual object as possible. So magnification on the radiograph is ordinarily not a good thing.

Size distortion is the misrepresentation of the true size of the image as compared to the object.

The best relationship to produce the least magnification is to have the object as close to the film as possible and to have the x-ray tube as far away from the film as possible. In the technical distance terms, it is best to have a short object-image distance (OID), and a long source-image distance (SID).

For the least magnification use a short OID, and a long SID.

Divergent rays were discussed in Chapter 2. These occur because the x-ray beam takes the shape of a cone. If the beam is directed straight at the patient, the photons in the center of the beam are perpendicular to the patient but the photons at the edges of the beam reach the patient at an angle.

Because of these divergent rays, placing the object farther away from the film causes the object's shadow or image on the film to be larger than it is when the object is placed very close to the film (Fig. 3–3). Placing the x-ray tube closer to the object also causes the image of the object to be larger than it is when the tube is placed farther away from the object.

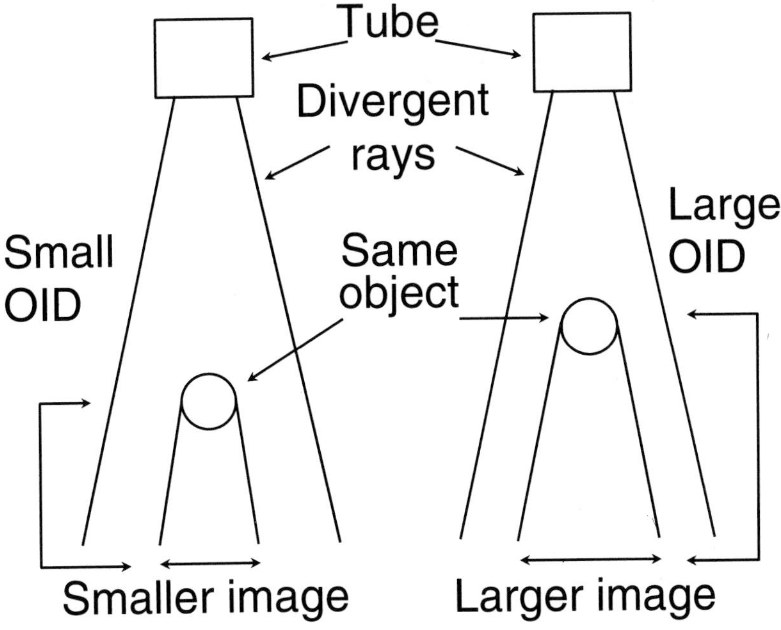

FIGURE 3–3. Image size differs with different OIDs.

PERFORM ACTIVITY 3.B

OBJECT-IMAGE DISTANCE (OID)

The object image distance (OID) is ***the major factor*** controlling magnification. The least magnification is produced when the object is placed close to the film. Magnification increases as the object is moved farther away from the film, so an OID of 10 inches will produce more magnification than an OID of 5 inches.

Proper positioning of the patient's body will help avoid too much magnification. If the patient is lying on his or her abdomen face down (prone), then the patient's spine is far away from the film. The spine would be magnified on the radiograph, and that wouldn't be good if that is the structure the radiologist is interested in seeing. By turning the patient over to lie on his or her back (supine), the spine is moved closer to the film and will appear much less magnified on the radiograph. It is important to learn the anatomy of the body, and then learn how to position the patient's body to put the structure being radiographed closest to the film.

Always try to put the object or structure of interest close to the film to avoid magnification.

Figure 3–4 shows some radiographs with magnification due to a large object-image distance (OID).

PERFORM ACTIVITY 3.C

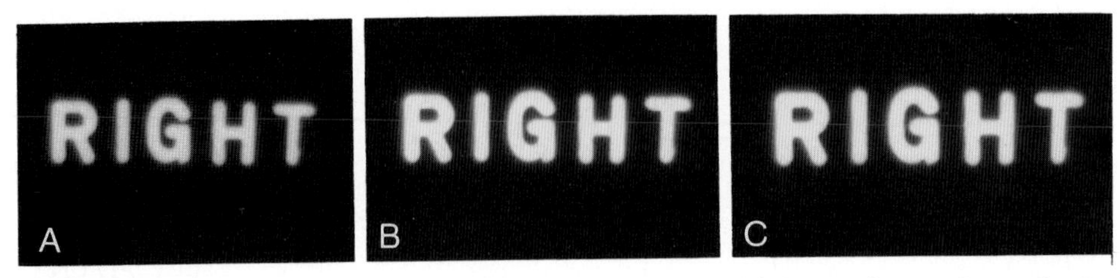

FIGURE 3–4. (*A*) Radiograph with no OID. (*B*) Radiograph with a 3-inch OID produces an image that is a little larger than radiograph *A*. (*C*) Radiograph with a 6-inch OID produces an image that is a little larger than radiograph *B*.

SOURCE-IMAGE DISTANCE (SID)

A long source-image distance (SID) will produce the least magnification or size distortion. Size distortion increases as the x-ray tube is moved closer to the object, so a SID of 50 inches will produce more magnification than a SID of 60 inches.

A long source-image distance produces the least magnification.

Even though it sounds like it should be better to use a very long source-image distance (SID), the distance between the x-ray tube and film isn't varied too much in standard clinical situations. The most commonly used SIDs are 72 inches or 40 inches. The 40-inch distance is usually used for radiographs exposed when the patient is lying on the x-ray table with the film in the Bucky tray or on the table top. This standard distance is used even though a moderate amount of magnification is produced. This amount of magnification is acceptable and expected. The longer distance of 72 inches is used when the image needs to be more precisely the size of the object. For example, the 72-inch distance is used for chest radiographs so that a minimal amount of magnification of the heart will appear on the radiograph.

In nonstandard situations the source-image distance (SID) can vary quite a bit, and this can make a noticeable difference in the size distortion on the radiograph. Figure 3–5 shows radiographs with magnification due to a short SID.

PERFORM ACTIVITY 3.D

The object-image distance and source-image distance work together to produce the total amount of size distortion. In nonstandard clinical situations, the radio-

FIGURE 3–5. (*A*) A radiograph with a 20-inch SID. (*B*) A radiograph with a 40-inch SID produces an image that is a little smaller than radiograph *A*. (*C*) A radiograph with a 60-inch SID produces an image that is a little smaller than radiograph *B*.

grapher may be unable to get the object as close to the film as possible. For instance, if a patient lying flat on the x-ray table were unable to straighten his or her knee and had to keep it bent, the knee would be up off the table and have an increased object-image distance (OID). The radiographer can compensate for this by increasing the source-image distance (SID) above the standard 40 inches. This increase will help to offset the magnification caused by the large object-image distance (OID).

CALCULATING MAGNIFICATION

In some clinical situations it is important for the radiologist to know the amount of magnification produced on a radiograph. This is especially important during pelvimetry exams, angiograms, and mammography. The image size, object size, magnification factor, and percent of magnification can all be calculated.

These factors will be used as a starting point for all the following examples:

Actual object length = 8 inches
Source-image distance = 72 inches
Object-image distance = 6 inches

Image and Object Size

When referring to "size," this is either the **length** of the image or object, or the **width** of the image or object.

Since the proportion below, used to calculate the image or object size, uses the unit of SOD, it is first necessary to calculate the SOD, which is 72 minus 6. The SOD is 64. Then insert the known factors into the proportion.

$$\frac{\text{Image size}}{\text{Object size}} = \frac{\text{SID}}{\text{SOD}}$$

$$\frac{\text{Image size}}{8} = \frac{72}{64}$$

Cross-multiply and solve the equation:

$$\text{Image size} \times 64 = 72 \times 8$$

$$\text{Image size} \times 64 = 576$$

$$\text{Image size} = \frac{576}{64}$$

$$\text{Image size} = 9 \text{ inches long}$$

If any of the other three factors in the proportion—object size, SID, or SOD—were the unknown factors, they could be calculated using the same formula.

Magnification Factor

The magnification factor tells the radiographer how much larger the image will appear as compared to the object. If the magnification factor is 1.5, the image will be 1.5 times longer and 1.5 times wider than the object. A 1.5 times magnification of an object that is 4 inches long will cause the image to be 6 inches long ($4 \times 1.5 = 6$).

There are two ways to calculate the magnification factor.

1. Divide the source-image distance by the source-object distance.

$$\text{Magnification factor} = \frac{\text{SID}}{\text{SOD}}$$

$$\text{Magnification factor} = \frac{72}{64}$$

$$\text{Magnification factor} = 1.125$$

2. Divide the image size by the object size.

$$\text{Magnification factor} = \frac{\text{Image size}}{\text{Object size}}$$

$$\text{Magnification factor} = \frac{9 \quad \text{(9-inch-long image)}}{8 \quad \text{(8-inch-long object)}}$$

$$\text{Magnification factor} = 1.125$$

If the magnification factor is 1.125, the image would be 1.125 times longer and 1.125 times wider than the actual object. The image length or width can then be calculated by multiplying the object length or width by the magnification factor. And 8 inches (the actual object length) times 1.125 is 9 inches (the image length).

The magnification factor tells the radiographer how much ***longer*** and ***wider*** the image will be compared to the object's actual length and width. This is not the same as the area of the image. Area is calculated by multiplying the length of an object by the width. If the length of the image is 2 times the length of the object, and the width of the image is 2 times the width of the object, the area of the image grows by 4 times (Fig. 3–6).

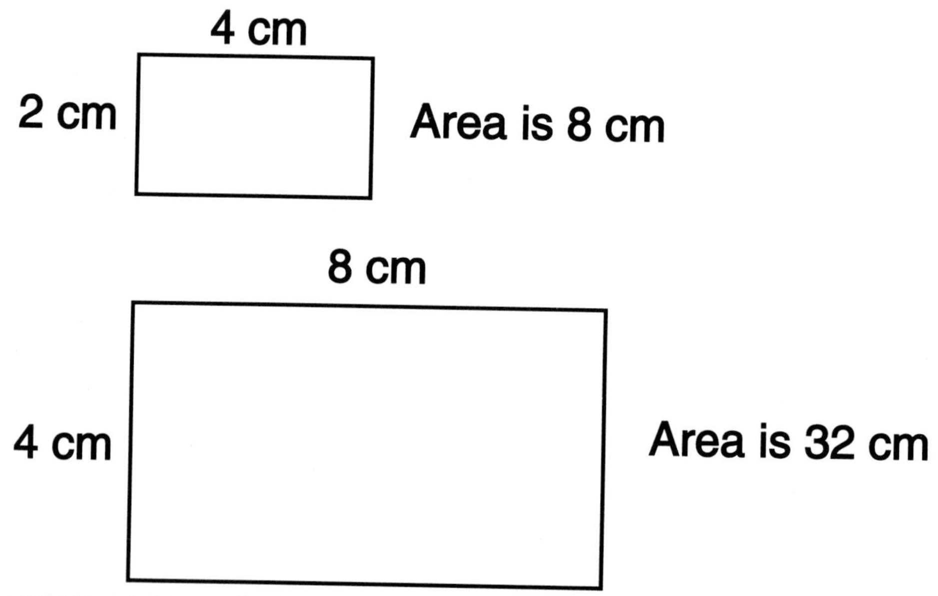

FIGURE 3–6. If the magnification factor is 2, the length of the image grows twice as large as the length of the object, and the width of the image grows twice as large as the width of the object. The area of the image grows 4 times larger than the area of the object.

Percent of Magnification

The percent of magnification is calculated by subtracting the object size (length or width) from the image size (length or width), dividing this answer by the object size (length or width), and then multiplying the result by 100.

$$\frac{\text{Image size} - \text{Object size}}{\text{Object size}} \times 100$$

To solve this, both the image and object sizes must be known. In our last example, the image was 9 inches long and the object was 8 inches long.

$$\frac{9-8}{8} \times 100$$

$$\frac{1}{8} \times 100$$

$$.125 \times 100$$

The percent of magnification is 12.5%.

PERFORM ACTIVITY 3.E

PERFORM ACTIVITY 3.F

DISTANCE AND THE FOUR RADIOGRAPHIC QUALITIES

The four radiographic qualities of density, contrast, recorded detail, and distortion were described in Chapter 1. In Figure 1 – 2, all the factors affecting these four radiographic qualities were listed on a chart. Refer to this chart now, and you will see that object-image distance (OID) and source-image distance (SID) are listed as factors that affect distortion.

Look at the factors that affect recorded detail. SID and OID are listed as affecting recorded detail. As the SID is increased by moving the x-ray tube away from the film, the recorded detail is increased; and as the OID is increased by moving the object away from the film, the recorded detail is decreased.

Source-image distance (SID) is listed as a factor that affects density. Whenever the SID is increased or decreased from the standard, the amount of radiation used for that radiograph needs to be adjusted. This adjustment is calculated with the density maintenance formula, which will be discussed in Chapter 6.

Object-image distance (OID) is listed as a factor that affects both density and contrast. This effect occurs only in the air-gap technique, which will be discussed in Chapter 10.

PERFORM ACTIVITY 3.G

SUMMARY

The distance from the x-ray tube to the film is the source-image distance (SID), or the focus-film distance (FFD). The distance from the object to the film is the object-image distance (OID) or object-film distance (OFD). The distance from the x-ray tube to the object is the source-object distance (SOD), or focus-object distance (FOD).

These distances control the amount of size distortion or magnification. Magnification causes the image to appear larger than the object. The least amount of magnification is achieved with a short object-image distance and a long source-image distance. The image size, object size, magnification factor, and percent of magnification can all be calculated.

PERFORM ACTIVITY 3.H

CHAPTER 4

SHAPE DISTORTION

CHAPTER OUTLINE

OBJECTIVES

At the end of this chapter you should be able to:

- Define shape distortion and explain how it differs from size distortion.
- List the three types of shape distortion.
- Differentiate between the x-ray beam and the central ray.
- Define the term **object**.
- Describe the ideal relationship between the central ray, object, and film that will produce the least amount of distortion.
- Describe how foreshortening occurs.
- Explain how foreshortening of the image can be avoided when the object is at an angle in relation to the film.
- Describe how elongation occurs.
- Explain why it is important that the central ray be placed directly over the structure of interest.
- Explain how elongation can be used to the radiographer's advantage.
- Describe superimposition.
- Describe how spatial distortion occurs.
- Explain the importance of the direction of the central ray when using spatial distortion to improve the image.

In Chapter 3 you learned about size distortion, which is also called magnification. Size distortion occurs when the image is larger than the actual size of the object. The cause of size distortion is a long object-image distance (OID) or a short source-image distance (SID).

Size distortion is only one part of the problem of distortion. Another type of distortion is called shape distortion. When shape distortion occurs, the image appears to be a different shape when compared with the shape of the object. The image could appear to be stretched out of shape or squashed together when compared with the object.

There are three types of shape distortion: foreshortening, elongation, and spatial distortion. In this chapter you will learn how each of these occurs, how to recognize these distortions on the radiograph, and how each type of distortion can be avoided. Shape distortion isn't always a bad thing. Elongation and spatial distortion are sometimes used intentionally to enhance the appearance of a part of the body on the radiograph.

TYPES OF SHAPE DISTORTION

Shape distortion is defined as the misrepresentation of the true shape of the image as compared to the object. It is sometimes called true distortion.

Shape distortion is the misrepresentation of the true shape of the image as compared to the object.

There are three types of shape distortion. The first type is called foreshortening. In foreshortening the image appears squashed together. On a radiograph with foreshortening a bone appears to be shorter and thicker than it actually is.

Another type of shape distortion is called elongation. In elongation the image appears stretched out when it is compared with the object. On the radiograph an elongated bone appears longer and thinner than it actually is.

The third type of shape distortion is called spatial distortion. In spatial distortion there is a misrepresentation of the three-dimensional relationship of the structures within the body part being examined. On the radiograph body parts may appear separated when they are not separated in the actual body.

Shape distortion occurs when the relationship of the direction of the x-ray beam, the position of the film, and the position of the part varies somehow from what is considered ideal.

PERFORM ACTIVITY 4.A

COMPONENTS OF THE IDEAL RELATIONSHIP

To produce the least amount of shape distortion, the radiographer needs to use the ideal relationship between the positions of the x-ray beam or central ray, the film, and the object.

The Central Ray

The x-ray beam that is directed at the patient is in the shape of a cone. If the beam is directed straight at the patient's body, the photons (or x-rays) at the edge of the cone of radiation would hit the patient's body at an angle. The photons in the center of the beam would be perpendicular to the body. The photon in the exact center of the beam is called the **central ray** (Fig. 4–1). The angle of the x-ray beam is always measured at the central ray rather than at the edges of the beam.

X-ray tubes can usually be angled 360 degrees, but most tubes have a stop or "detent," which lets the radiographer know when the tube is positioned so the central ray is perpendicular to the Bucky tray or x-ray table top. The tube can also have a stop to let the radiographer know when the central ray is exactly horizontal for

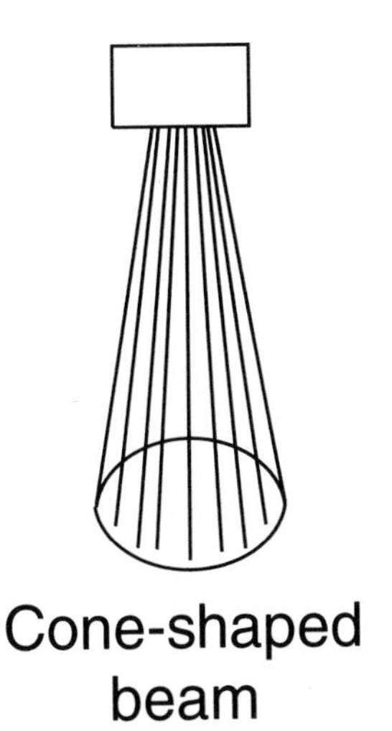

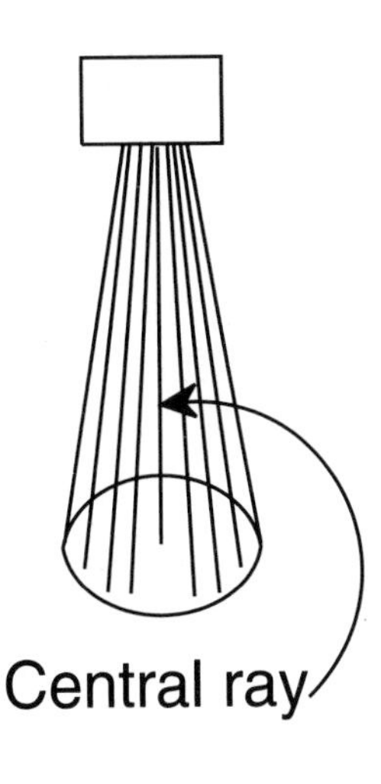

FIGURE 4–1. Cone-shaped beam and the central ray.

upright or cross-table lateral radiography. The stops are there so that the central ray isn't accidentally at an angle when it is supposed to be perpendicular to the film.

The Film and Film Holder

The image is usually recorded on a film. The film is placed inside a device called a cassette, and the cassette is placed where the radiation will exit from the patient's body. The cassette with the film in it can be placed in several different locations depending on how the patient is being positioned. Sometimes the cassette is placed in the Bucky tray, which is located just under the x-ray table top. The cassette could also be placed on the table top, or in a special device used for upright radiography. The cassette is sometimes placed directly under the patient's body. Some of these locations are more prone to producing shape distortion than others.

The Object

The object is the body part that the radiographer is trying to image on the radiograph. The radiographer may be trying to produce an image of a whole section of the patient's body such as the abdomen, or just one part inside of the abdomen. If the area of interest is just one part of the abdomen like the kidney, then that part is referred to as the object.

PRODUCING THE IDEAL RELATIONSHIP

The ideal relationship is produced by placing the object parallel to the film, the central ray perpendicular to the object, and the central ray perpendicular to the film. The central ray should also be placed over the center of the object (Fig. 4–2).

Variations from the ideal relationship can produce the three types of shape distortion: foreshortening, elongation, and spatial distortion.

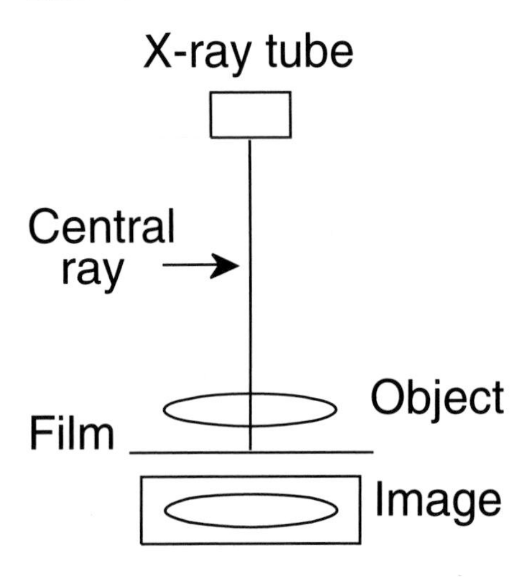

FIGURE 4–2. Ideal relationship of the central ray, object, and film.

FORESHORTENING

Foreshortening occurs when the object is at an angle and the central ray is perpendicular to the film (Fig. 4–3). With foreshortening the image will appear squashed together when compared with the object, like a car that was in the middle of a three-car wreck. Minute detail in the object may not be seen on the image.

Foreshortening produces an unequal magnification of the parts of the object. With a tilt or angle of the object in relation to the film, each part of the object will lie at a different object-image distance, so each part will be magnified a different amount on the image.

> **Foreshortening occurs when the object is angled but the central ray remains perpendicular to the film.**

If a radiograph is taken of a fractured bone, the radiologist needs to be able to tell how far apart the broken bone fragments are. The fracture space can be seen well on an image taken with the ideal central ray, object, film relationship. If the image is

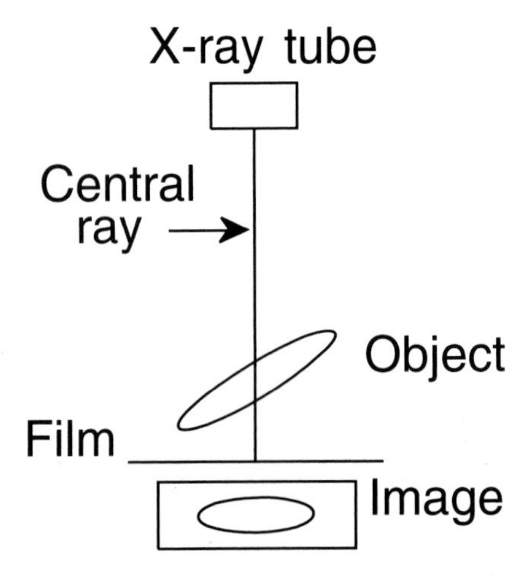

FIGURE 4–3. Foreshortening of the image.

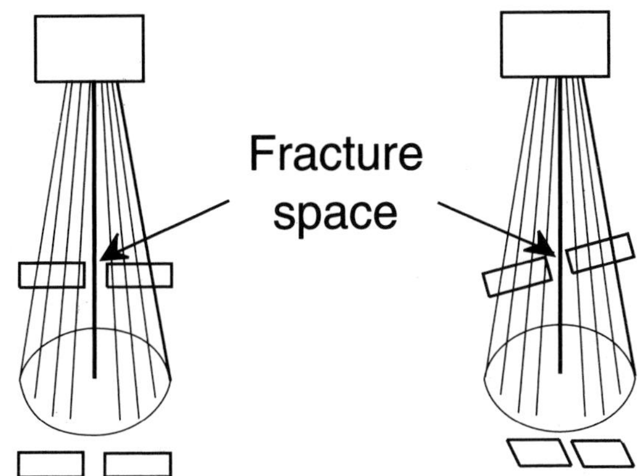

FIGURE 4–4. Foreshortening of the image distorts the separation of a fracture.

foreshortened, the radiologist will be unable to judge the space between the fracture fragments correctly. If the fracture is very small, it can even be hidden in a foreshortened image (Fig. 4–4).

In clinical situations where it is impossible to achieve the ideal central ray, object, and film relationship, the body part may lie at an angle to the central ray and film, and the image would be foreshortened. In this case the radiographer can sometimes avoid a foreshortened image by turning or angling the x-ray tube so the central ray will be perpendicular to the object. Placing the central ray perpendicular to the object helps to improve the image even if the central ray is not also perpendicular to the film. The image will appear less foreshortened because some elongation occurs since the central ray is perpendicular to the object but not to the film.

Figure 4–5 shows radiographs that demonstrate foreshortening.

PERFORM ACTIVITY 4.B

ELONGATION

Elongation is a type of distortion that occurs when the object is parallel to the film but the central ray is angled (Fig. 4–6). Elongation can also occur if the central ray is

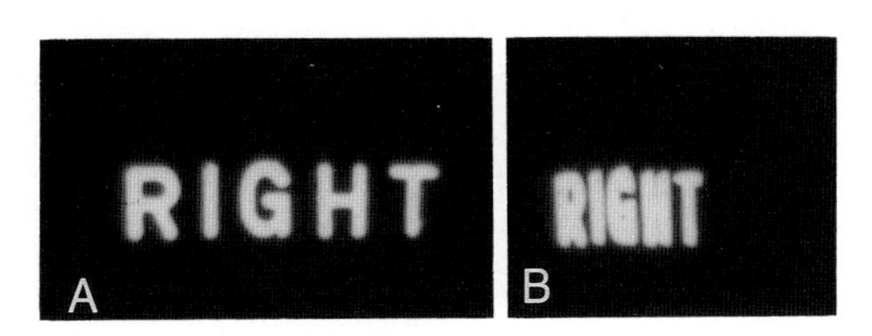

FIGURE 4–5. (*A*) Good image. (*B*) Foreshortening of the image.

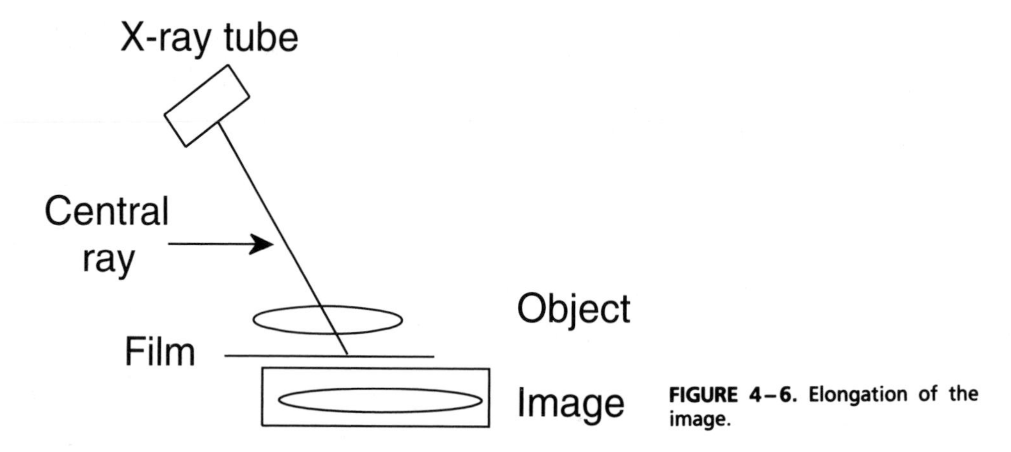

FIGURE 4–6. Elongation of the image.

perpendicular to the object but the object is not parallel to the film. With elongation, the image appears to be stretched out of shape when compared with the object, like when a piece of taffy is pulled on from both ends. Figure 4–7 shows radiographs that demonstrate elongation.

Although elongation can produce shape distortion in the image, sometimes this shape distortion can actually help the radiographer image body parts that would ordinarily be hidden. A good example of this is the tilt or axial view of the sigmoid colon taken during a barium enema.

The sigmoid colon, which is right near the rectum, is S-shaped and twists around in the body. If a radiograph is taken during a barium enema with the patient lying flat on the x-ray table and the central ray perpendicular to the film, the parts of the sigmoid will lie on top of each other in the image. If the radiographer angles the central ray, the sigmoid colon will appear elongated on the image. The twisted parts of the sigmoid colon will then be seen separated on the image (Fig. 4–8).

PERFORM ACTIVITY 4.C

Beam Centering

Another consideration with elongation concerns divergent rays. Because the x-ray beam is cone-shaped, when the beam is directed straight at the patient's body, the photons at the edge of the beam are at a slight angle compared with the photons at the center of the beam. Therefore on every radiograph, especially ones on a large film, there is some elongation of the image at the edges of the film. Because of this it is important to keep the structure of interest directly under the central ray to avoid the slight elongation that may occur if the structure is placed at the edge of the beam. This is especially important when the joint space is required to be "open" on the radiograph (Fig. 4–9).

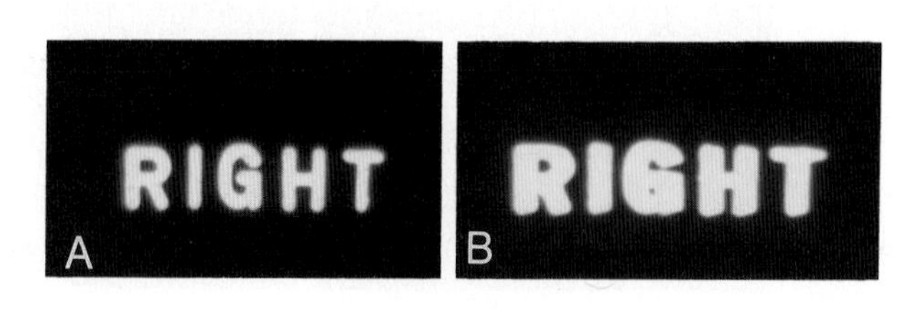

FIGURE 4–7. (*A*) Good image. (*B*) Elongation of the image.

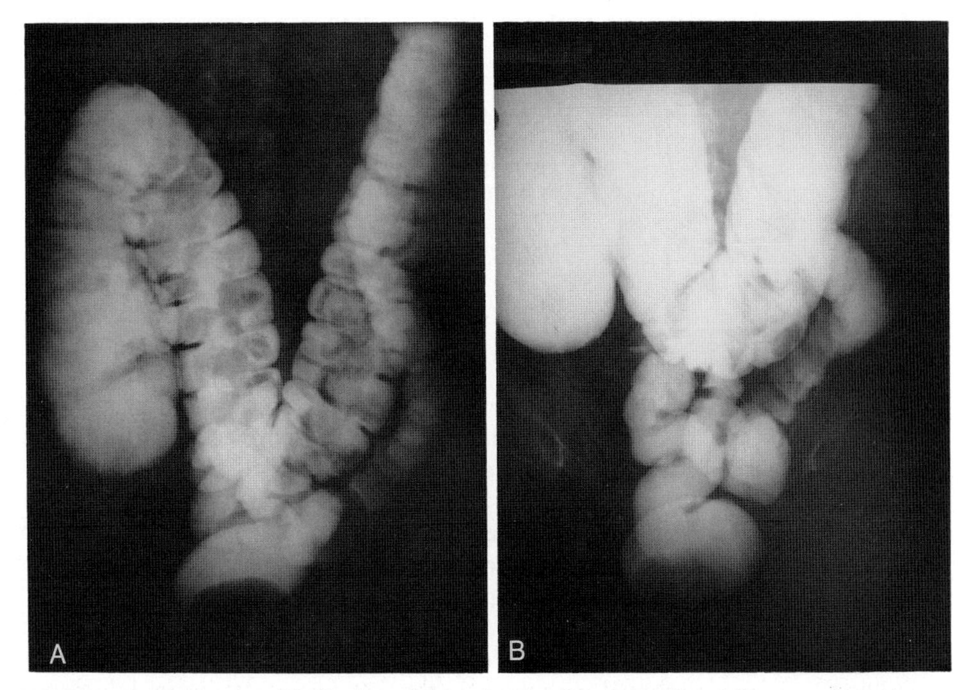

FIGURE 4–8. (*A*) PA colon. (*B*) Tilt view of the colon showing elongation of the recto-sigmoid area.

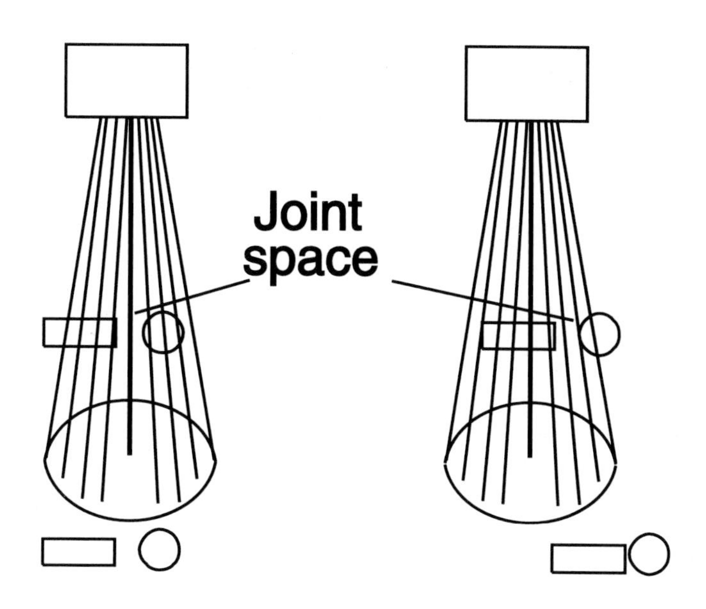

FIGURE 4–9. The central ray must be placed directly over a joint space to demonstrate the space or joint opening on a radiograph.

Place the central ray directly over the structure of interest to minimize shape distortion.

PERFORM ACTIVITY 4.D

SPATIAL DISTORTION

Spatial distortion occurs when the central ray is at an angle but the object and film are parallel to each other. In spatial distortion the three-dimensional relationship between several body parts is distorted on the image by a different elongation of each part.

If two body parts lie on top of each other in the image, they are **superimposed**. If the radiographer is taking a radiograph of the whole abdomen, with the patient lying on the table face up, the x-ray photons from a perpendicular beam would enter the patient's abdomen in the front, go through the entire abdomen, and exit from the back. The photons would then enter the film, which is where the image is formed. The film is only about .01 inch thick, so the contents of the entire abdomen are presented on a thin film and appear to be on top of each other. This is called **superimposition** (Fig. 4–10).

If a radiographer were trying to produce an image of the right kidney, the ribs, liver, and fat may be seen on the image of the kidney. If several body parts are superimposed in the image, none of these parts is seen clearly as individual structures. Sometimes this is not a problem, but when it is necessary to avoid superimposition, the radiographer can either turn the patient's body so the parts will be separated and not be superimposed, or angle the x-ray beam. Angling the beam produces spatial distortion.

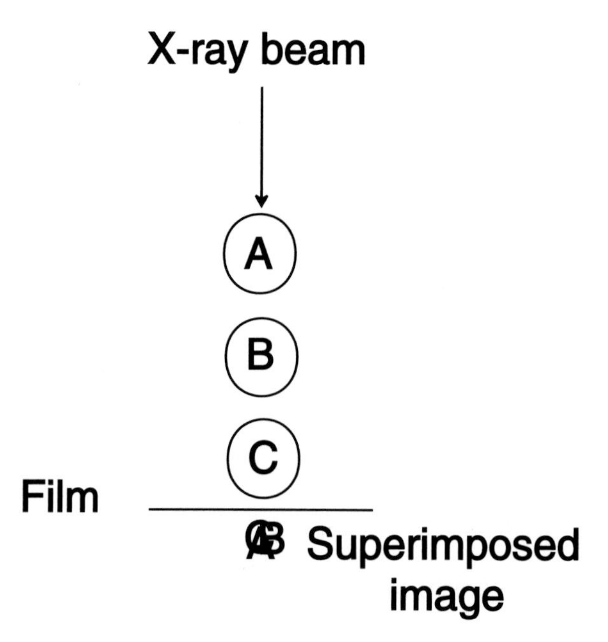

FIGURE 4–10. Superimposition of parts A, B, and C.

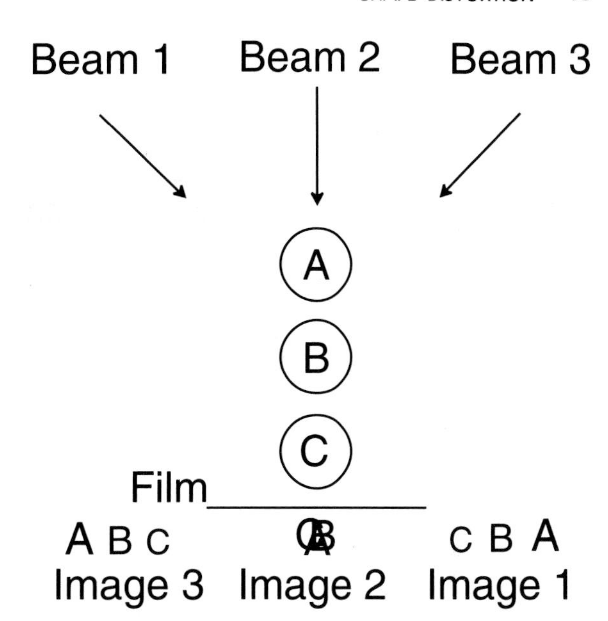

FIGURE 4–11. Spatial distortion of parts A, B, and C with an angle of the beam.

If the central ray is directed at an angle to two body parts that lie on top of each other in the body but at different distances from the film, the two body parts would not be superimposed but would appear separated on the image. Both body parts would be elongated, but the object with the largest object-image distance would be more elongated. This part will lie in a different spot on the image than the part with less object-image distance. Thus, on the image it would look as though the two parts were not actually on top of each other in the patient. The two parts would be spatially (in space) distorted on the image (Fig. 4–11).

In spatial distortion the three-dimensional relationship of body parts is distorted by an angle of the central ray.

Spatial distortion can be used to the radiographer's advantage. A good example is the problem of trying to see the clavicle as a separate structure on the image. The clavicle is located in the superior aspect of the chest. If a radiograph is taken of this area with the patient flat on the table face up and the central ray perpendicular to the film, the clavicle will appear superimposed over the top of the chest on the radiograph. A small fracture of the clavicle might be hidden by this superimposition. By angling the central ray toward the patient's head, the clavicle, which has more object-image distance than the chest, appears above the chest on the radiograph, and it is seen as a separate structure. Figure 4–12 shows two clavicle radiographs, one taken with the central ray perpendicular to the clavicle and one with the central ray angled toward the head. The fracture is only seen on the radiograph with the central ray angle.

The direction of the angle of the central ray is important when the radiographer is trying to use spatial distortion to separate structures. In the above example, with an angle of the central ray toward the patient's head, the clavicle appears above the chest on the radiograph. It is seen higher than it really is in the body. With an angle of the central ray toward the patient's feet, the clavicle will be projected lower in the pa-

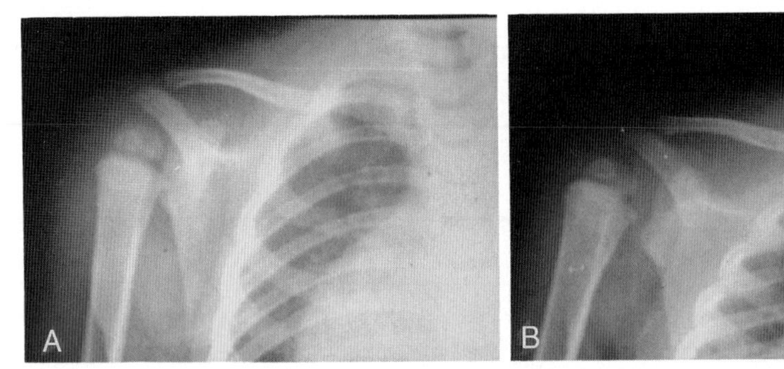

FIGURE 4–12. *(A)* AP clavicle with no central ray angle. *(B)* The same clavicle with a 10-degree angle toward the head demonstrates a fracture that is hidden in radiograph *A*.

tient's chest than it really is in the body. This would superimpose the clavicle over the middle part of the chest and would not improve the image of the clavicle.

An object with a large object-image distance will appear to move on the radiograph, in the same direction as the central ray angle. This relocation on the image is spatial distortion.

PERFORM ACTIVITY 4.E

SUMMARY

The ideal relationship between the central ray, object, and film produces the least shape distortion. The central ray should be placed directly over the structure of interest. The central ray should be positioned perpendicular to the object and to the film. The object and film should be parallel to each other.

Foreshortening occurs when the object is at an angle, but the central ray is kept perpendicular to the film. Elongation occurs when the object is parallel to the film, but the central ray is angled. Spatial distortion occurs when two objects would normally appear superimposed in the image but appear as separate structures due to an angle of the central ray.

PERFORM ACTIVITY 4.F

Distortion Section Review Activities

PERFORM ACTIVITY 4.G

PERFORM ACTIVITY 4.H

PERFORM ACTIVITY 4.I

SECTION III

THE PRIMARY EXPOSURE FACTORS

CHAPTER 5

mAs AND RECIPROCITY

CHAPTER OUTLINE

OBJECTIVES

At the end of this chapter you should be able to:

- Define mA and explain its relationship to density.
- Define time and explain its relationship to density.
- Define mAs and explain its relationship to density.
- Describe the relationship of mA, time, and mAs to: (a) contrast, (b) recorded detail, and (c) distortion.
- Convert a time quantity expressed in milliseconds to either a fraction or a decimal equivalent and convert a time quantity expressed as a fraction or decimal to its equivalent in milliseconds.
- Calculate the mAs with the time stated in either fractions, decimals, or milliseconds.
- Given two of these factors: mA, time, or mAs, calculate the unknown factor.
- Change the mA, time, or mAs in order to control density.
- Describe the reciprocity law by explaining how two different sets of mA and time stations can equal the same mAs.
- Use the reciprocity law to control motion, to use the small focal spot, and to use a breathing technique.
- Use a mAs chart to find the mA, time, or mAs.

Before each and every x-ray exposure the radiographer has to set certain exposure factors on the x-ray control panel. How these factors are set determines the finished quality of the radiograph, so their proper selection is very important. If the radiograph has to be repeated because the exposure factors were selected improperly, the patient gets an unnecessary extra dose of radiation.

This section of the book deals with the primary exposure factors of milliamperage, exposure time, and kilovoltage. Together with the source-image distance, they are the primary factors that determine the photographic properties of density and contrast.

In this chapter you are going to learn about two of the primary exposure factors: milliamperage and exposure time, and their relationships to the quality of the radiograph. You will do some calculations of the mAs, which is a unit derived by combining milliamperage and exposure time. You will also learn how to manipulate the mA and time according to the reciprocity law, and learn how to read a mAs chart.

DENSITY

In Chapter 1, the four radiographic qualities were discussed: density, contrast, recorded detail, and distortion. Density is the overall blackness of a radiograph. The blackness of a radiograph is controlled by the amount or quantity of x-rays used to produce the image. The radiograph will be blacker or more dense if a larger amount of x-rays is used to produce it.

Density is the overall blackness of the radiograph.

The Densitometer

A device called a densitometer can measure the density of a small area on a radiograph. Figure 5–1 shows a picture of a densitometer. The densitometer displays a number corresponding to the amount of radiographic density it measures. A high number will be displayed when a black area on the radiograph is measured, meaning a lot of radiographic density is present in that area. A low number means the area measured was gray or white and that area did not have much radiographic density.

PERFORM ACTIVITY 5.A

MILLIAMPERAGE (mA)

Two exposure factors directly control the quantity of x-rays produced and therefore the amount of radiographic density. These are milliamperage and exposure time.

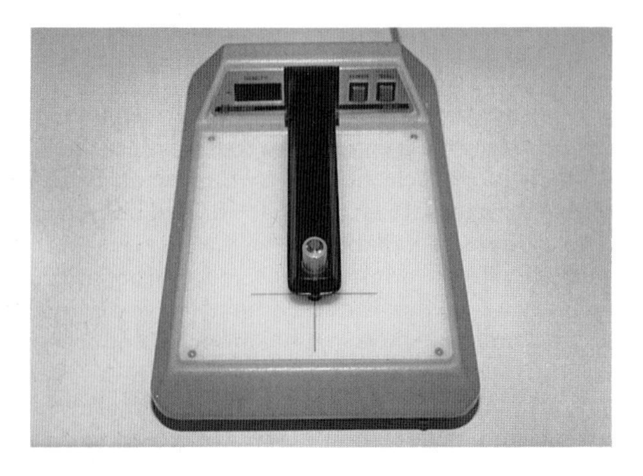

FIGURE 5–1. A photograph of a densitometer.

Table 5–1. Typical mA Stations on a Control Panel

Small Focal Spot (mA)	Large Focal Spot (mA)
25	300
50	400
100	500
200	600
	800
	1000
	1200

The milliamperage, or mA, is a measure of the quantity of current passing through the x-ray tube at the time of the exposure. The milliamperage is set by the radiographer on the control panel, and this setting determines the quantity of x-rays produced during the exposure. The mA setting determines how hot the filament of the x-ray tube gets. The heat of the filament controls how many electrons the filament releases, and the number of electrons released determines the amount of x-rays that are produced during an exposure. Table 5–1 shows the typical mA settings available on control panels.

There is a nice, easy-to-understand *direct* relationship between the mA and the quantity of x-rays produced. If the mA is increased, the quantity of x-rays produced is increased, and if the mA is decreased, the quantity of x-rays produced is decreased. The relationship is so direct and dependable that if the mA is doubled, the amount of x-rays produced is doubled. If the mA is cut in half, the amount of x-rays produced is cut in half.

Direct relationship:
Increase in mA = Increase in quantity of x-rays produced
Decrease in mA = Decrease in quantity of x-rays produced

The density or blackness of a radiograph is controlled by the quantity of x-rays in the beam, and since mA controls this quantity, there is also a direct relationship between mA and density. If the mA is increased, the density is increased, and if the mA is decreased, the density is decreased.

Direct relationship:
Increase in mA = Increase in density on the radiograph
Decrease in mA = Decrease in density on the radiograph

Figure 5–2 shows three radiographs taken with everything the same but the mA. As the mA is increased, the density or blackness of the radiograph changes. In clinical practice, it would not take many x-rays to produce an image of a small patient. A lower quantity of x-rays and therefore a small mA setting could be used. For a larger patient the mA setting could be increased in order to increase the amount of x-rays.

In routine radiography, using well-chosen techniques, milliamperage has no effect on contrast, recorded detail, or distortion. The only thing the mA controls or changes is the quantity of x-rays produced, and that controls or changes only density. Milliamperage cannot affect contrast because it does not change the energy of the

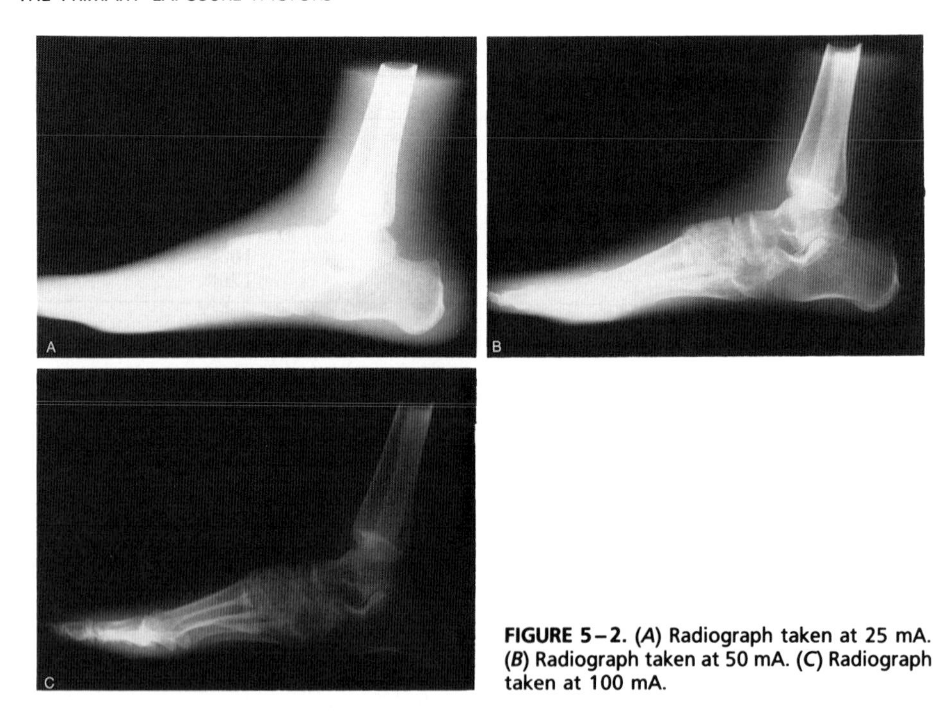

FIGURE 5–2. (*A*) Radiograph taken at 25 mA. (*B*) Radiograph taken at 50 mA. (*C*) Radiograph taken at 100 mA.

x-rays in the beam. It changes the amount of x-rays equally in the entire beam, so as it produces more or fewer x-rays in the low-energy part of the beam, it also produces more or fewer x-rays in the medium and high-energy part of the beam. A change in the mA does not change any of the distances used during the exposure, or the film and screen system used, so mA cannot affect recorded detail or distortion. It only changes one radiographic quality and that is the density.

mA affects only density.

PERFORM ACTIVITY 5.B

EXPOSURE TIME (s)

Another exposure factor the radiographer must set on the control panel before every x-ray exposure is the exposure time. The exposure time controls the length of the x-ray exposure by determining how long the current (mA) will be passing through the x-ray tube.

Exposure time determines the length of the x-ray exposure.

Since the mA controls the quantity of x-rays produced, the time also controls the quantity of x-rays produced because the time determines how long the mA will be working. Since mA has a direct relationship with density, time also has a *direct* relationship with density. If the time is increased, the density will increase, and if the time is decreased, the density will decrease.

Direct relationship:
Increase in time = Increase in density on the radiograph
Decrease in time = Decrease in density on the radiograph

Figure 5–3 shows three radiographs taken with everything the same but the time. As the time is increased, the density increases. If the time is doubled, the density doubles, and if the time is cut in half, the density is cut in half.

You have already learned that in routine radiography, using well-chosen techniques, mA controls only density and does not affect contrast, recorded detail, or distortion. Since time controls how long the mA is working, it is easy to see that time also controls only density and does not affect contrast, recorded detail, or distortion.

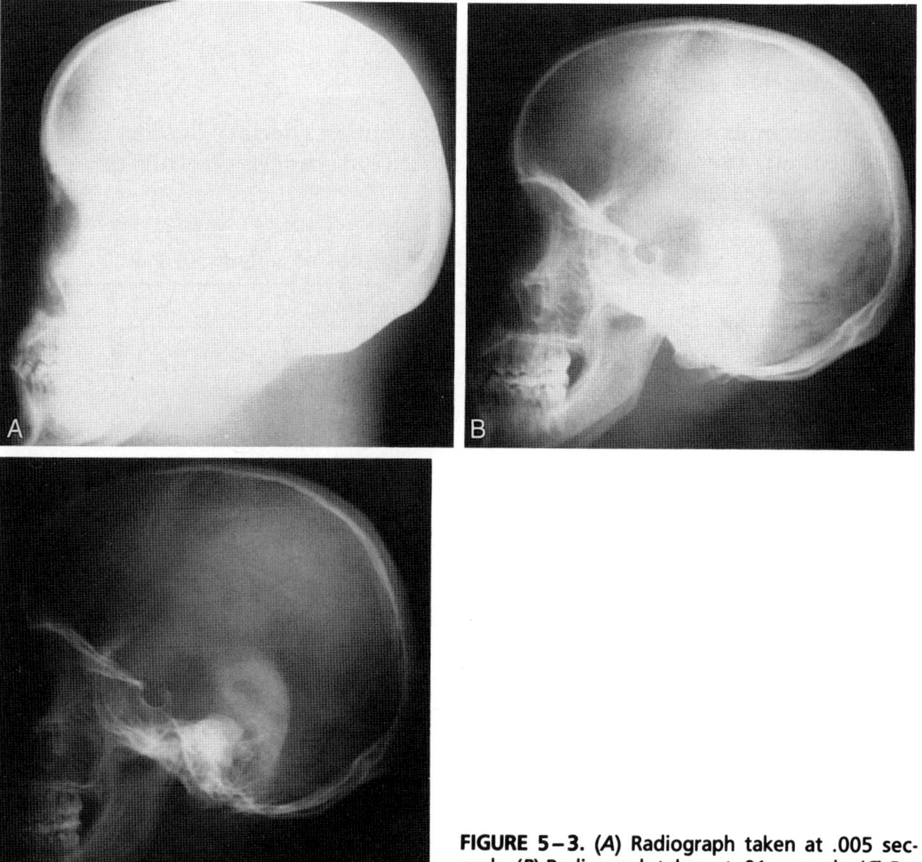

FIGURE 5–3. (*A*) Radiograph taken at .005 seconds. (*B*) Radiograph taken at .01 seconds. (*C*) Radiograph taken at .02 seconds.

Exposure time affects only density.

If the density on a radiograph needs to be adjusted, either the mA or time can be changed. In clinical practice it is better to change the time than the mA in order to change density. You will see the reason for this later.

PERFORM ACTIVITY 5.C

Time Stations

There is a significant problem for new x-ray students with the timer selections on x-ray equipment. The same problem that occurred with the Tower of Babel also occurred with the timer. According to the Bible, the Tower of Babel was a tower built to reach heaven, but which stopped short when God caused the builders to speak a multitude of different languages.

Time stations on a control panel can be stated in fractions, decimals, or milliseconds depending on the type of x-ray unit and the manufacturer. Table 5–2 shows some of the typical settings for the timer with the three different "languages." Most people are familiar with calculations involving fractions and decimals, but milliseconds is a new term.

Milliseconds

Milliseconds need to be converted to a fraction or a decimal in order to perform calculations. The prefix "milli-" in front of a word changes it to 1000 times smaller. A

Table 5–2. Typical Time Stations on a Control Panel

Time in fractions			
1/120	1/10	1/2	2
1/60	3/20	3/5	3
1/40	1/5	2/3	4
1/30	1/4	3/4	6
1/20	1/3	4/5	
1/15	2/5	1	
Time in decimals			
.005	.03	.20	.70
.007	.035	.25	1
.01	.05	.30	2
.015	.07	.35	3
.02	.10	.40	4
.025	.15	.50	6
Time in milliseconds			
1.0	4.0	16.0	64.0
1.2	5.0	20.0	80.0
1.6	6.4	25.0	100.0
2.0	8.0	32.0	125.0
2.5	10.0	40.0	150.0
3.2	12.5	50.0	

millisecond is 1000 times smaller than a second. One thousand milliseconds equals 1 second.

To change milliseconds to a fraction, put the number of milliseconds in the numerator and 1000 in the denominator.

$$2 \text{ milliseconds} = \frac{2}{1000} \text{ seconds}$$

$$50 \text{ milliseconds} = \frac{50}{1000} \text{ seconds}$$

$$400 \text{ milliseconds} = \frac{400}{1000} \text{ seconds}$$

To change milliseconds to a decimal, put a decimal point to the right of the number of milliseconds, move it three places to the left and fill in any empty spaces with zeros. The thousandth place in the decimal system is the third place, which is why the decimal point is moved three places.

10 milliseconds = .01 seconds
350 milliseconds = .35 seconds
1500 milliseconds = 1.5 seconds

PERFORM ACTIVITY 5.D

MILLIAMPERE-SECONDS (mAs)

If the two exposure factors of mA and time are put together they form a new unit called milliampere-seconds (mAs). The mAs represents the total quantity of x-rays produced in an x-ray beam because it takes into account both the quantity of x-rays produced by the mA and the length of time the x-rays are produced.

mAs represents the total quantity of x-rays produced in a beam.

The mAs is the product of the mA and time and is calculated by multiplying the mA by the time.

500 mA × .01 second = 5 mAs
200 mA × 1/5 second = 40 mAs
300 mA × 50 msec = 15 mAs

Be careful! When the time is stated in milliseconds, the millisecond number must always be converted to a fraction or decimal before it is multiplied by the mA.

To calculate the mAs, multiply the mA by the time.

On some control panels, technologists must set only the mAs and do not select the mA and time separately. On others, the mA and time are selected separately and the mAs is not shown. The mAs is not known until it is calculated. Some technologists prefer to think in terms of mA and time and others prefer to think in terms of mAs. Students need to become adept with both ways of thinking.

PERFORM ACTIVITY 5.E

mA and time control only density and do not affect contrast, recorded detail, or distortion. So the unit of mAs, composed of the mA and time, also controls only density and does not affect contrast, recorded detail, or distortion. There is a direct relationship between mA and density and time and density. So there must also be a direct relationship between mAs and density. If the mAs changes, the density must also change. If the mAs is decreased by 30%, the density will be decreased by 30%.

Direct relationship:
Increase in mAs = Increase in density on the radiograph
Decrease in mAs = Decrease in density on the radiograph

Figure 5–4 shows radiographs taken with different mAs settings. As the mAs is increased, the density is increased.

PERFORM ACTIVITY 5.F

Changing the Density with mAs

If the density on a radiograph needs to be changed because the radiograph is too dark or too light, totally new mA and time stations could be used for the repeat radiograph, or just the mA station or just the time station could be changed.

If the mA station is kept the same and only the time setting is changed, a whole new mAs is produced and the density on the radiograph will be changed.

400 mA × .01 second = 4 mAs
400 mA × .025 second = 10 mAs
400 mA × .05 second = 20 mAs

If the time setting is kept the same and only the mA station is changed, a whole new mAs is produced and the density on the radiograph will be changed.

200 mA × .02 second = 4 mAs
300 mA × .02 second = 6 mAs
500 mA × .02 second = 10 mAs

PERFORM ACTIVITY 5.G

The direct relationship between density and mAs is very useful in clinical practice. If a radiograph turns out too dark or dense, the radiograph must be repeated with a decrease in density. This is done very easily by decreasing the mAs, which can be accomplished by decreasing the mA or the time. If the radiograph is judged to be just a little too dark, the density might only need to be decreased by 30%. If it is very

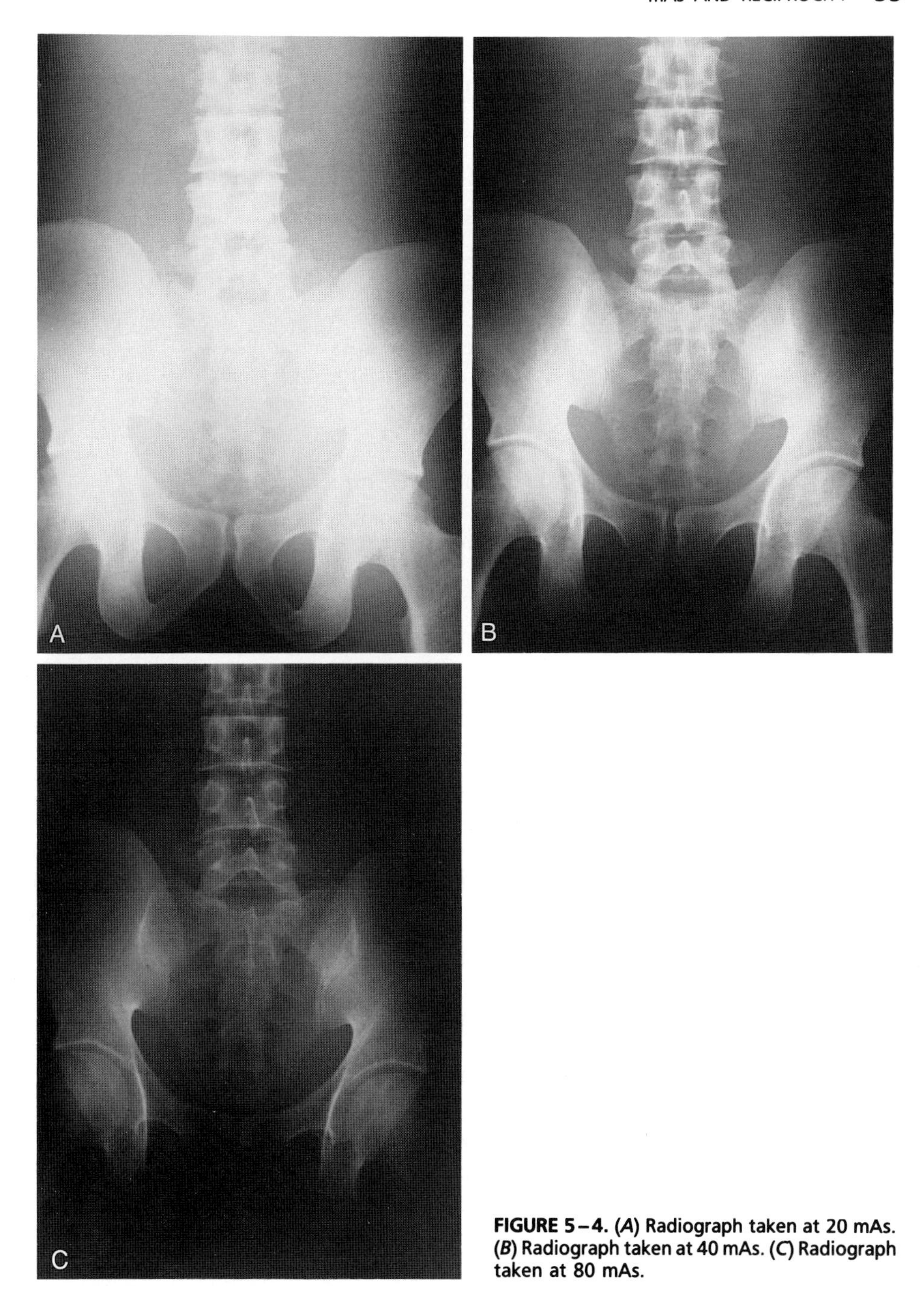

FIGURE 5–4. (*A*) Radiograph taken at 20 mAs. (*B*) Radiograph taken at 40 mAs. (*C*) Radiograph taken at 80 mAs.

dark, the density might need to be decreased by 50% or even more. It usually requires at least a 30% change in mAs to see a visible change in density on the radiograph. The judgment of how dark or light a radiograph appears is very difficult at first and is a skill students acquire as they progress in clinical education.

Calculating the Unknown Factor

In an algebraic formula containing three factors, if two of the factors are known, the other one can be calculated. The following equation can be used to calculate any unknown factor:

$$\text{mA} \times \text{time} = \text{mAs}$$

To calculate mAs:

$$200 \text{ mA} \times .05 \text{ second} = \text{mAs}$$
$$200 \times .05 = 10 \text{ mAs}$$

To calculate mA:

$$\text{mA} \times .05 \text{ second} = 10 \text{ mAs}$$
$$\text{mA} = \frac{10}{.05}$$
$$\text{mA} = 200$$

To calculate time:

$$200 \text{ mA} \times \text{time} = 10 \text{ mAs}$$
$$\text{time} = \frac{10}{200}$$
$$\text{time} = .05$$

This capability is very useful in clinical situations. For example, what if you knew you wanted to use 15 mAs on a patient with the 600-mA station, and you needed to know what time to set on the control panel in order to get 15 mAs?

$$600 \text{ mA} \times \text{time} = 15 \text{ mAs}$$
$$\text{time} = \frac{15}{600}$$
$$\text{time} = .025$$

PERFORM ACTIVITY 5.H

RECIPROCITY LAW

Now here's a dilemma. If the control panel is set at 500 mA and .02 second, 10 mAs would be produced. If it is set at 100 mA and .10 second, 10 mAs would also be produced. The total quantity of x-rays produced has not changed between the two different settings because the mAs is exactly the same. And the density on the two radiographs should be exactly the same.

This is an example of the reciprocity law, which says that a variety of different mA and time settings could produce the same mAs and therefore the same density

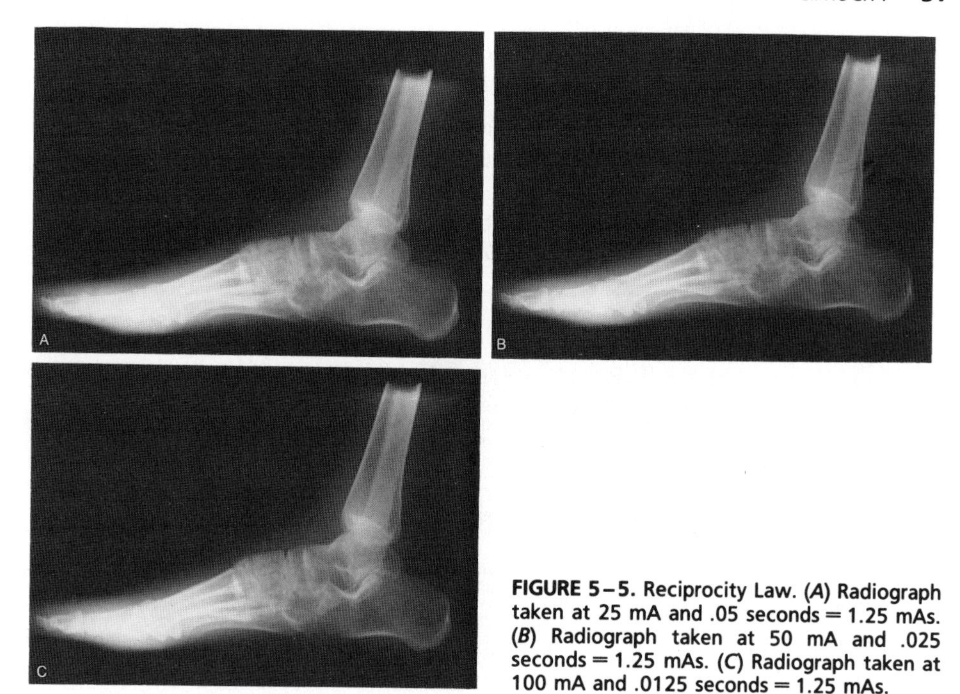

FIGURE 5–5. Reciprocity Law. (*A*) Radiograph taken at 25 mA and .05 seconds = 1.25 mAs. (*B*) Radiograph taken at 50 mA and .025 seconds = 1.25 mAs. (*C*) Radiograph taken at 100 mA and .0125 seconds = 1.25 mAs.

(Fig. 5–5). This law works well most of the time, except at very low or very high time settings.

Here are some examples:

$$400 \text{ mA} \times .05 \text{ second} = 20 \text{ mAs}$$

$$200 \text{ mA} \times .10 \text{ second} = 20 \text{ mAs}$$

$$300 \text{ mA} \times \frac{1}{15} \text{ second} = 20 \text{ mAs}$$

$$50 \text{ mA} \times \frac{2}{5} \text{ second} = 20 \text{ mAs}$$

$$500 \text{ mA} \times 40 \text{ msec} = 20 \text{ mAs}$$

$$800 \text{ mA} \times 25 \text{ msec} = 20 \text{ mAs}$$

Technique charts usually show a specific mA and time setting that should be used on a body part. The charts ordinarily work well and can be depended on most of the time. But a good radiographer also has the ability to use different settings from those the technique chart calls for depending on variables that can occur in clinical practice. There are three instances in clinical practice when the reciprocity law can be used. These are to control motion, to use a small focal spot, and to use the breathing technique.

Control of Motion

If a patient moves during an x-ray exposure the radiograph will appear blurry (Fig. 5–6). The recorded detail of the anatomy on the radiograph won't be sharp and the radiograph would need to be repeated, causing more radiation exposure to the patient.

The possibility of motion blur on a radiograph can be reduced by using a short time setting on the control panel. For example, 300 mA and .5 second is 150 mAs.

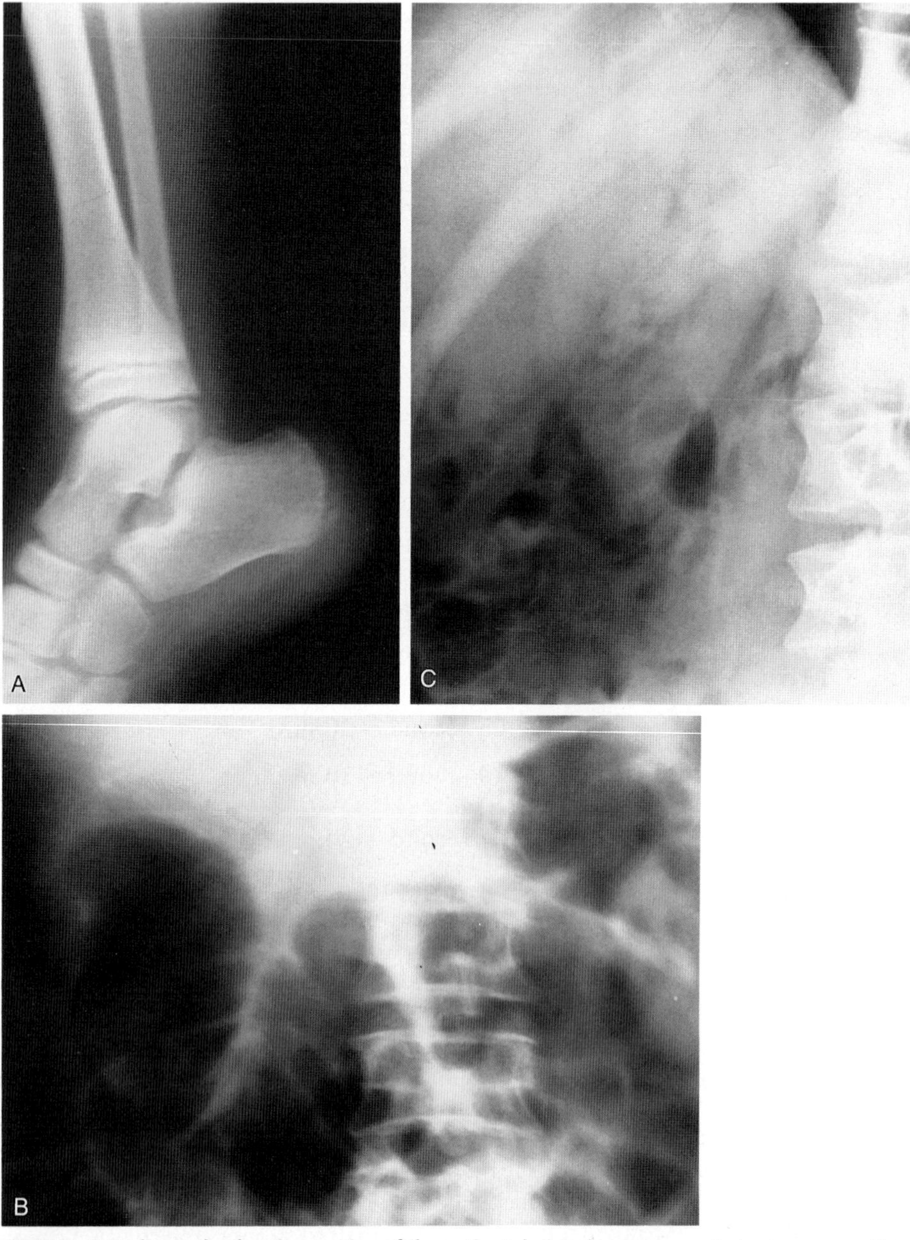

FIGURE 5–6. Radiographs showing motion of the patient during the exposure. A short exposure time helps control motion.

But 600 mA and .25 second is also 150 mAs. Two radiographs taken with these factors should look exactly the same, but with the higher mA of 600 and the shorter time of .25 second, the patient would have less chance of moving during the exposure.

Short time reduces the chance of motion blur.

A good technique is established to use a high mA station so that a short time can be used. This helps eliminate the chance of motion on the radiograph. It is often better in clinical practice to use a high mA station and change the time rather than the mA when the density needs to be changed.

PERFORM ACTIVITY 5.I

The Small Focal Spot

As learned in Chapter 2, the focal spot size is determined by which filament in the x-ray tube is heated. A small focal spot is achieved when the small filament is heated and a large focal spot is achieved when the large filament is heated. Heating of the different sizes of filaments causes either a small or large area on the anode of the x-ray tube to be hit with electrons. This area on the anode is the actual focal spot.

The small focal spot is used to enhance recorded detail. A small focal spot produces better recorded detail than a large focal spot, and this makes the image appear sharper.

A small focal spot improves recorded detail.

On some x-ray control panels the radiographer must set the focal spot independently from the mA station. On other x-ray units, the focal spot and the mA station are both set at the same time because they are linked together on the same control panel button or dial. On both types of units the smaller mA stations produce a small focal spot and the larger mA stations produce a large focal spot. A small focal spot cannot be obtained with a high mA station.

A setting of 50 mA and .2 second will produce 10 mAs. This mA station would be in the small focal spot range; 500 mA and .02 second will also produce 10 mAs, but this high mA station would be in the large focal spot range.

The small focal spot cannot be used on every radiograph because the small filament cannot produce the higher mA that should be used for most of the radiographic exams performed. Chests, abdomens, spines, skulls, and gastrointestinal (GI) work all require a high mAs and therefore a high mA station to produce enough density on the radiograph because these are large body parts. Trying to heat the small filament and get a high mA can cause the filament wire to burn out and break.

In clinical settings the small focal spot is usually used on small body parts like hands, wrists, feet, and noses. The small focal spot is used to enhance the recorded detail on these parts.

A smaller mA station is required when using the small focal spot. The ability to calculate the unknown factor in the formula mA $\times$ time = mAs is useful here. First figure out what mAs is necessary for the exposure. Then divide the mAs by the highest mA that is in the small focal spot range. The answer is the exposure time. If that time station is not available on the control panel, find an mA and time combination that will produce the mAs necessary and still use a small focal spot. This might take some trials before the right combination is found. The highest mA station that is in the small focal spot range should be used to keep the exposure time short and reduce the possibility of motion on the radiograph.

PERFORM ACTIVITY 5.J

The Breathing Technique

How many times so far in your clinical education have you told patients to hold their breath? This is done to control the motion of the patient during the exposure. It prevents the image from becoming blurry due to the motion. The breathing technique flips this theory and purposely produces motion on a radiograph.

As the patient breathes, his or her ribs and lungs move. If a radiograph of the chest area is exposed while the patient is breathing, the ribs and bronchial markings of the lungs that are seen on chest radiographs would appear blurry. By purposely blurring these parts, the other structures in the chest area are seen better.

If a low mA station and a long time is used, the patient would have more opportunity to breathe during the exposure and blur out the ribs and bronchial markings. This special selection of a low mA with a long time is called the breathing technique.

A low mA with a long time produces the breathing technique.

Most radiographers use a breathing technique during sternum exams, and when performing a lateral view of the thoracic spine. Also a transthoracic humerus radiograph, which is a lateral humerus exposed through the chest, is enhanced with the breathing technique (Fig. 5–7). In these instances the sternum, thoracic spine, and humerus are seen better because the ribs and bronchial markings of the lungs are blurred on the radiograph.

PERFORM ACTIVITY 5.K

mAs CHARTS

Most technologists do not walk around at work with calculators in their pockets; so in order to be able to calculate all the different mAs values or to find the unknown factor, departments often have mAs charts posted near the x-ray rooms. The ability to read a mAs chart makes life easier.

Table 5–3 shows a partial mAs chart. To find the mAs produced by a particular mA and time station, it is necessary to find where the mA and time intersect on the chart. Try it. First find the 50-mA spot on the top of the chart and keep a finger on it. Then on the left side of the chart, find the .10 time spot and put another finger on that. Slide the finger on the mA spot down and the finger on the time spot over until

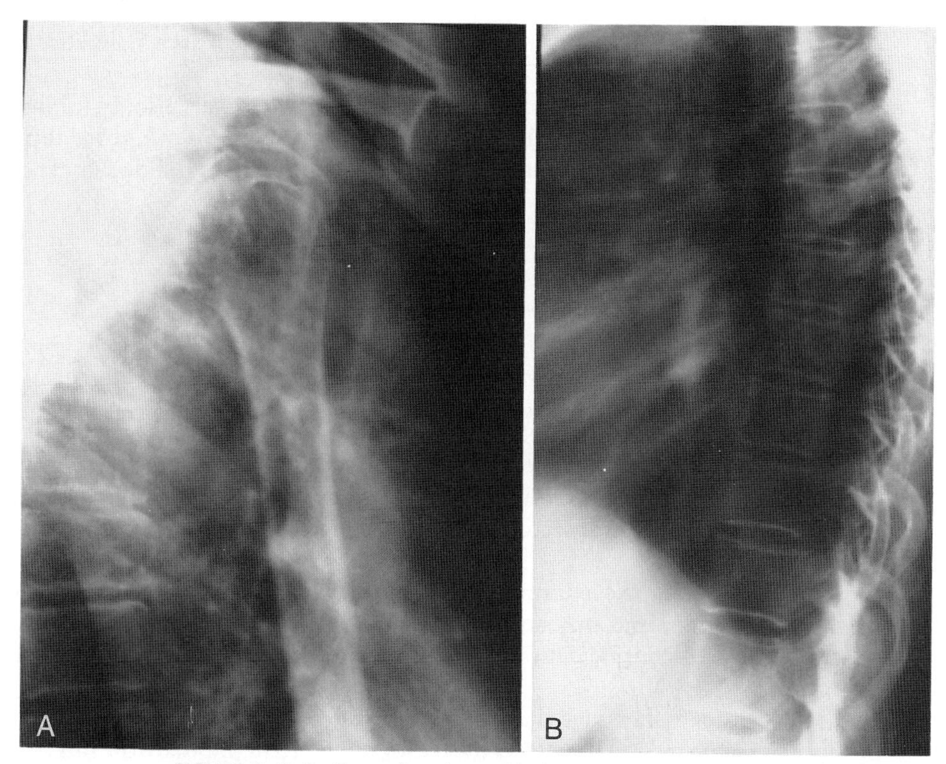

FIGURE 5–7. Radiographs taken with the breathing technique.

Table 5–3. mAs Chart

Time (ms)	Time (fraction)	Time (decimal)	25 mA	50 mA	100 mA	200 mA	300 mA	400 mA	500 mA	600 mA
5	—	.005	.125	.250	.50	1.0	1.5	2.0	2.5	3.0
7	—	.007	.175	.350	.70	1.4	2.1	2.8	3.5	4.2
8.3	1/120	.0083	.207	.414	.828	1.65	2.48	3.33	4.16	5.0
10	—	.010	.25	.50	1.0	2.0	3.0	4.0	5.0	6.0
15	—	.015	.375	.75	1.5	3.0	4.5	6.0	7.5	9.0
16.6	1/60	.0166	.417	.834	1.66	3.33	4.98	6.66	8.30	9.96
20	—	.020	.50	1.0	2.0	4.0	6.0	8.0	10.0	12.0
25	1/40	.025	.625	1.25	2.5	5.0	7.5	10.0	12.5	15.0
30	—	.030	.750	1.5	3.0	6.0	9.0	12.0	15.0	18.0
33.3	1/30	.0333	.834	1.66	3.33	6.66	9.99	13.3	16.6	20.0
35	—	.035	.875	1.75	3.5	7.0	10.5	14.0	17.5	21.0
40	—	.040	1.0	2.0	4.0	8.0	12.0	16.0	20.0	24.0
50	1/20	.050	1.25	2.5	5.0	10.0	15.0	20.0	25.0	30.0
66.6	1/15	.0666	1.66	3.32	6.66	13.2	19.9	26.4	33.3	40.0
100	1/10	.10	2.5	5.0	10.0	20.0	30.0	40.0	50.0	60.0

the two fingers meet. They should meet on the chart where it says 5, because 50 mA and .10 second is 5 mAs.

Figuring out any unknown factor is very easy with the chart also. If, for instance, 5 mAs with the 50-mA station is required, it is easy to find 50 mA at the top of the chart, slide a finger down until it meets with the number 5, then slide a finger over to the left to read the time.

PERFORM ACTIVITY 5.L

SUMMARY

Milliamperage (mA) is the current in the x-ray tube at the time of the exposure. The exposure time determines how long the mA will be working. Time can be stated in fractions, decimals, or milliseconds. mA multiplied by time forms a unit called the mAs.

Time, mA, and mAs determine the quantity of x-rays produced and the density on the radiograph. Time, mA, and mAs are all directly proportional to density. They should be used to control density. They do not affect contrast, recorded detail, or distortion.

The reciprocity law says that two sets of different mA and time selections can produce the same mAs. This allows the radiographer to manipulate the mA and time to control motion by using a short exposure time, use the small focal spot by selecting a small mA station, and use the breathing technique by selecting a long exposure time with a low mA.

PERFORM ACTIVITY 5.M

CHAPTER 6

THE INVERSE SQUARE LAW

CHAPTER OUTLINE

OBJECTIVES

At the end of this chapter you should be able to:

- Describe the changes in radiation intensity at the film as the distance between the x-ray tube and film is increased or decreased.
- State the inverse square law and its formula.
- Use the inverse square law formula to calculate the new radiation intensity when the SID is increased or decreased.
- Use the inverse square law rule of thumb to calculate the new radiation intensity when the SID is doubled or cut in half.
- Explain what happens to density on a radiograph as the SID is increased or decreased.
- State the density maintenance formula.
- Use the density maintenance formula to calculate the new mAs when the SID is increased or decreased.
- Use the density maintenance formula rule of thumb to calculate the new mAs that will maintain film density when the SID is doubled or cut in half.
- Estimate the new mAs when the SID is increased or decreased.

The radiation intensity, or strength of the x-ray beam when it reaches the film, is a major factor in radiography. The intensity of the beam determines how dense or black the radiograph will appear. The radiation intensity is influenced by milliampere-seconds (mAs), which was discussed in Chapter 5, and kilovoltage (kVp), which will be discussed in Chapter 7.

The intensity of the beam at the film is also influenced by the distance between the x-ray tube and film, which is the source-image distance (SID). This distance helps determine the density on the radiograph. The effect of the distance between the x-ray tube and film on the density of the radiograph will be the focus of this chapter.

The inverse square law, which enables the radiographer to calculate the intensity of the beam at the film when the distance between the x-ray tube and the film changes, will be presented first. After learning how distance changes the intensity of the beam, you must learn how to change the exposure factors to produce a radiograph with the proper density when the distance between the x-ray tube and film changes. This is done by using the density maintenance formula. This formula is used often in nonstandard clinical situations like portable x-ray, surgery, trauma, or emergency cases, so the concepts and calculations are important.

THE INVERSE SQUARE LAW

When you were a child, did you ever play under the water sprinkler on a hot day in the summer? Think about the type of sprinkler that remains stationary and sprays water from its center into a circular area. If you stand far away from it, you won't get wet, but as you move closer and closer you get wetter and wetter.

The x-ray beam acts similarly to the water sprinkler. If you move closer to the source of an x-ray beam or the source of the x-ray beam is moved closer to you, the radiation becomes more intense or stronger at your body. And if the source of the x-ray beam is moved farther away, the radiation becomes less intense at your body. In this instance the amount of radiation coming from the x-ray tube does not change, but the distance between you and the x-ray tube changes and that causes the amount of radiation reaching you to be more or less intense.

Now think about pulling your car into a parking spot that is perpendicular to a building. At nighttime, the light from your headlights on the building gets smaller as the car gets closer to the building. As the area of light gets smaller, the light on the building appears brighter.

The x-ray beam acts similarly to the headlights. As it is moved closer to a film the beam covers a smaller area on the film. As the x-ray tube is moved closer to the film, the same amount or quantity of radiation used at the farther distance is now confined to a smaller area, and the radiation is more intense at the closer distance. As the x-ray tube is moved farther away from the film the beam covers a larger area. The same amount or quantity of radiation used at the closer distance is now spread out and covers a larger area, and the radiation is less intense at the farther distance. So both the size of the radiation area and the intensity of radiation change as the distance between the x-ray tube and film changes (Fig. 6–1).

PERFORM ACTIVITY 6.A

The intensity of radiation coming from the x-ray tube is measured in a unit called the roentgen or coulombs per kilogram. This unit can be made 1000 times smaller and it is then called a milliroentgen.

The distance between the x-ray tube and film is the source-image distance (SID). There is an inverse relationship between the SID and the radiation intensity at the film. If the SID increases, the radiation intensity at the film decreases. And if the SID decreases, the radiation intensity at the film increases. The new radiation intensity after any SID change can be calculated with the inverse square law formula. The inverse square law states

The intensity of radiation is inversely proportional to the square of the distance from the source of radiation.

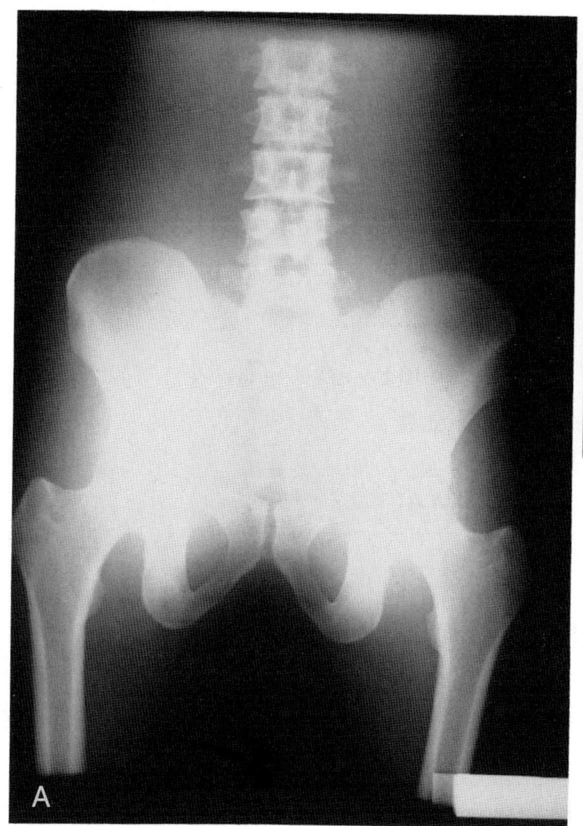

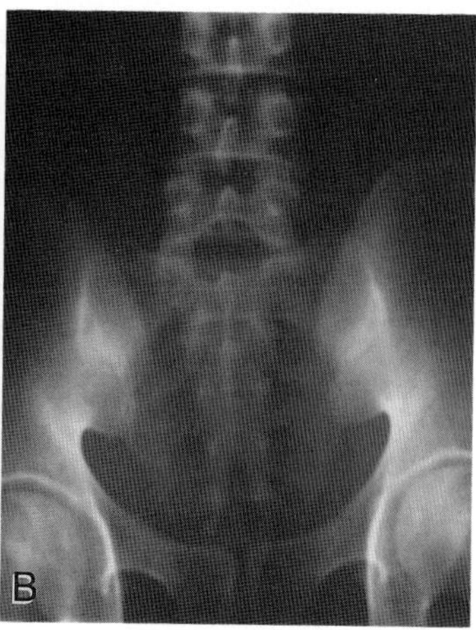

FIGURE 6–1. (*A*) Radiograph was taken at a 72-inch SID. (*B*) Radiograph was taken at a 36-inch SID without changing the collimation field size or exposure factors. The x-ray beam covers a smaller area as it is moved closer to the film. It also becomes more intense.

The inverse square law formula is

$$\frac{I_1}{I_2} = \frac{D_2^2}{D_1^2}$$

I_1 = the original intensity of radiation
I_2 = the new intensity of radiation after the distance changes
D_2^2 = the new distance squared
D_1^2 = the original distance squared

Calculating the New Intensity

Usually the unknown factor is the new intensity. For example, what if the original amount of radiation intensity at the film is 100 mR (milliroentgens) when the x-ray tube is at a 40-inch distance from the film. If the x-ray tube had to be moved to a 72-inch distance from the film, the amount of radiation intensity at the film changes. The radiation intensity at the film would be less if the x-ray tube is moved farther away. The same amount of radiation used at the original distance would be spread over a larger area becoming less intense. To calculate the new intensity

$$\frac{100}{I_2} = \frac{72^2}{40^2}$$

First square the distances,

$$\frac{100}{I_2} = \frac{5184}{1600}$$

then cross-multiply,

$$5184 \times I_2 = 160{,}000$$

then solve the equation:

$$I_2 = \frac{160{,}000}{5184}$$

$$I_2 = 30.86 \text{ mR}$$

The new radiation intensity is 30.86 mR.

PERFORM ACTIVITY 6.B

Rule of Thumb for Calculating Radiation Intensity

The change in radiation intensity after a change in SID is more than what might be expected. Students often make the mistake of thinking that if the source-image distance is doubled, the radiation intensity is cut in half. When the SID is doubled, the area of radiation at the film grows by 4 times because both the length of the radiation and the width of the radiation are doubled. This spreads the radiation over an area which is four times larger than the original area and this reduces the radiation intensity. When the SID is doubled, the radiation area increases by four times, but the radiation intensity decreases by four times (Fig. 6–2).

The following is a rule of thumb that is helpful to remember.

If the source-image distance is doubled, the radiation intensity at the film becomes four times less; and if the source-image distance is cut in half, the radiation intensity at the film becomes four times greater.

If the radiation intensity at a 36-inch SID is 50 mR, the radiation intensity at a 72-inch SID would be four times less or 12.5 mR. If the radiation intensity at an 80-inch SID is 70 mR, the radiation intensity at a 40-inch SID would be 280 mR.

PERFORM ACTIVITY 6.C

Measuring Radiation Intensity

The amount of radiation intensity can be measured with a device called an ionization chamber. When using an ionization chamber, the arrangement for an ordinary x-ray exposure is used, except the ionization chamber is placed at the location where the film would usually be placed. Then an exposure is made by exposing the ionization chamber to radiation. The ionization chamber measures the number of milliroent-

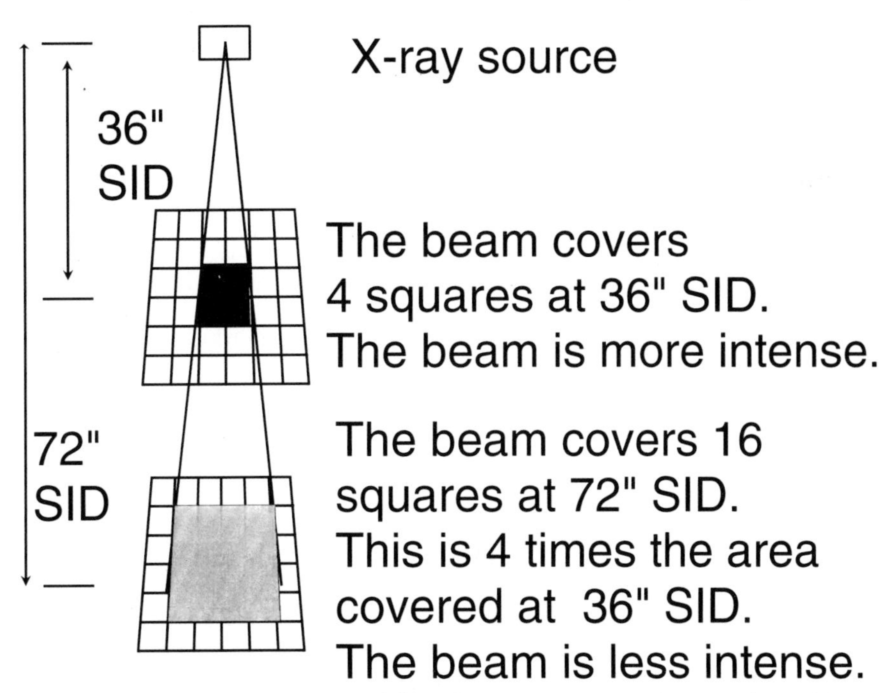

FIGURE 6–2. The radiation area is smaller and the radiation is more intense at a 36-inch SID. If the SID is doubled to 72 inches, the area of radiation is 4 times larger, but the radiation intensity is 4 times less than it was at the 36-inch SID.

gens it receives. The reading on the ionization chamber corresponds to the amount of radiation that reaches it.

PERFORM ACTIVITY 6.D

THE DENSITY MAINTENANCE FORMULA

There is another formula, derived from the concept of the inverse square law, which is very useful to the radiographer in clinical practice. This formula, called the density maintenance formula, allows the radiographer to calculate the new exposure factors to be used when the distance between the x-ray tube and film changes.

The radiation intensity at the film determines the amount of density on the radiograph. If two radiographs are taken with the same amount of radiation but with different source-image distances, the intensity of the radiation at the film is different for each exposure and therefore the density on each radiograph is also different (Fig. 6–3).

If the density on the film was satisfactory before the distance changed, it won't be acceptable at the new distance because the radiation intensity has changed. When the SID changes, the intensity also changes. The mAs needs to be increased or decreased to compensate for the distance change.

If the source-image distance decreases, the radiation intensity at the film increases, and then the mAs needs to be decreased to maintain the same density as be-

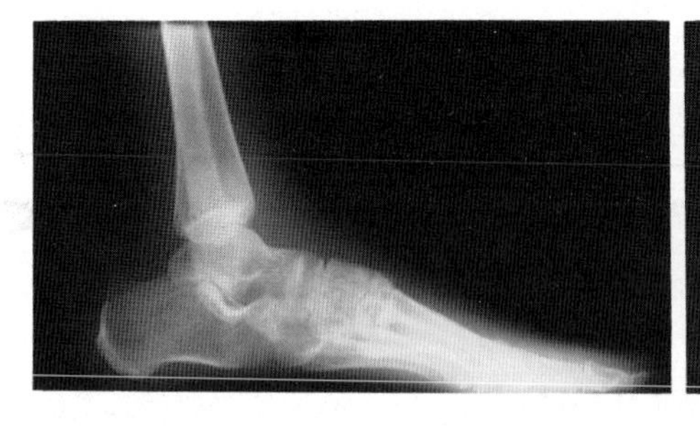
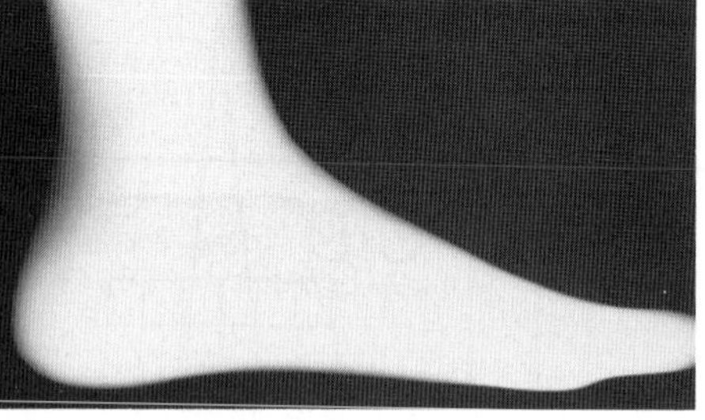

FIGURE 6–3. (*A*) Radiograph taken at a 40-inch SID and 1.25 mAs. (*B*) Radiograph taken at a 72-inch SID and 1.25 mAs.

fore the distance change. Conversely, if the source-image distance increases, the radiation intensity at the film decreases, and then the mAs needs to be increased to maintain the density. The amount of increase or decrease of the mAs can be calculated with the density maintenance formula. The density maintenance formula states

The new mAs equals the old mAs multiplied by the new distance squared and divided by the old distance squared.

The formula is

$$\text{New mAs} = \frac{\text{Old mAs} \times \text{New distance}^2}{\text{Old distance}^2}$$

Calculating the New mAs with the Density Maintenance Formula

Assume that 1.25 mAs was used to produce a good radiograph at an original 40-inch SID. Then the SID was changed to 72 inches for a repeat radiograph. The radiographer needs to know what mAs to use at the new 72-inch SID to produce another good radiograph.

$$\text{New mAs} = \frac{1.25 \times 72^2}{40^2}$$

First square the distances.

$$\text{New mAs} = \frac{1.25 \times 5184}{1600}$$

Then solve

$$\text{New mAs} = \frac{6480}{1600}$$

$$\text{New mAs} = 4.0$$

In this example the mAs must be increased from 1.25 to 4.0 because the SID was

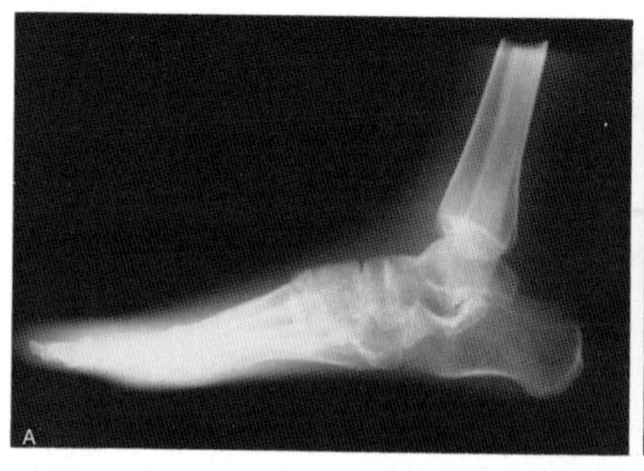

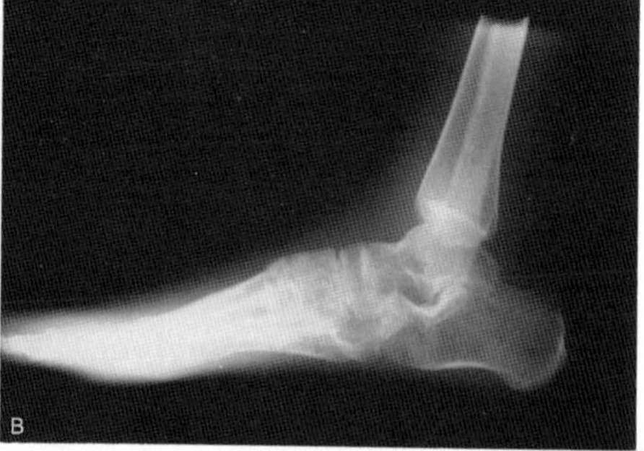

FIGURE 6–4. (*A*) Radiograph taken at a 40-inch SID and 1.25 mAs. (*B*) Radiograph taken at a 72-inch SID and 4 mAs.

increased, which decreased the radiation intensity at the film. The two radiographs, the one with a 40-inch SID and 1.25 mAs, and the one taken with a 72-inch SID and 4.0 mAs should have the same density (Fig. 6–4).

PERFORM ACTIVITY 6.E

PERFORM ACTIVITY 6.F

The density maintenance formula can also be used to calculate the new mA or exposure time. Instead of inserting mAs into the formula, either the mA or exposure time could be inserted and a new mA or exposure time can be calculated.

It isn't too useful in clinical situations to calculate the new mA station because the mA station should be standard for the exam being performed. Usually a high mA should be used. This allows the use of a short exposure time, and short exposure times limit motion on the radiograph. So if a radiographer is already using a high mA station, that should not be changed.

The new time can be calculated when the source-image distance changes instead of the new mAs. Then the radiographer would know what new time to use after one calculation rather than having to calculate the new mAs first and then the new time. In the example used to calculate the new mAs, assume that the original 1.25 mAs was achieved by using 50 mA and .025 second.

$$\text{New time} = \frac{.025 \times 72^2}{40^2}$$

$$\text{Time} = \frac{.025 \times 5184}{1600}$$

$$\text{New time} = \frac{130}{1600}$$

$$\text{Time} = .08$$

The new exposure time of .08 multiplied by 50 mA equals 4.0 mAs, which is the same mAs calculated in the original problem.

PERFORM ACTIVITY 6.G

Rule of Thumb for Calculating Exposure Factors

A rule of thumb can be used to calculate the new mAs when the SID is doubled or cut in half. The rule of thumb makes the calculations easier.

If the source-image distance is doubled, the mAs needs to be increased by 4 times. If the source-image distance is cut in half, the mAs needs to be decreased by 4 times.

If 1 mAs is used at a 36-inch SID, a mAs of 4.0 could be used at a 72-inch SID. The two radiographs would display the same density (Fig. 6–5). If an exposure time of .10 second is used at an 80-inch SID, an exposure time of .025 second could be used at a 40-inch SID. These two radiographs would also display the same density.

PERFORM ACTIVITY6.H

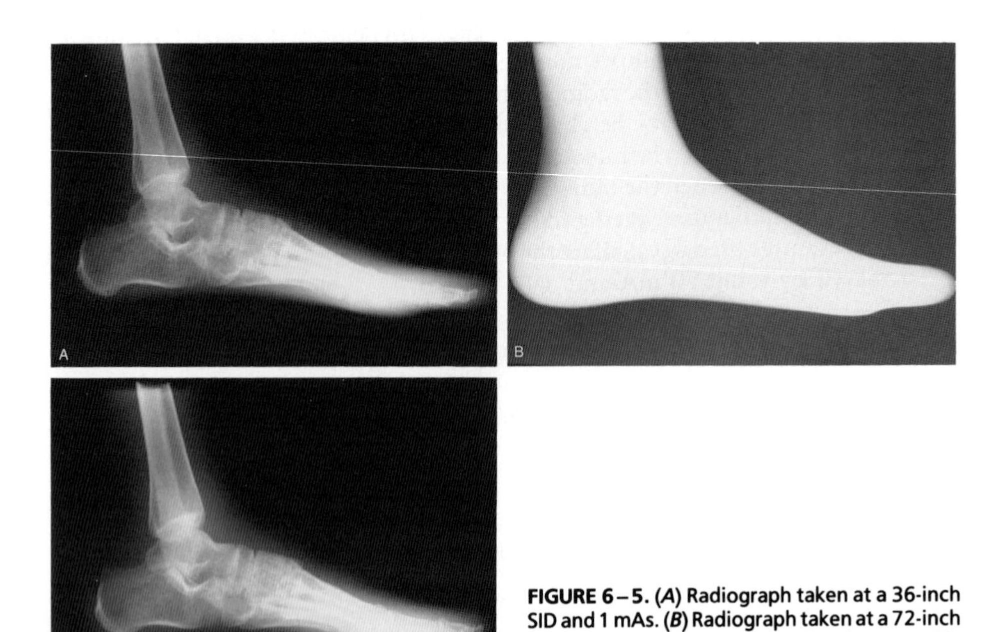

FIGURE 6–5. (*A*) Radiograph taken at a 36-inch SID and 1 mAs. (*B*) Radiograph taken at a 72-inch SID and 1 mAs. (*C*) Radiograph taken at a 72-inch SID and 4 mAs, which is 4 times the mAs used for Radiograph *A*.

Clinical Use

In clinical practice, the most commonly used source-image distances are 40 inches and 72 inches. A change of the source-image distance from 40 to 72 inches isn't an exact double of the distance. So the rule of thumb is used in this instance as an estimate.

A simple chart (Table 6–1) can help the radiographer calculate the new mAs quickly.

If a radiographer used 15 mAs at a 40-inch SID and then had to change the SID, the new mAs could be calculated using the chart. If the distance changed to 49 inches, the old mAs of 15 could be multiplied by 1.5 to get the new mAs of 22.5. And if the distance changed to 56 inches, the old mAs of 15 could be multiplied by 2 to get the new mAs of 30.

For distances falling in between the numbers, the mAs can be estimated first and then calculated. Learning to estimate the new mAs before calculating it with the density maintenance formula is helpful as a cross-check for the math.

If the new distance falls in between the numbers on the chart, a ballpark figure can be estimated. For example, 52 inches falls between the 49- and 56-inch distances on the chart. So before the new mAs at the 52-inch distance is calculated, it can be estimated at somewhere between 22.5 and 30. The answer after calculating is 25 mAs.

PERFORM ACTIVITY 6.1

SUMMARY

If the distance between the x-ray tube and film, which is the source-image distance (SID), is changed, the radiation intensity at the film changes. If the SID is increased, the radiation intensity at the film is decreased. And if the SID is decreased, the radiation intensity at the film is increased. The new radiation intensity after the distance changes can be calculated using the inverse square law.

Table 6–1. Chart for Determining New mAs

Distance Change (Inches)		
From	**To**	**Multiply old mAs by**
40	49	1.5
40	56	2
40	72	3.2
40	80	4
Distance Change (Inches)		
From	**To**	**Divide old mAs by**
72	59	1.5
72	51	2
72	40	3.2
72	36	4

To maintain film density when the source-image distance and thus the radiation intensity is changed, the density maintenance formula is used. This tells the radiographer the new mAs or new time to be used when the SID is changed. If the SID is increased, the mAs or time must be increased. If the SID is decreased, the mAs or time must be decreased.

The relationships between SID, radiation intensity, and film density are clinically important. The radiographer must be able to calculate the technique changes required, and should also be able to estimate the required changes.

PERFORM ACTIVITY 6.J

CHAPTER 7

RADIOGRAPHIC CONTRAST

CHAPTER OUTLINE

OBJECTIVES

At the end of this chapter you should be able to:

- Define radiographic contrast.
- Differentiate between high radiographic contrast and low radiographic contrast.
- Differentiate between short and long scale contrast.
- Define subject contrast.
- List the two factors that control tissue density.
- Explain why different body components absorb x-rays differently.
- Define the term differential absorption.
- Explain how body components of varying thickness can cause radiographic contrast.
- Describe the types of patients whose radiographs will display low and high radiographic contrast.
- Explain how the addition of contrast media to a patient's body enhances the radiographic image.
- List the most commonly used contrast media and indicate whether the media increase or decrease tissue density.
- State the exposure factor that is the controlling factor for radiographic contrast.
- Explain why kVp causes a heterogeneous x-ray beam.
- Describe how the photon energy, radiographic contrast, and scale of contrast vary as the kVp is changed.
- Describe the production of scattered radiation and its effect on radiographic contrast.
- Explain how kVp affects the production of scattered radiation.
- Define the term attenuation.

Until now we have been discussing factors that affect the radiographic qualities of distortion and density. These are usually easier for students to understand and see on a radiograph than the quality of contrast, which is the subject of this chapter.

The amount of radiographic contrast is judged by the number of gray shades or tones present on the radiograph. There can be too little contrast when the radiograph appears very gray, or too much contrast when there are only a few gray shades and the radiograph appears mostly black and white.

The judgment of the correct amount of contrast on a radiograph is somewhat subjective. If each person in a group of radiographers and radiologists were asked to judge acceptable contrast on a radiograph, there might be conflicting opinions. Within a certain range, it is all right if the contrast varies a little. Beyond that range the radiograph will be unacceptable.

Many factors that are under the radiographer's control influence the amount of radiographic contrast. The concept of contrast will be presented first in this chapter. Then subject contrast, which is caused by the composition of the patient's body, will be discussed. Subject contrast can be enhanced by the use of contrast media. The chapter will finish with the exposure factor of kilovoltage (kVp), which has a major influence on contrast. Radiographic contrast is affected by the amount of scattered radiation that falls on the film. Kilovoltage is one factor that determines how much scattered radiation is produced.

RADIOGRAPHIC CONTRAST

Radiographic contrast is judged by the number of gray tones present on a radiograph. Suppose you wanted to paint your bedroom walls gray. You would probably first look at a color chart at the paint store. This chart has sample blocks of the colors of gray paint carried by the store. The blocks on the color chart range from a very light gray that is almost white to a very dark gray that is almost black. Depending on the paint store, there may be many shades of gray in between the white and black to choose from or only a few shades.

The shades of gray on a radiograph are similar to the shades of gray on the paint color chart. A radiograph will ordinarily have several areas that appear very white and several areas that appear very black. The radiograph will also have some areas that appear as varying shades of gray. The number of gray tones or shades that fall between the extremes of black and white determines how much radiographic contrast the radiograph has.

Density refers to the *overall* blackness of the radiograph. The definition of radiographic contrast is the degree of *difference* between adjacent densities on a radiograph. So with contrast, the various densities of small sections of the radiograph are being compared. For a body part to be seen on a radiograph as a distinct and separate entity, it must display a contrasting shade of black, white, or gray compared to the structures surrounding it.

Radiographic contrast is the degree of difference between adjacent densities on a radiograph.

High and Low Contrast

If the colors of black and white are adjacent to each other, they display a high amount of contrast. However, if two similar shades of gray are next to each other, their dif-

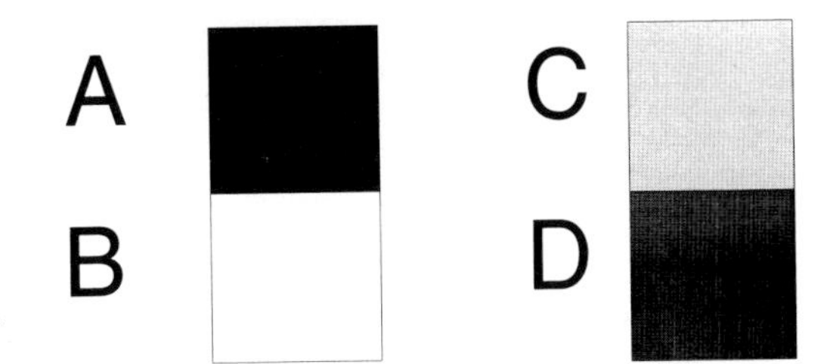

FIGURE 7–1. Blocks *A* and *B* show high contrast; Blocks *C* and *D* show low contrast.

ferences might not be so apparent. They would display a low amount of contrast (Fig. 7–1).

If a radiograph is mostly black and white and has just a few gray shades, the radiograph would display a **high contrast** image. If a radiograph has black-and-white tones and many shades of gray, the radiograph would display a **low contrast** image. Figure 7–2 shows a radiograph with high contrast and one with low contrast.

A high contrast image appears very black and white.
A low contrast image has many shades of gray.

Contrast Scales

The image on a radiograph containing the various shades of gray is called a **gray scale image**. If a radiograph has just a few shades of gray and appears mostly black and white, it has high contrast. This would also be called **short scale contrast**. A radiograph with many shades of gray and fewer blacks and whites has low contrast. This would also be called **long scale contrast**.

Short scale contrast = high contrast
Long scale contrast = low contrast

To remember this, think of evenly spaced blocks of black, white, and gray placed in a row. If just a few shades of gray had to be inserted between the black and white

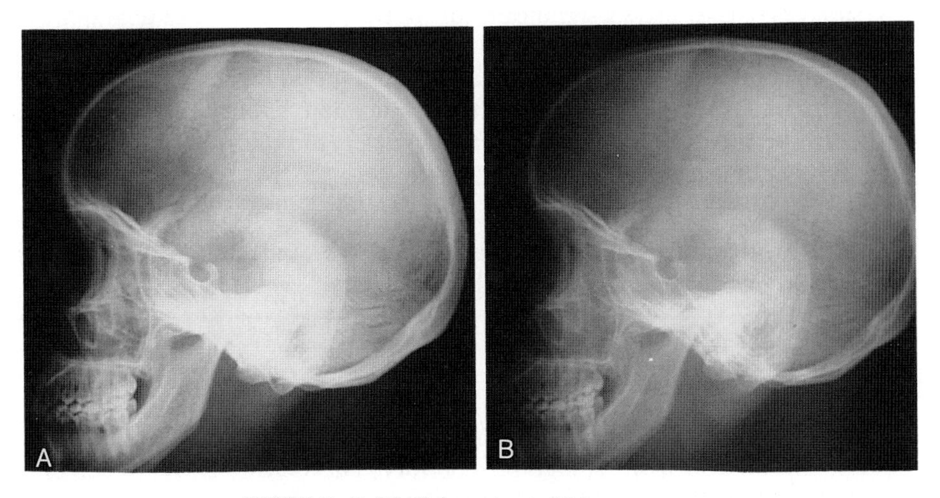

FIGURE 7–2. (*A*) High contrast. (*B*) Low contrast.

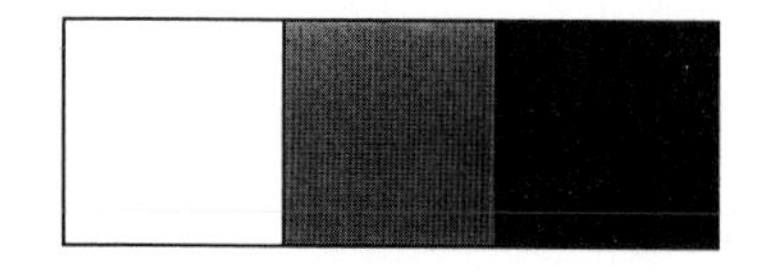

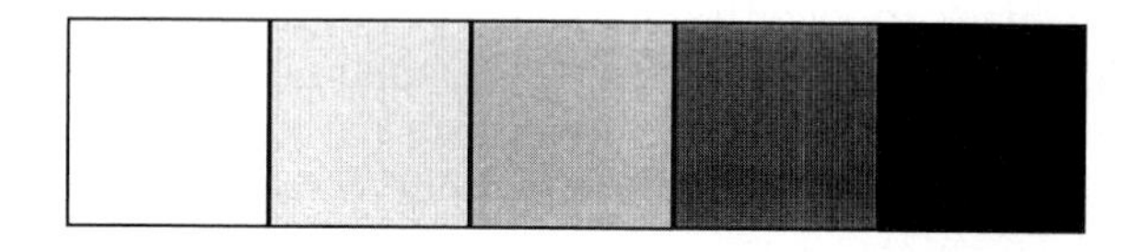

FIGURE 7–3. Short scale contrast shows very few shades of gray; long scale contrast shows many shades of gray.

blocks, this would take up a *short* distance. If many gray shades had to be fit in between the black and white blocks, this would take up a *long* distance (Fig. 7–3).

Short scale contrast = black and white = high contrast
Long scale contrast = many gray shades = low contrast

PERFORM ACTIVITY 7.A

SUBJECT CONTRAST

Subject contrast plays a significant role in the production of radiographic contrast. Subject contrast is contrast caused by the differences in the composition of the patient's body parts. The patient is the subject of the radiographic image, which is why this type of contrast is called subject contrast. Subject contrast is caused by the tissue density differences, atomic number differences, and thickness differences of the patient's body parts.

Subject contrast is the radiographic contrast caused by the differences in the composition of the patient's body tissues.

Tissue Density Differences

A person's body is made up of a variety of tissues, each having a unique density. Do not confuse this with radiographic density. This density is **tissue density**. Tissue density depends on the average atomic number of the body tissue and how compact or close together the atoms in the tissue are. The atoms in bone are very compact. The atoms in air in the patient's lungs are not very compact at all.

The number of protons in an atom determines its atomic number, and in a stable atom the number of electrons equals the number of protons. An atom with a high atomic number has a large number of protons and electrons, and an atom with a low atomic number has a small number of protons and electrons.

When photons from the primary x-ray beam enter the patient's body, their energy can be absorbed by the electrons in the patient's body. If the photons enter a part of the body where the atoms are very compact and have a high average atomic number as in bone, it is likely that the photons will be absorbed because there are many electrons present. The absorbed photons are stopped by the electrons and cannot go through the patient's body to put density on the film.

If the photons enter a body part with a lot of air as in the lungs, the atoms are not very compact, the average atomic number is lower, and fewer electrons are present. In this instance, it is likely that the photons would not be absorbed or stopped by the electrons. The photons would go right through this body part and put density on the film.

The area of the film under the air would receive a lot of radiation, and this part of the film would appear very dense or black after development. The area of the film under the bone would receive very little radiation and this part of the film would appear white after development. The black-and-white areas on the radiograph would display a contrast, and in this case a high contrast.

Considering all the tissues in the patient's body, each would absorb x-ray photons differently depending on the tissue density, which is determined by the average atomic number and how compact the atoms are in each tissue. This phenomenon is called **differential absorption**. Figure 7–4 lists some components of the body in order according to their ability to absorb radiation and the type of radiographic density they would display. Depending on the body part being radiographed, any number of these components could be present on the radiograph (Fig. 7–5).

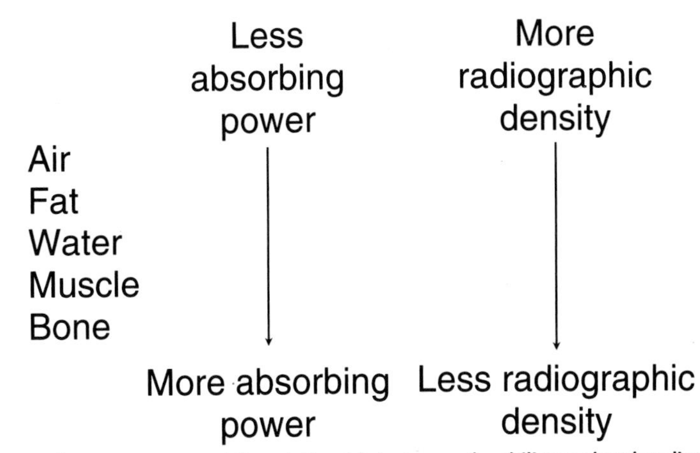

FIGURE 7–4. Body components and the relationship between the ability to absorb radiation and radiographic density.

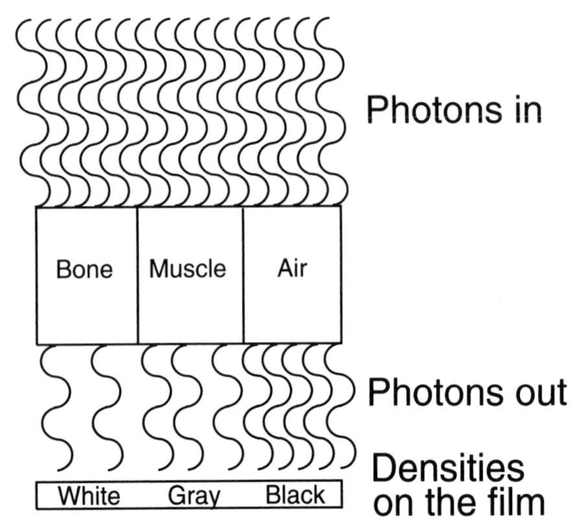

FIGURE 7–5. Different parts of the body display varying radiographic density because they absorb x-rays differently depending on the atomic number and how compact the atoms are in the body part.

Thickness Differences

With tissue density differences a variety of body tissues are considered. The topic of thickness differences considers the *same* type of body tissue, but a variety of thicknesses of it.

If it were possible to take a radiograph of a section of only muscle that is 2 inches thick across its whole surface, the radiograph would display approximately the same shade of gray because the x-ray photons would be absorbed about equally over the whole section of muscle. If it were possible to take a radiograph of just muscle again, but with different thicknesses of muscle, such as a 2-inch section and a 5-inch section, the radiograph would display two different shades of gray.

If the same amount and quality of radiation enters both thicknesses of muscle, more x-ray photons will be absorbed as the radiation passes through the 5-inch piece of muscle than when it passes through the 2-inch piece. There are more electrons present in the thicker piece of muscle to stop the x-ray photons. This causes a difference in the amount of radiation reaching the film under the different pieces of muscle. The area under the thicker 5-inch section of muscle would be a lighter shade of gray on the radiograph than the area under the 2-inch piece of muscle (Fig. 7–6).

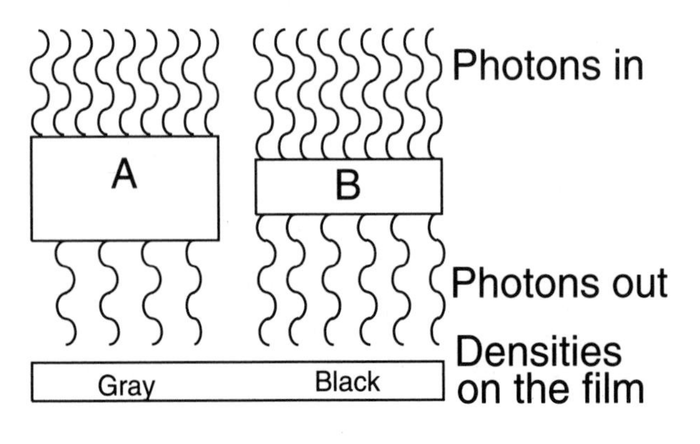

FIGURE 7–6. In Block *A*, the thick part lets little radiation through. In Block *B*, the thin part lets more radiation through. The two parts would display contrast on a radiograph.

Clinical Application

In clinical settings radiographers have little control over subject contrast. Patients come in all different shapes and sizes. In the same work day, a radiographer will probably serve several patients who are very muscular and in good physical shape, some who are very sick and whose bodies have begun to deteriorate, some whose bodies have a high fat content, and some whose body parts are swollen due to injury or water retention.

Patients who are in good physical shape usually display the highest subject contrast. Their muscles are strong, they have only a little fat content, and their bones are dense.

Patients whose bodies have deteriorated due to disease will ordinarily display less subject contrast. Their muscles have lost strength and their consistency becomes more like fat. On a radiograph of this patient the fat and muscle densities look more alike and subject contrast decreases.

Many diseases involve a demineralization of bone. Bones that have lost minerals because of disease become less dense and x-ray photons pass through them more easily. The bones will appear gray on the radiograph rather than white and they will blend in more with their surrounding body tissues (Fig. 7–7).

Patients who have retained water in their bodies will display a decrease in subject contrast. The water surrounds all the body tissues, causing their tissue densities to become more alike. The additional water absorbs some of the x-ray photons, which decreases density. Water also causes an increase in the amount of scattered radiation produced in the patient's body. This increased scatter will hit the film and decrease radiographic contrast (Fig. 7–8).

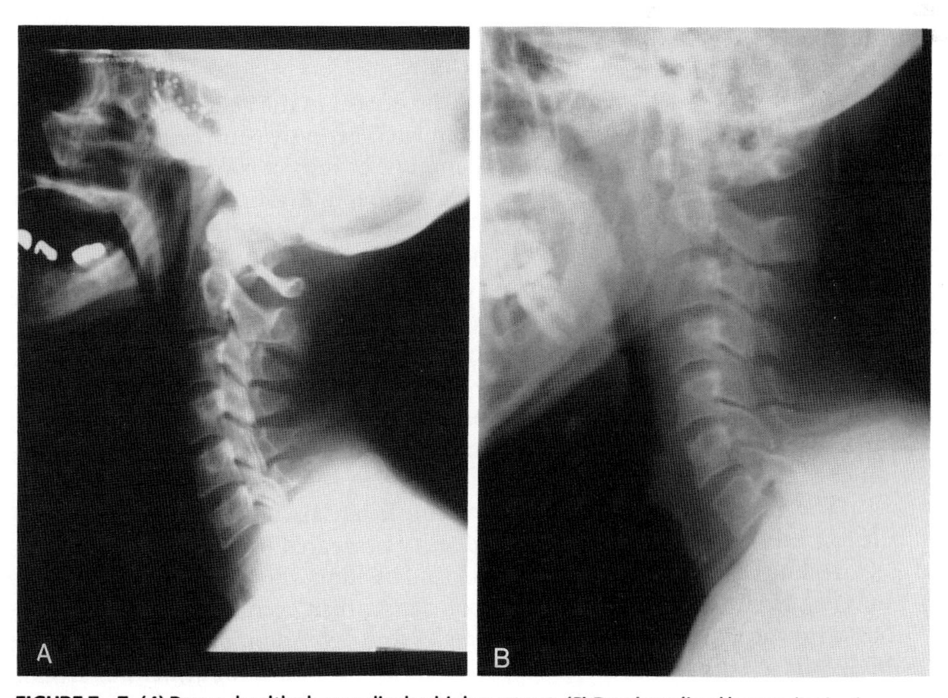

FIGURE 7–7. (*A*) Dense, healthy bones display high contrast. (*B*) Demineralized bones display low contrast.

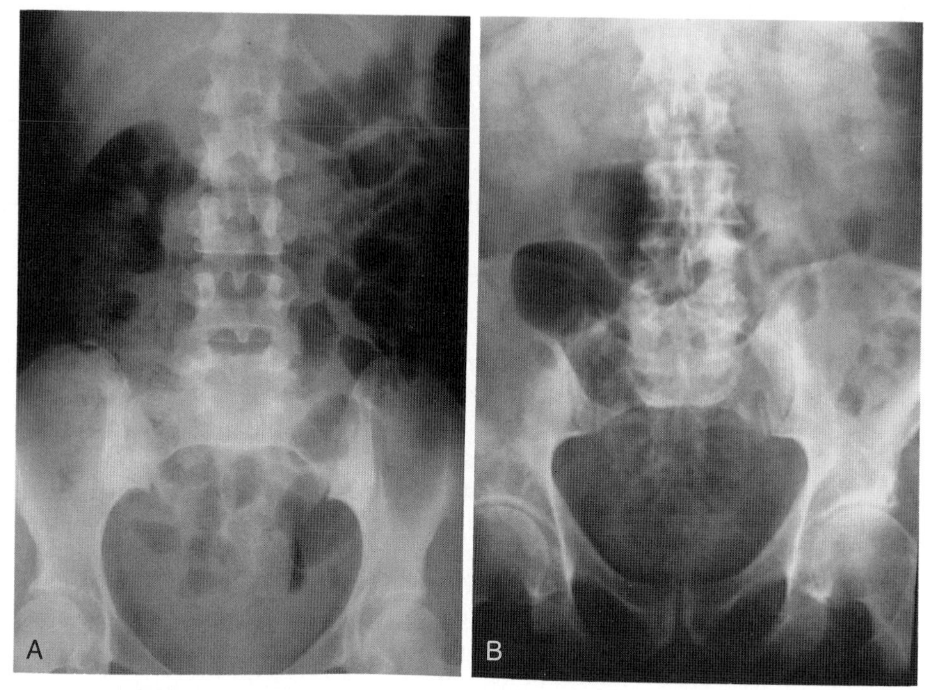

FIGURE 7–8. (*A*) Good contrast. (*B*) Poor contrast due to water retention.

PERFORM ACTIVITY 7.B

Contrast Media

The tissue density and composition of the organs in the abdomen are very similar. Also the thickness of these organs is similar. The liver, pancreas, spleen, stomach, kidneys, and bowel will display a low amount of subject contrast. These organs are not always seen as distinct entities on a radiograph. A plain radiograph of the abdomen may show the outline of some of the structures depending on the patient. For a healthy patient, the radiographer might see the outline of the liver, which is large and dense, and the outline of the kidneys, which are surrounded by a contrasting layer of fat. However, if the patient's body has deteriorated, has a high fat content, or the patient has retained water, these structures are difficult to see as separate entities.

Adding contrast media to a body part changes its tissue density. Then the body part will display a different density on a radiograph compared to its surrounding structures. Contrast media is used often in clinical situations, especially in the abdomen.

The most common types of contrast media are air, iodine, and barium. Adding air to a body part decreases its tissue density compared to the structures around it.

Iodine has an atomic number of 53, and barium, which is a metal, has an atomic number of 56. These materials are much denser than even the densest bone, which has an average atomic number between 12 and 13. Adding iodine or barium to a body part greatly increases its tissue density compared to the structures around it.

Barium and air are used in the gastrointestinal tract. Iodine is used in other body parts such as the kidneys and gall bladder. Figure 7–9 shows radiographs of patients who have had contrast media added to their body.

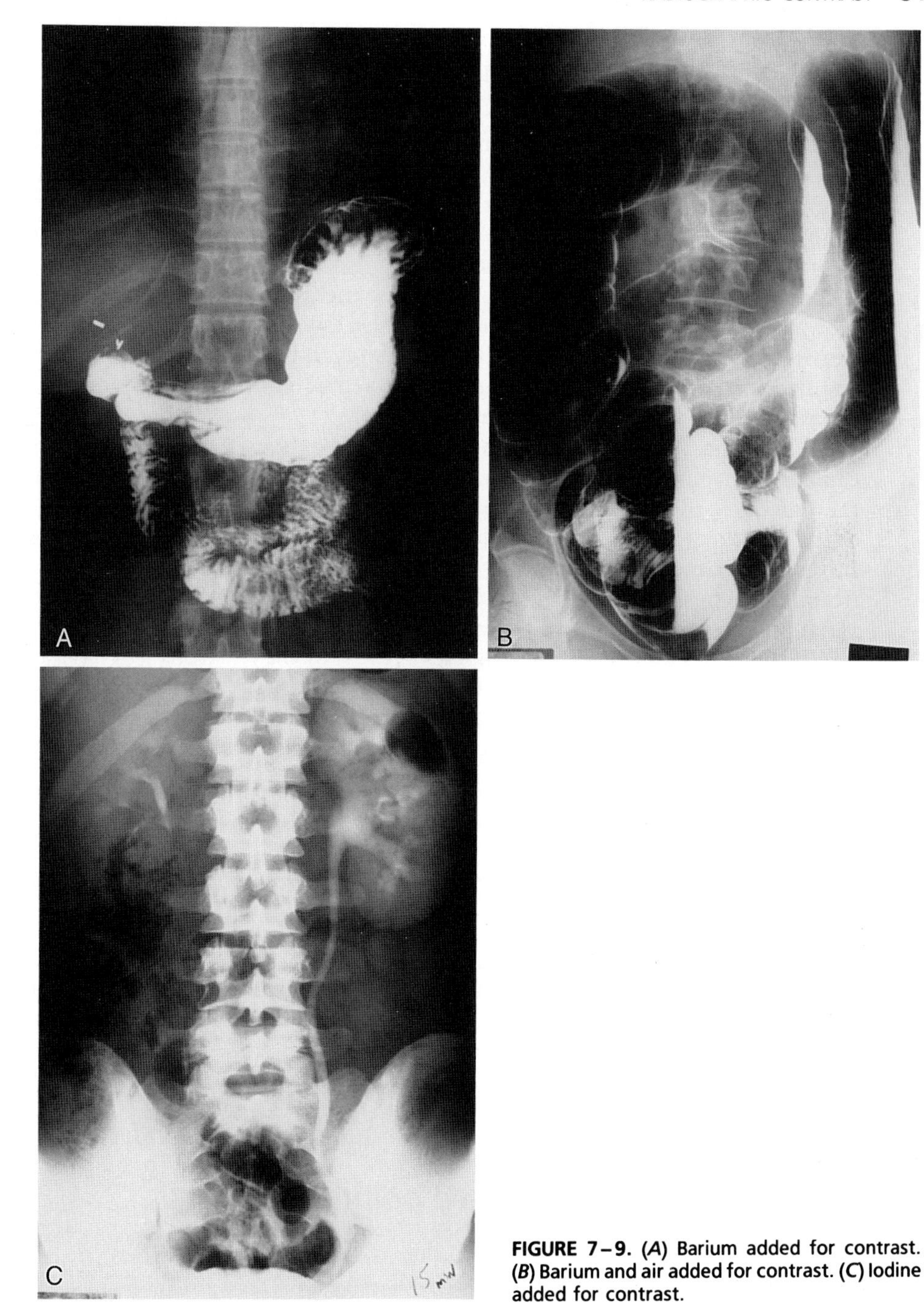

FIGURE 7–9. (*A*) Barium added for contrast. (*B*) Barium and air added for contrast. (*C*) Iodine added for contrast.

KILOVOLTAGE (kVp)

There are other factors besides subject contrast that affect radiographic contrast. In Chapter 5 we discussed the primary exposure factors of milliamperage (mA) and time. Another very important exposure factor is kVp. Kilovoltage (kVp) is the main controlling factor for radiographic contrast. This factor must be set on the control panel by the radiographer before every x-ray exposure. The kVp selected has a major influence on the quality of the radiograph.

kVp is the controlling factor for radiographic contrast.

Chapter 2 discussed the production of x-rays in detail. When x-rays are produced, electrons are released from the filament of the x-ray tube. These electrons shoot over to the anode, stop suddenly when they hit the anode, and give up energy in the form of x-rays. The kinetic energy (energy of motion) of the electrons is changed into x-ray energy at the anode.

If an electron has a high amount of kinetic energy, it has the potential to give up more energy at the anode than an electron with a low amount of kinetic energy. If an electron gives up a high amount of kinetic energy, it produces a photon with a high amount of energy. And if an electron gives up a low amount of kinetic energy, it produces a photon with a low amount of energy.

kVp is the factor that determines the energy of the x-ray photons produced because it determines the amount of kinetic energy each electron has as it moves from the filament to the anode. Kilovoltage is produced in the form of a wave over the time of the exposure (Fig. 7–10). The "p" in kVp stands for peak. The kVp that is set on the control panel is the maximum or peak kilovoltage reached. Kilovoltage varies from zero to this maximum and back to zero several times during the exposure. This variation gives each electron a different amount of energy as it travels to the anode.

If the radiographer selects a high kVp, most of the electrons will have a lot of kinetic energy as they move toward the anode and a large percentage of the photons produced in the x-ray beam will have a lot of energy. If the radiographer selects a low kVp, the electrons have less kinetic energy and a large percentage of the photons produced will have a low amount of energy.

High kVp = high photon energy
Low kVp = low photon energy

Photons with a low energy because of a low kVp are absorbed more easily by the atoms in the patient's body. Differential absorption increases, and this creates an image with high contrast (short scale), which is mostly black and white.

When photons have a high energy, they penetrate through body tissues more easily. The different tissues of the body are all penetrated more equally. Differential

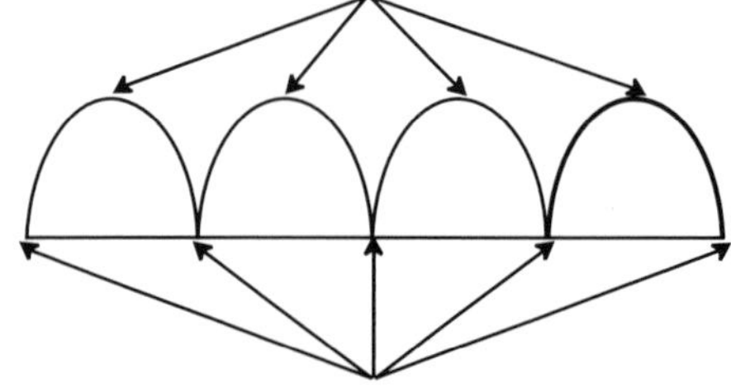

FIGURE 7–10. kVp fluctuates during the exposure. This produces an x-ray beam in which the photons have many different energies.

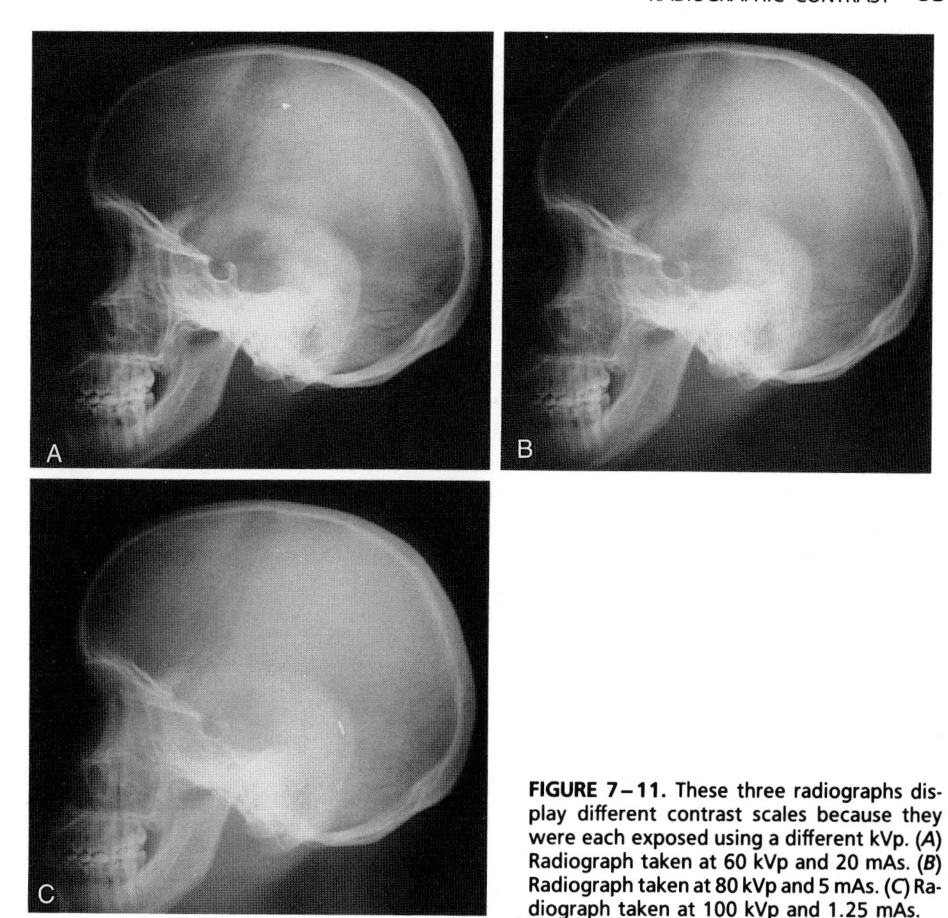

FIGURE 7–11. These three radiographs display different contrast scales because they were each exposed using a different kVp. (*A*) Radiograph taken at 60 kVp and 20 mAs. (*B*) Radiograph taken at 80 kVp and 5 mAs. (*C*) Radiograph taken at 100 kVp and 1.25 mAs.

absorption decreases, and the image will have a low contrast (long scale), which is many gray tones. Figure 7–11 shows radiographs with varying contrast because they were all taken with different kVp settings. The density looks about the same because the mAs was adjusted according to the 15% rule, which will be discussed in the next chapter.

High kVp = high photon energy = low contrast = long scale
Low kVp = low photon energy = high contrast = short scale

Most control panels have two controls for kilovoltage. One is a major kVp control and one is a minor kVp control. The major kVp control changes the kVp by a unit of 10, and the minor kVp control changes the kVp by a unit of 1 or 2. kVp settings on control panels usually range from 40 kVp to 120 kVp.

SCATTERED RADIATION PRODUCTION

Primary radiation (radiation from the x-ray tube) enters the patient's body and some of it is absorbed by the atoms in the body depending on the tissue density and thickness of the body parts. The radiation that gets through the patient's body is called exit radiation or remnant radiation. Exit radiation hits the film and is recorded as density on the radiograph when the film is developed. Besides exiting through the patient's body or being absorbed by the body parts, primary radiation can also be scattered.

Scattered radiation is produced when a primary x-ray photon collides with an atom in the patient's body, bounces off the atom, and changes its original direction. When the photon collides with the atom, it also loses some of its energy.

Since the photon has changed its direction, it could take several new paths. It could bounce directly back at the x-ray tube, it could fly out the sides of the patient's body, or it could exit through the patient's body and hit the film from a different direction than it would have if it had remained a primary photon. It is in the patient's body where most scattered radiation originates.

Scattered radiation that hits the film puts density on the film. This is unwanted density that degrades the image quality. This unwanted density is sometimes referred to as **fog**, because it appears as a blanket of grayness on the image. The fog makes the individual and distinct gray shades of the image blend in with each other so that they cannot be seen as separate structures. The image will appear very gray and have low contrast. Figure 7–12 shows a radiograph with good contrast and one in which the image is obscured by too much scattered radiation.

Scattered radiation lowers radiographic contrast.

PERFORM ACTIVITY 7.C

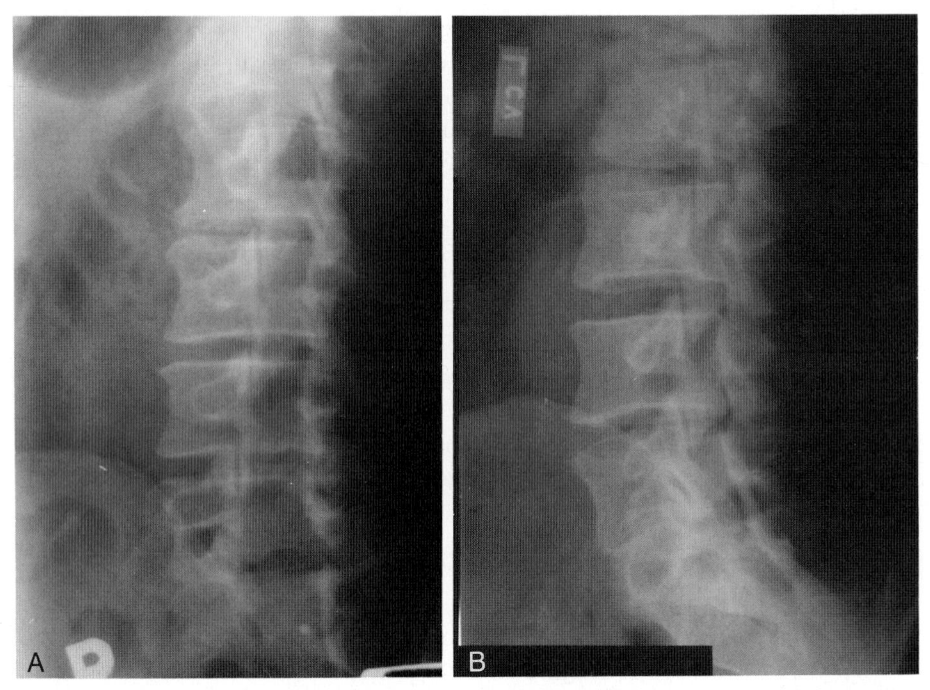

FIGURE 7–12. (*A*) Good contrast. (*B*) The image is obscured by too much scattered radiation.

Kilovoltage is the exposure factor that determines how much scattered radiation is produced. A low kVp beam has more photons with low energy and those are more easily absorbed by the atoms of the patient's body. A photon that has already been absorbed cannot be scattered. A high kVp beam has more photons with higher energy, and these photons are more easily scattered by the patient's body.

High kVp = more scattered radiation = low contrast image
Low kVp = less scattered radiation = high contrast image

Three things can happen to the primary x-ray photons as they enter the patient's body. They can be absorbed, they can be scattered, or they can pass through and hit the film. As the x-ray photons are absorbed or scattered, the radiation intensity of the original beam is reduced. The reduction of radiation intensity by absorption or scattering as the beam passes through matter is called **attenuation** (Fig. 7–13).

There are several radiographic devices that help control the amount of scattered radiation reaching the film. The most important of these devices are the grid and the collimator. They will be discussed in Chapters 9 and 10.

SUMMARY

Radiographic contrast is the degree of difference between adjacent densities on a radiograph. A high contrast radiograph will appear mostly black and white with few grays. This is called short scale contrast. A low contrast radiograph will display many shades of gray and few blacks and whites. This is called long scale contrast.

Subject contrast is caused by the composition of the patient's body parts. Subject contrast is the number of different tissue densities and tissue thicknesses in the patient's body. Each body tissue will display a different radiographic density depending on how x-rays passed through it and thus will contrast with each other on the radiograph. If the patient's body parts are very similar in tissue density and thickness, contrast media can be added to the body to increase subject contrast.

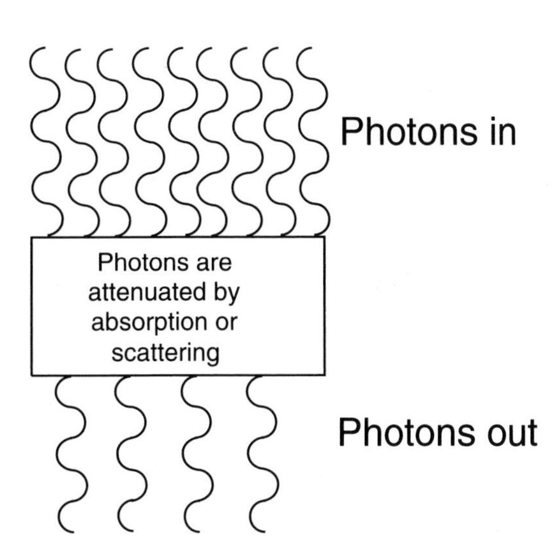

FIGURE 7–13. Attenuation is the reduction of beam intensity by absorption or scattering of the photons in the beam as the beam passes through matter.

Kilovoltage (kVp) is the exposure factor that controls radiographic contrast. A high kVp beam will produce a radiograph with low contrast, and a low kVp beam will produce a radiograph with high contrast. A high kVp beam produces more scattered radiation than a low kVp beam. Scattered radiation reduces radiographic contrast.

PERFORM ACTIVITY 7.D

CHAPTER 8

mAs AND kVp RELATIONSHIP

CHAPTER OUTLINE

OBJECTIVES

At the end of this chapter you should be able to:

- Define optimum kVp.
- List the optimum kVp for commonly radiographed body parts.
- State the controlling factor for density and for contrast.
- State the relationship of mAs to density and to contrast.
- State the relationship of kVp to density and to contrast.
- Describe and calculate the 15% rule.
- Apply the 15% rule to control radiographic contrast.
- Apply the 15% rule to control motion.
- Calculate 15% rule changes in the 60 to 90 kVp range.

Chapter 5 discussed two important exposure factors, milliamperage (mA) and exposure time, that produce the unit of mAs when the mA is multiplied by the time. Chapter 7 discussed another important exposure factor: kilovoltage (kVp). Along with the source-image distance (SID) they are the primary exposure factors and used together they have a very significant effect on radiographic quality.

The relationship between the primary exposure factors of mAs and kVp is the subject of this chapter. In this chapter you will learn about optimum kVp, which is the exposure factor that should be selected first by the radiographer. You will also learn how to calculate the 15% rule and apply the rule to control contrast and motion. The 15% rule expresses the relationship between mAs and kVp.

OPTIMUM kVp

Kilovoltage is the exposure factor that determines the **quality** of the x-ray beam. The quality of the beam is determined by the penetrating power of the beam. A beam produced with a high kVp will have a high average photon energy. A beam produced with a low kVp will have a low average photon energy. A high kVp beam will be able to penetrate through the patient's body more easily than a low kVp beam.

A primary consideration when the radiographer selects the exposure factors to set on the control panel is the kVp, because the kVp controls the quality of the beam and its penetrating power. The kVp selected should be the **optimum kVp** for the body part being examined.

Optimum kVp is the kVp that will be able to penetrate the body part, produce sufficient radiographic contrast, and produce an acceptable level of scattered radiation.

Penetration of the Part

In order to make an acceptable radiographic image, the part must be penetrated, which means the photons in the beam must have enough energy so that some of the photons will go through the matter in the body part and affect the film. Figure 8 – 1 shows a series of radiographs of the skull with an attempt to penetrate the skull with 40 kVp. This low kVp would never produce a beam with the ability to penetrate through a skull.

Table 8 – 1 shows the optimum kVp for the most commonly radiographed body

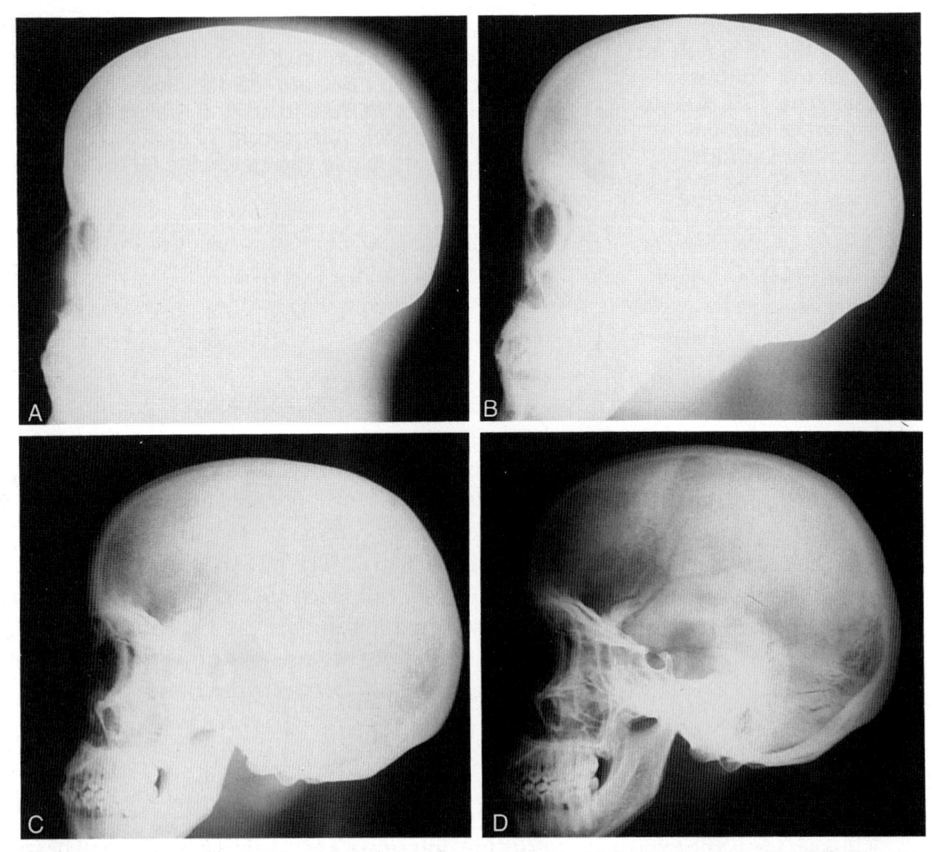

FIGURE 8 – 1. Four radiographs of the skull are taken at 40 kVp with increasing mAs. The skull cannot be penetrated at 40 kVp no matter how much the mAs is increased. (*A*) Radiograph taken at 40 kVp and 40 mAs. (*B*) Radiograph taken at 40 kVp and 80 mAs. (*C*) Radiograph taken at 40 kVp and 160 mAs. (*D*) Radiograph taken at 40 kVp and 320 mAs.

Table 8–1. Optimum kVp for Common Body Parts

Small extremities	55–60
Large extremities	65–70
Skull	80
Abdomen with barium	110
Abdomen without barium	70
Chest with grid	110
Chest without grid	80
Spine	80
Pelvis and hip	70
Shoulder	70
Ribs	70

parts. If the radiographer uses the optimum kVp, that kVp will always be able to penetrate through the body part. In general, a thick and dense body part must be penetrated with a higher kVp than a thin and less dense body part. Small extremities like hands and feet can usually be penetrated with 55 to 60 kVp, whereas 65 to 70 kVp is usually selected for larger extremities like the knee and elbow.

Figure 8–2 shows two skull radiographs taken with different kilovoltage. Look closely at the center of the radiograph where the bones of the skull are more dense, and notice the differences in penetration and demonstration of the anatomy.

Optimum kVp will always be able to penetrate the part.

Sufficient Radiographic Contrast

Determination of the best radiographic contrast is somewhat subjective. A high contrast radiograph, one which appears mostly black and white with few grays, is produced with a kVp that is lower than the optimum kVp. At first glance a high contrast radiograph may appear to be pretty and pleasing to the eye. But a closer examination of the whiter areas of the image will show that some of the anatomical parts were not demonstrated well because they were not penetrated.

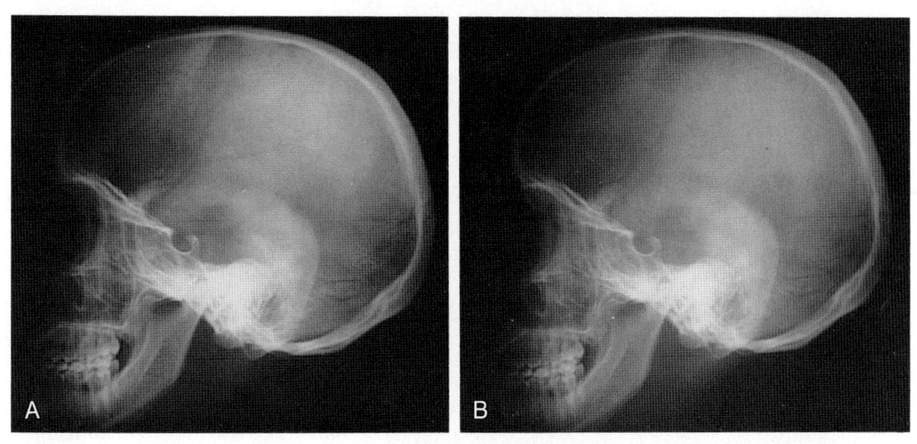

FIGURE 8–2. (*A*) Radiograph taken at 70 kVp. (*B*) Radiograph approximately the same density as radiograph *A* but taken at 80 kVp, the optimum kVp; Radiograph *A* is a little underpenetrated.

A low contrast radiograph, one which is very gray, is produced with a kVp that is higher than the optimum kVp. A high kVp produces a lot of scattered radiation on the radiograph, which is what causes the very gray image. On a very gray image, it is difficult to see the separate shades of gray produced by the patient's different body parts, so some of the patient's anatomy may be obscured.

A radiograph with a sufficient amount of contrast, one that includes blacks, whites, and an average amount of gray shades, is produced with optimum kVp. Each gray shade is seen as separate from the surrounding shades of gray. These subtle differences demonstrate anatomy that may not be seen on a high contrast or very low contrast image.

Figure 8 – 3 shows three radiographs, one with too much contrast, one with sufficient contrast, and one with too little contrast.

Optimum kVp provides sufficient contrast.

Scattered Radiation

The amount of scattered radiation produced in an x-ray beam is controlled by the kVp. A high kVp produces a lot of scatter. Scattered radiation degrades the image by

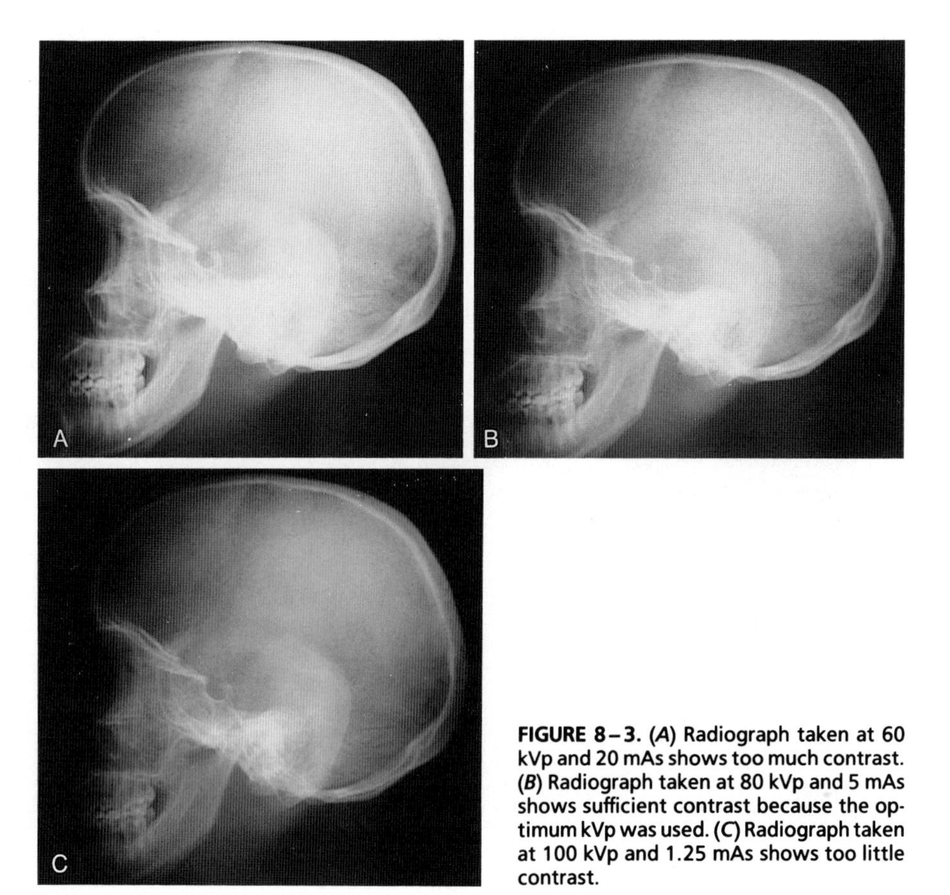

FIGURE 8 – 3. (*A*) Radiograph taken at 60 kVp and 20 mAs shows too much contrast. (*B*) Radiograph taken at 80 kVp and 5 mAs shows sufficient contrast because the optimum kVp was used. (*C*) Radiograph taken at 100 kVp and 1.25 mAs shows too little contrast.

placing an extra blanket of gray density on the film, which lowers the radiographic contrast.

If a radiographer uses the optimum kVp for each body part, the amount of scattered radiation produced is consistent. It will vary somewhat with different patients, but it is at least predictable. Then it becomes a standard decision whether or not to use a device to control scattered radiation.

If one time a radiographer used 60 kVp to radiograph a knee and the next time used 80 kVp, the contrast on the two radiographs would vary, the parts that were penetrated would vary, and the radiographer would need to use a grid to control scatter with the 80-kVp technique, but not with the 60-kVp technique. Thus it is better to use the optimum kVp for each body part.

Optimum kVp produces an acceptable amount of scattered radiation.

PERFORM ACTIVITY 8.A

mAs VERSUS kVp

When examining the same body part on small, medium, and large patients, the kVp could be adjusted for each patient in order to change the density of the radiograph because kVp affects density. Since kVp also changes the penetrating ability of the beam, the radiograph contrast, and the amount of scattered radiation produced, adjustment of the kVp is not a good idea.

mAs controls density by only changing the quantity of radiation produced. A variation in the mAs does not change the penetrating ability of the beam, the radiographic contrast, or the amount of scattered radiation produced. mAs only controls density and does not affect contrast.

The milliamperage determines how many electrons will be released by thermionic emission at the cathode of the x-ray tube, and this determines the quantity of x-rays produced. Exposure time determines how long the thermionic emission will take place. So together, mA and time determine the *quantity* of x-ray photons, which will be produced in the x-ray beam.

Kilovoltage determines the *quality* of the x-ray beam by determining its penetrating power. A variation in the kVp changes the energy of the photons in the beam. A change in the mAs does nothing to the energy of the photons. A change in the mAs only produces an increase or decrease in the number of photons of all energies.

mAs controls the quantity of radiation in the beam.
kVp controls the quality of radiation in the beam.

Refer to Figure 1 – 11, the chart showing the factors that affect each of the four radiographic qualities. mAs is listed as the controlling factor for density, and kVp is listed as the controlling factor for contrast. Looking at the list of the other factors that affect density, you should see kVp listed as affecting density, but you will not see mAs as a factor that affects contrast.

This is important to remember when thinking about exposure factors. mAs can-

Table 8-2. The Effect of Changing mAs and kVp on Density and Contrast (Compare each change to the original factors)

Original	Change 1	Change 2	Change 3	Change 4
5 mAs	10 mAs	5 mAs	5 mAs	10 mAs
70 kVp	70 kVp	80 kVp	60 kVp	80 kVp
Density	Increases	Increases	Decreases	Increases
Contrast	No change	Decreases	Increases	Decreases

not affect contrast because mAs does nothing to the energy of the photons in the beam. It only changes the quantity of the photons produced. So mAs affects density by making the whole radiograph more or less black or dense.

kVp changes the energy of the photons in the beam. It controls the contrast on the radiograph by changing the penetrating power of the beam. A beam that is more penetrating will be able to put more density on the radiograph than one that is less penetrating. So while mAs only controls density, kVp controls contrast but also affects density.

mAs controls density.
kVp controls contrast.
kVp affects density.

Suppose a radiographer produces a radiograph and then repeats the radiograph with variations in the kVp and mAs settings. Density will be affected when the kVp and mAs are changed, but contrast is only affected when the kVp is changed. Table 8-2 shows the effect of variations in the mAs and kVp on density and contrast.*

THE 15% RULE

There are only a few times in clinical situations when the mAs and optimum kVp can be varied slightly. These instances are when the contrast needs to be changed or when the radiographer wants to help control motion of the patient.

If a radiograph taken at 10 mAs and 80 kVp is of good quality, the mAs can be increased a little and the kVp decreased a little and the radiograph will still display the same density as the original radiograph and be acceptable. The mAs could also be decreased and the kVp increased from the original factors and the radiograph will display the same density as the original radiograph and still be acceptable. This range of acceptable exposure factors is called **exposure latitude**.

When using exposure latitude to change the factors from the optimum there is a definite method. If the kVp is increased the mAs has to be decreased, and if the mAs is increased the kVp has to be decreased.

*The discussions in this book refer to routine radiography using well-chosen techniques. mAs is said by some authors to affect contrast. This occurs only under extreme conditions. If the mAs chosen were so high or so low that the entire radiograph was only one shade, either black or white, there would be no contrast since contrast is the difference in densities on the radiograph.

To maintain film density:
If the kVp is decreased, increase the mAs.
If the kVp is increased, decrease the mAs.

The 15% rule helps the radiographer determine exactly how much the mAs and kVp should be changed. If the kVp is changed by 15%, the mAs should be changed by a factor of 2. If the kVp is increased by 15%, the mAs should be divided by 2. If the kVp is decreased by 15%, the mAs should be multiplied by 2.

If the kVp is increased by 15%, the mAs should be cut in half.
If the kVp is decreased by 15%, the mAs should be doubled.

In the following examples assume that the original radiograph was taken at 80 kVp and 5 mAs.

Example 1: Increasing the kVp

80 kVp × .15 = 12
80 kVp + 12 = 92 (the new kVp)
5 mAs/2 = 2.5 mAs (the new mAs)

Example 2: Decreasing the kVp

80 kVp × .15 = 12
80 kVp − 12 = 68 (the new kVp)
5 mAs × 2 = 10 mAs (the new mAs)

The three sets of exposure factors are

1	2	3
80 kVp 5 mAs	92 kVp 2.5 mAs	68 kVp 10 mAs

The density on the radiographs taken with each of these three sets of exposure factors will be approximately the same, but the contrast will be different (Fig. 8–4). The radiograph from exposure 3 with the lowest kVp will have the highest contrast, while the radiograph from exposure 2 with the highest kVp will have the lowest contrast. The radiograph from exposure 1, using the optimum kVp, will have the best contrast.

PERFORM ACTIVITY 8.B

Using the 15% Rule to Control Contrast

The 15% rule can be applied in clinical situations to control contrast. Suppose a radiographer made an exposure of the abdomen at 80 kVp and 20 mAs. The radio-

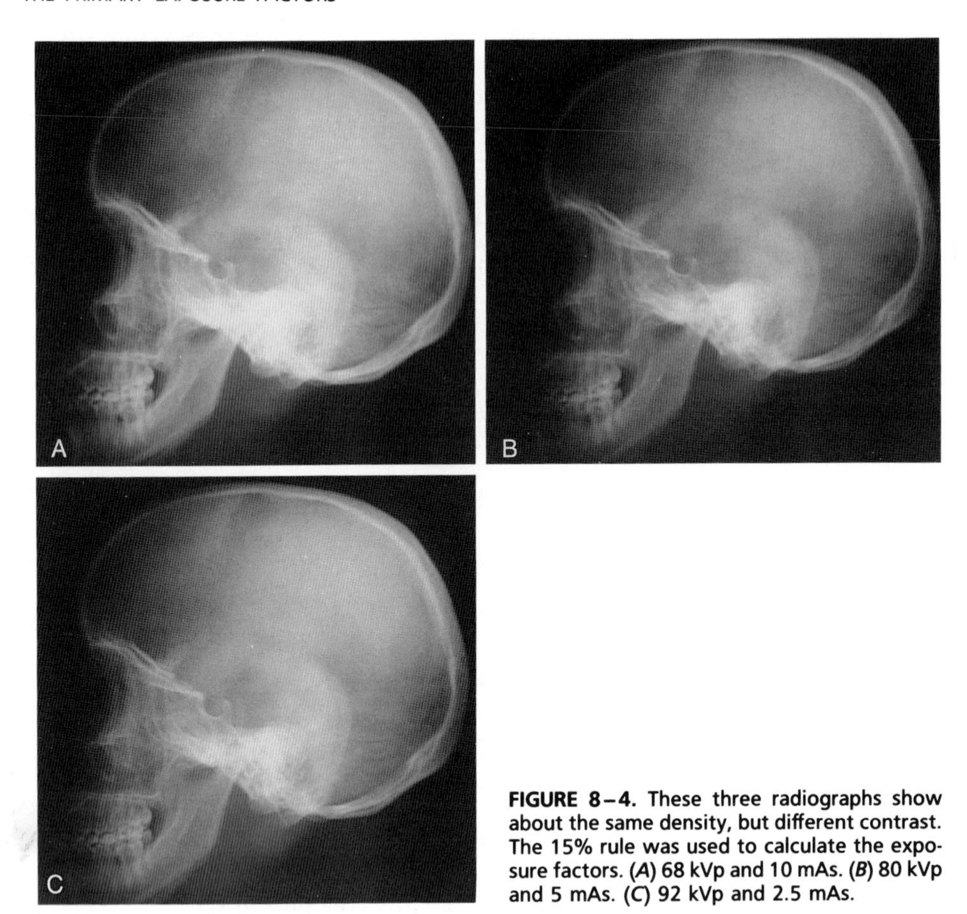

FIGURE 8–4. These three radiographs show about the same density, but different contrast. The 15% rule was used to calculate the exposure factors. (*A*) 68 kVp and 10 mAs. (*B*) 80 kVp and 5 mAs. (*C*) 92 kVp and 2.5 mAs.

graph showed adequate density, but the contrast was too low. The contrast would be increased by using a lower kVp. In this case the mAs would have to be increased if the kVp is lowered.

$$80 \text{ kVp} \times .15 = 12$$
$$80 \text{ kVp} - 12 = 68 \text{ kVp (the new kVp)}$$
$$20 \text{ mAs} \times 2 = 40 \text{ mAs (the new mAs)}$$

The two radiographs would have approximately the same density, but the contrast would be higher with the lower kVp.

Using the 15% Rule to Control Motion

The 15% rule can also be applied in clinical situations to control motion. Suppose a radiographer made an exposure of the skull on an uncooperative patient at 80 kVp and 20 mAs. The 20 mAs was achieved by using 500 mA at .04 second. The radiograph produced was blurry as a result of motion of the patient and it needed to be repeated. The radiographer would want to avoid motion on the second exposure.

Applying the 15% rule, the radiographer could increase the kVp and decrease the mAs. The decrease in the mAs can be achieved by reducing the exposure time. This decrease in time would lessen the chance of having motion on the repeat radiograph.

80 kVp × .15 = 12
80 kVp + 12 = 92 (the new kVp)
20 mAs/2 = 10 (the new mAs)
10/500 mA = .02 (the new and shorter exposure time)

The two radiographs would have approximately the same density, but the contrast would be lower on the repeat radiograph taken with the higher kVp and shorter time. The chance of motion is less on the second exposure.

PERFORM ACTIVITY 8.C

PERFORM ACTIVITY 8.D

Exposure Latitude

Exposure latitude gives the radiographer room for small errors. The exposure factors can vary a little from what would be the perfect factors, and the radiograph will still be acceptable. The small range of factors cannot be exceeded or the radiograph will not be acceptable.

The 15% rule cannot be applied in every situation, because there are times when the range of exposure latitude would be exceeded. If the original kVp chosen is not the optimum kVp, and this kVp is at the upper or lower end of the acceptable range, a further adjustment of the kVp using the 15% rule will place the kVp above or below the acceptable range. A very low kVp may not be sufficient to penetrate the part, and a very high kVp may produce too much scattered radiation.

Suppose a radiographer chose 60 kVp to expose a radiograph of the skull. Since 80 kVp is the optimum kVp for skull radiography, the radiograph may be acceptable with 60 kVp because of exposure latitude, although some parts of the skull are not penetrated well at 60 kVp. If the radiographer reduces the kVp further according to the 15% rule, the new kVp would not penetrate the skull (Fig. 8–5).

60 kVp × .15 = 9
60 kVp − 9 = 51 kVp not enough to penetrate

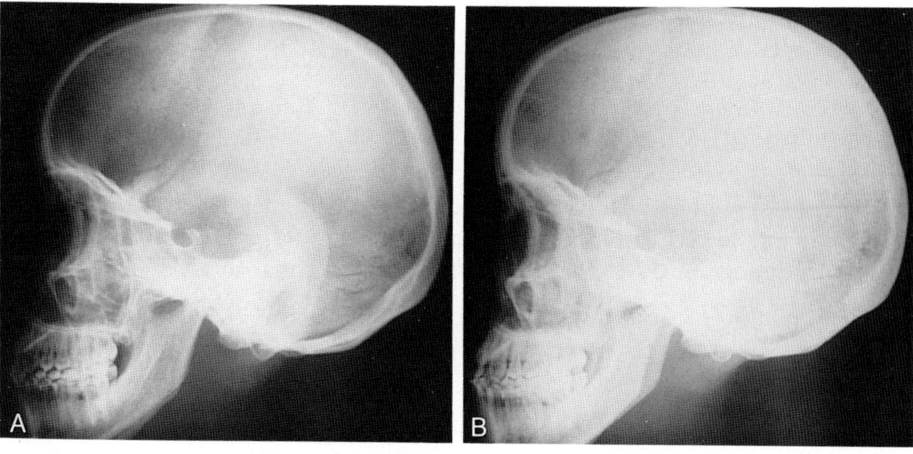

FIGURE 8–5. (*A*) Radiograph taken at 60 kVp and 20 mAs. (*B*) Radiograph taken at 51 kVp and 40 mAs. The skull is not penetrated well at 50 kVp.

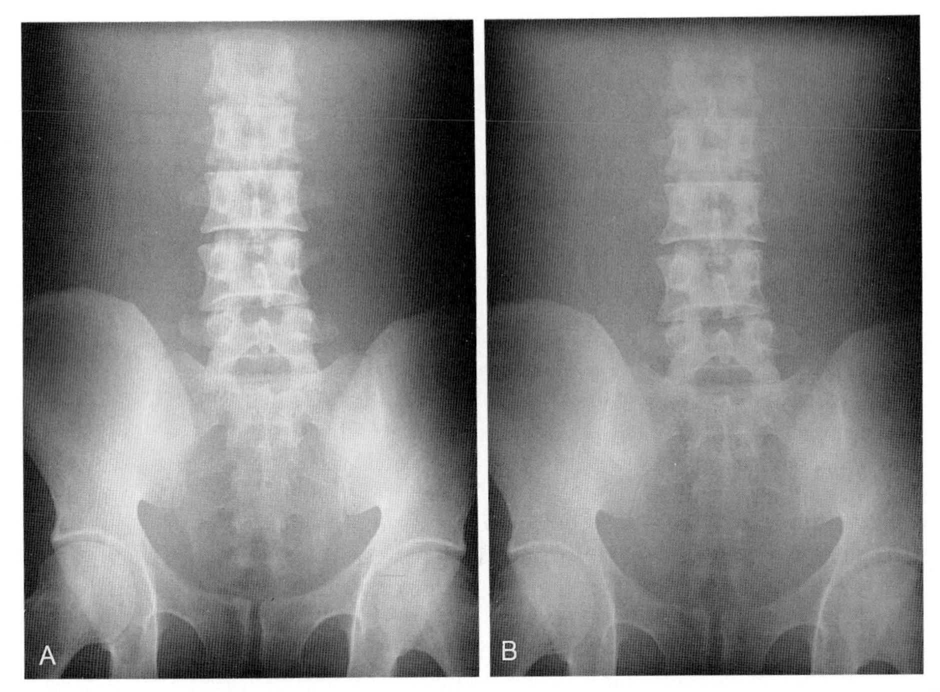

FIGURE 8–6. (*A*) Radiograph taken at 80 kVp and 12.5 mAs. (*B*) Radiograph taken at 92 kVp and 6.25 mAs produces too much scattered radiation.

Suppose a radiographer chose 80 kVp to penetrate an abdomen radiograph. This kVp is already above the optimum kVp of 70. If the radiographer increases the kVp further according to the 15% rule, the new kVp would produce too much scattered radiation (Fig. 8–6).

$$80 \text{ kVp} \times .15 = 12$$
$$80 \text{ kVp} + 12 = 92 \quad \text{too much scatter production}$$

The 15% rule can only be applied over a small range of kVp changes. About 10 kVp above or below the optimum kVp is the acceptable tolerance range. A variation of more than 10 kVp above or below the optimum kVp will usually produce an unacceptable radiograph.

THE 60 TO 90 kVp RANGE

Since most radiographers do not have calculators in their pockets at work, there is a simple way to perform most of the calculations necessary for the 15% rule. Within the kVp range of 60 to 90, a 10-kVp change is equal to a 15% change.

60 kVp	70 kVp	80 kVp	90 kVp
×.15	×.15	×.15	×.15
9	10.5	12	13.5

Multiply any kVp between 60 and 90 by 15% and the answer will fall between 9 and 13.5. This is close enough to the round number of 10 to make a rule of thumb. If the original kVp is between 60 and 90, add or subtract 10 kVp and either double the mAs or cut the mAs in half. These calculations can all be done easily and quickly in clinical situations.

In the 60 to 90 kVp range, a change of 10 kVp is equal to a 15% change.

Using the rule of thumb to increase contrast when the original factors are 80 kVp at 7 mAs, decrease the kVp to 70 and increase the mAs to 14. Using the rule of thumb to control motion when the original factors are 80 kVp at 7 mAs, increase the kVp to 90 and decrease the mAs to 3.5 by cutting the exposure time in half.

Look again at Table 8 – 1, which lists the optimum kVp for commonly radiographed body parts. Most of the numbers on the list fall between 60 and 90 kVp, so this rule of thumb will be useful.

PERFORM ACTIVITY 8.E

SUMMARY

mAs controls density and kVp controls contrast. kVp affects density, but mAs does not affect contrast.

The optimum kVp should be used most of the time because it will always be enough to penetrate the body part, it will produce a sufficient level of contrast, and it will produce an acceptable amount of scattered radiation.

The 15% rule can be applied to control motion or change contrast. If the kVp is increased by 15%, the mAs can be cut in half by reducing the exposure time. This will help control motion. If the kVp is reduced by 15%, the mAs must be doubled. This will increase contrast because a lower kVp is used.

For faster calculation within the commonly used 60 to 90 kVp range, a change of 10 kVp is equal to a 15% change.

PERFORM ACTIVITY 8.F

Primary Exposure Factors Section Review Activities

PERFORM ACTIVITY 8.G

PERFORM ACTIVITY 8.H

PERFORM ACTIVITY 8.I

SECTION IV

CONTROL OF SCATTERED RADIATION

CHAPTER 9

GRIDS AND THE BUCKY

CHAPTER OUTLINE

OBJECTIVES

At the end of this chapter you should be able to:

- Compare the energy and direction of scattered radiation to primary radiation.
- Describe the effect of scattered radiation on density and contrast.
- Differentiate between the construction of a focused, parallel, and crossed grid.
- Explain how a grid absorbs scattered radiation.
- Define grid ratio.
- List the most common grid ratios.
- State which grid ratio is the most efficient at absorbing scattered radiation.
- Define the term grid frequency.
- Describe how to avoid the five methods of producing grid cut-off.
- Describe the grid focusing distance and focal range.
- Differentiate between a grid and a Bucky.
- Explain how it is decided when a grid should be used and what type should be used.
- Calculate the new mAs to be used when changing from nongrid to grid, or when changing grid ratios.

This section, consisting of Chapters 9 and 10, discusses the subject of scattered radiation control. Scattered radiation reduces radiographic contrast by placing a layer of fog or grayness over the image.

The amount of scattered radiation that hits the film can be controlled by either preventing the production of scatter in the patient's body, or by preventing the scatter from reaching the film after it is produced in the patient's body. A device that prevents the production of scatter in the patient's body is the collimator. The collimator and several other devices and techniques to control scatter will be discussed in Chapter 10. The grid is the device that prevents scatter from reaching the film and is the subject of this chapter. The Bucky, which is used to move the grid during the exposure, will also be described.

SCATTERED RADIATION

Primary radiation is produced in the x-ray tube and is aimed toward the patient's body. When the photons in the beam enter the body they interact with the atoms in the patient's body. Sometimes the photons are absorbed by the components of the body, and sometimes they pass right through the patient's body and put density on the film. The photons can also be scattered.

Scattered radiation is produced when a primary photon hits an atomic particle, usually in the patient's body, and then the photon is deflected off the atomic particle. The primary photon is scattered. Scattering causes the primary photon to change its original direction and lose energy (Fig. 9–1). The new direction could cause the scattered radiation to bounce back toward the x-ray tube, shoot out of the patient's body in all directions, or hit the x-ray film.

Scattered radiation travels in a different direction from primary radiation and loses energy.

Scattered radiation that hits the film affects the film by putting density on it. This density is an extra density and it is not good for the image. Scatter puts a layer of gray equally over the whole image, making the image appear to have low contrast. The density distinctions between adjacent structures are muted, and some structures are hidden in the image. Scatter produces an image with a very long scale contrast and reduces the quality of the whole image.

Scattered radiation produces a low contrast image.

In 1913, Dr. Gustave Bucky invented a device called the grid. The grid is placed between the patient and the film. The grid absorbs scattered radiation and prevents the scatter from reaching and affecting the film. When a grid is used, radiographic contrast increases. Figure 9–2 shows a radiograph taken with and without a grid.

Using a grid increases radiographic contrast.

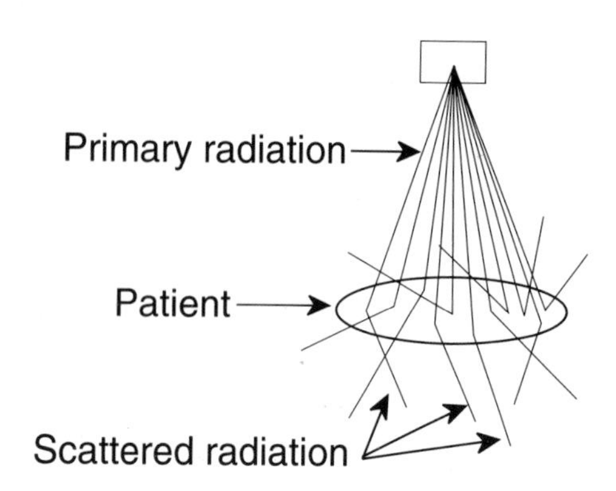

FIGURE 9–1. Primary radiation that changes its direction produces scattered radiation.

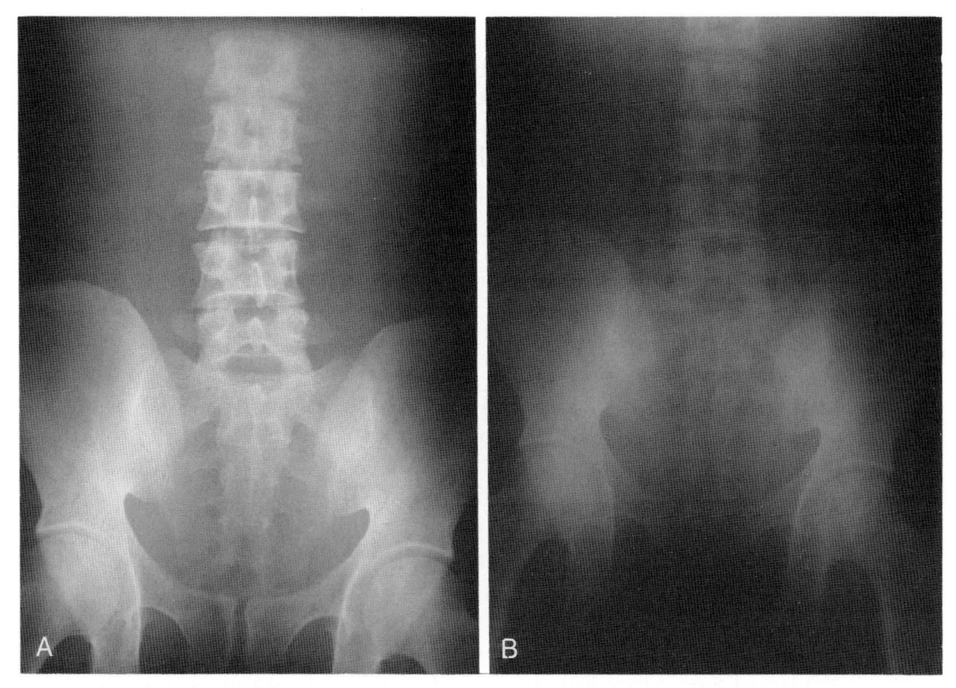

FIGURE 9–2. (*A*) Radiograph taken with a grid. (*B*) Radiograph taken without a grid.

GRID CONSTRUCTION

Grids are made to match the sizes of the cassettes and x-ray film. The grid is constructed of lead strips that are so thin that they are sometimes referred to as lead foil strips.

When the lead strips are assembled to make a grid, they are placed on edge next to one another. If the grid were assembled on top of a table, the strips would be placed side by side vertical to the table top (Fig. 9–3).

Each strip is separated from the other by a space called an **interspace**. The material used in the interspace can be a type of cardboard fiber, plastic, or aluminum. The interspace material should be **radiolucent**, which means it should not absorb the x-ray beam. The strips and interspaces are bound together and covered by aluminum or plastic to give the grid strength.

If a grid is made to match the size of a 14 × 17 inch cassette, the surface of the grid that measures 14 × 17 is called the **face** of the grid. A line, called the center line,

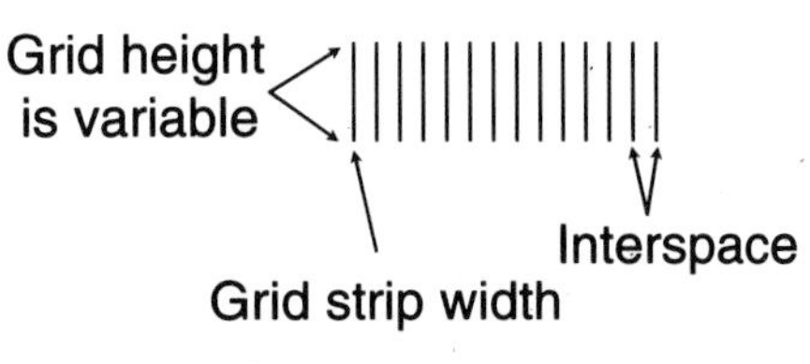

FIGURE 9–3. The height, width, and length of grid strips and the interspaces.

is usually drawn on the face of the grid, which lets the radiographer know the direction of the grid lines since they are hidden by the grid's cover. The direction of the grid lines is very important to know when using the grid so the problem of grid cutoff can be avoided. This problem will be discussed later in this chapter.

If the cover were not on the grid, the radiographer could look at the thin edge or side of the grid and see the vertically placed grid strips.

GRID PATTERNS

Focused Grid

The most common type of grid pattern in use is the **focused** grid. When the grid strips are placed on edge during the construction of a focused grid, they are not all placed parallel to each other. The strips in the very center of the grid are parallel to each other, but the strips at the sides of the grid are angled. The angle increases as the strips get closer to the sides of the grid (Fig. 9–4).

It's a pretty smart design, because the grid strips are aligned to match the way the primary photons emerge from the x-ray tube. The x-ray beam is cone-shaped, and the primary photons near the central ray are not at much of an angle when they reach the film. The photons at the edge of the film are at more of an angle.

When the x-ray beam hits the grid, the grid is supposed to let the primary photons through it and absorb the scattered photons. If the primary photons and grid strips are aligned, the primary photons will pass through the grid. Since scattered radiation travels in a changed direction from primary radiation, it is more probable that the scattered rays will be absorbed by the grid strips. The scattered rays will hit the grid from a different angle than the primary rays and may run right into the lead strips of the grid. The lead strips will then absorb the scattered photons. When a primary photon bounces off a part of the patient's body, it loses energy as it is scattered. Since the scattered rays have lost energy, it becomes easier for the lead strips to absorb the scatter (Fig. 9–5).

Primary radiation passes through a grid, whereas scattered radiation is absorbed by the grid.

Parallel Grid

A **parallel** grid is another design or pattern of a grid. This type of a grid is constructed the same way as a focused grid, but the grid strips are not placed at an angle. If the

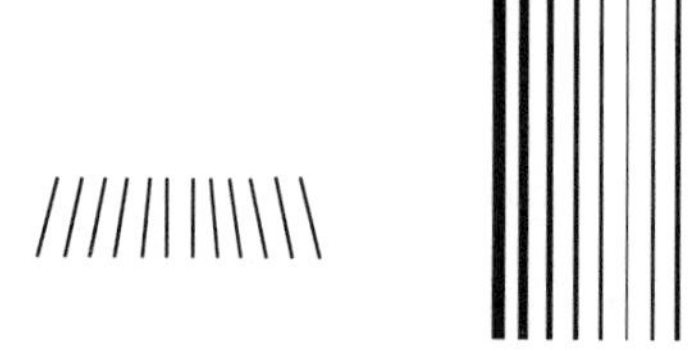

FIGURE 9–4. A focused grid pattern viewed from the edge and face.

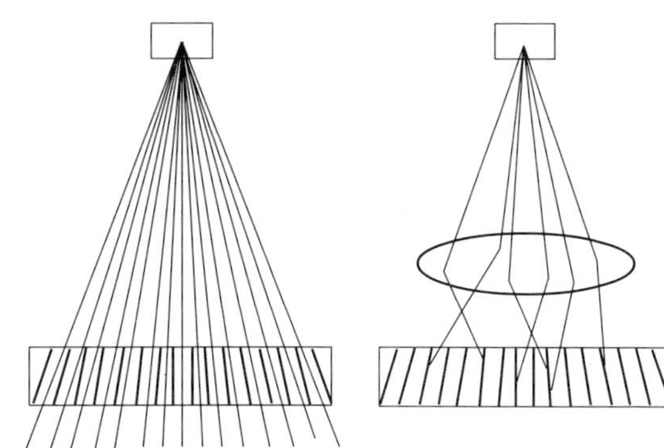

FIGURE 9–5. Primary radiation gets through a grid, and scattered radiation is absorbed.

grid were assembled on a table top, all the grid strips would be placed perpendicular to the table top and they would all be parallel to each other.

When looking at this type of grid from either the face or edge of the grid, the strips are parallel to each other (Fig. 9–6). This pattern does not match the way the x-ray beam emerges from the tube as well as the focused grid does.

Crossed Grid

The **crossed** grid is also called a criss-cross grid or a cross-hatch grid. It is a combination of two parallel grids. One parallel grid is placed on top of the other, but one of the grids is turned 90 degrees so that the lines of the two grids cross each other (Fig. 9–7). The crossed grid is the pattern that will absorb the most scattered radiation. It is not used often, though, because the x-ray tube cannot be angled at all when using it.

PERFORM ACTIVITY 9.A

GRID RATIO

The grid ratio is an important feature of the grid. The grid ratio is defined as the relationship between the height of the lead strips and the distance between the strips. Grid ratios vary from 5:1 to 16:1. The most common grid ratios are 5:1, 6:1, 8:1, 12:1, and 16:1.

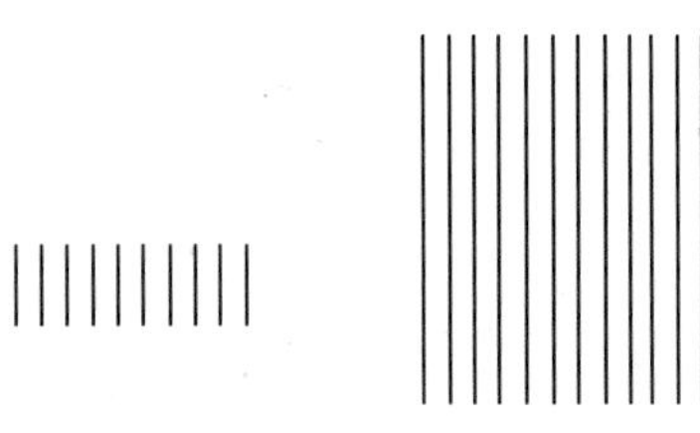

FIGURE 9–6. A parallel grid pattern viewed from the edge and face.

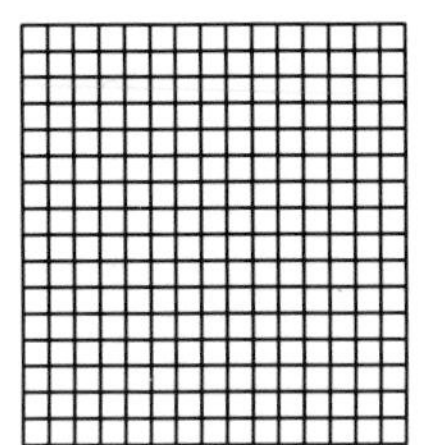

FIGURE 9–7. A crossed grid pattern.

Grid ratio is the height of the lead strips compared to the distance between the lead strips.

The grid ratio always ends with the number 1, so no matter what the actual measurements are of the height of the strips and interspace distance, the grid ratio must be converted to a certain number to 1. If the grid strips are .080 inch high, and the interspaces are .010 inch wide, the grid ratio is 8:1. The grid ratio is determined by setting up a proportion:

$$\frac{.080}{.010} = \frac{X}{1}$$

Cross-multiply:

$$.010X = .080$$
$$X = 8$$

The actual measurements of the height of the grid strips and the interspace distance are unimportant after the measurements have been converted to a grid ratio. The grid ratio is the way the radiographer determines how much scattered radiation the grid will absorb or "clean up." Most grids have a label that indicates the grid pattern and ratio.

A high-ratio grid (16:1) will absorb more scattered radiation than a low-ratio grid (5:1). A grid absorbs scattered rays that hit the grid strips. If the grid strips extend up higher from the surface of a grid as with a higher ratio grid, the strips will be able to capture the scattered rays sooner and thus absorb more of them (Fig. 9–8).

A high-ratio grid absorbs more scattered radiation than a low-ratio grid.

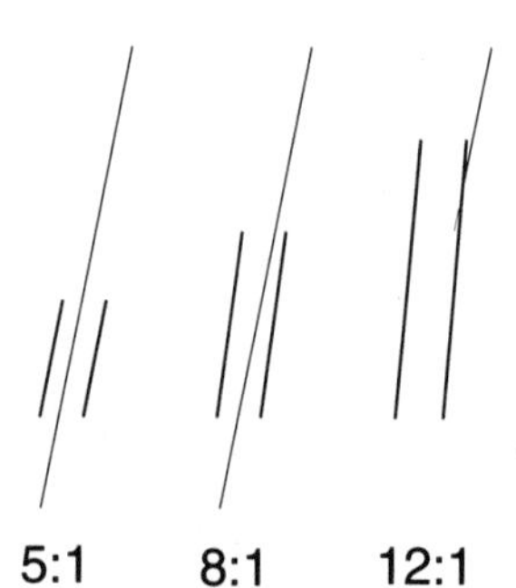

FIGURE 9–8. A scattered photon enters each of these grids at the same angle. It is absorbed by the higher ratio grid.

GRID FREQUENCY

The grid frequency is defined as the number of grid lines per inch. The usual range is from 60 to 110 lines per inch. A grid with more grid lines per inch is more efficient at absorbing scattered radiation because it has more lead in it.

Grid frequency is the number of grid lines per inch.

GRID CUT-OFF

A grid is designed to absorb the scattered radiation and allow the primary radiation to pass through it. However, if the grid is used incorrectly, the grid strips can absorb some of the primary radiation. This is called grid cut-off or grid striping. Grid cut-off usually results in a radiograph that is unacceptable.

Grid cut-off is the unwanted absorption of primary radiation by the grid.

A radiograph with grid cut-off will have areas that appear lighter or less dense than they should. Sometimes the image of the grid lines can be seen in these lighter areas. Grid cut-off is usually seen on the edges of the radiographs.

Because the focused grid is the most common grid pattern, it is important to learn how to use it correctly and avoid grid cut-off. Grid cut-off with a focused grid can occur in five general ways:

1. The wrong source-image distance is used.
2. The x-ray tube is angled against the grid lines.
3. The grid is angled in relation to the x-ray beam.
4. The x-ray tube is not centered so that the central ray is over the center of the grid.
5. The grid is used upside down.

Source-Image Distance (SID)

The SID used with a focused grid must fall within a certain range or the radiograph will display grid cut-off. The acceptable range is determined by the **grid focusing distance**. The grid focusing distance is an imaginary point in space above the face of a focused grid. If it were possible to extend the height of focused grid strips, they would converge or meet at a point somewhere above the face of the grid, and that point is called the grid focusing distance (Fig. 9–9).

The grid strips of a focused grid are angled so that they are aligned with the pattern of the x-ray beam. So if the x-ray tube is placed at a source-image distance corresponding to the grid focusing distance, this would be the best place to allow the primary rays to get through the grid.

In actual use, there is a tolerance range that extends a little bit above and below the grid focusing distance. This range, called the **focal range**, is the acceptable range of source-image distances that can be used with a focused grid. If the x-ray tube is placed either above or below the focal range, grid cut-off can occur (Fig. 9–10).

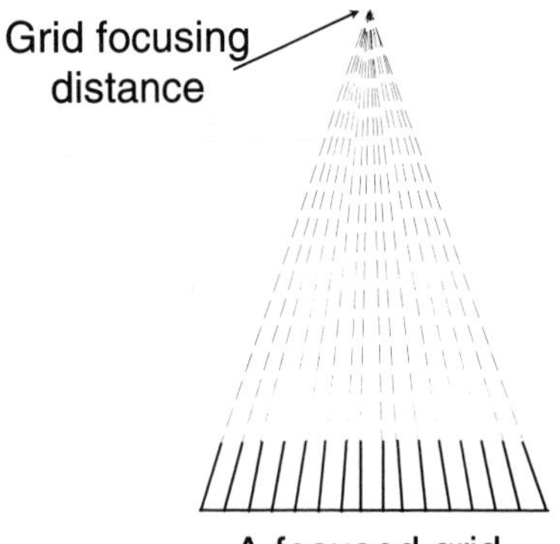

FIGURE 9–9. The grid focusing distance.

Use the SID within the grid's focal range to avoid grid cut-off.

PERFORM ACTIVITY 9.B

Angle of the X-ray Tube

Angling the x-ray tube against the grid lines will produce a noticeable grid cut-off. The line drawn down the center of the face of a grid indicates the direction of the placement of the grid lines in the grid. The x-ray tube can be angled either way in the direction of this line with no problem.

Angling the tube across the grid lines, perpendicular to the center line of the grid, will produce grid cut-off (Fig. 9–11).

To avoid grid cut-off do not angle the x-ray beam against the grid lines.

PERFORM ACTIVITY 9.C

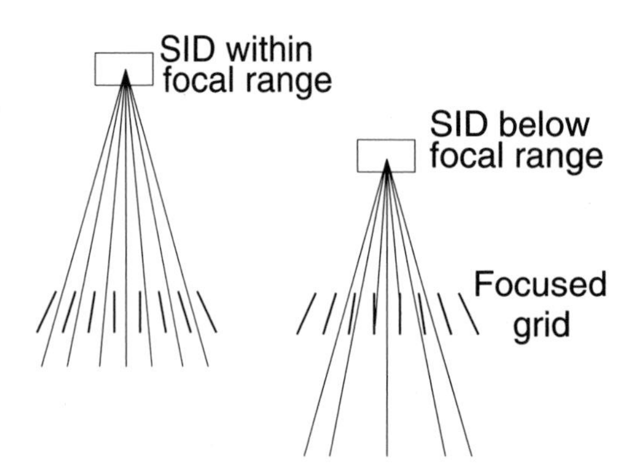

FIGURE 9–10. Grid cut-off produced by using an SID that is out of the focal range.

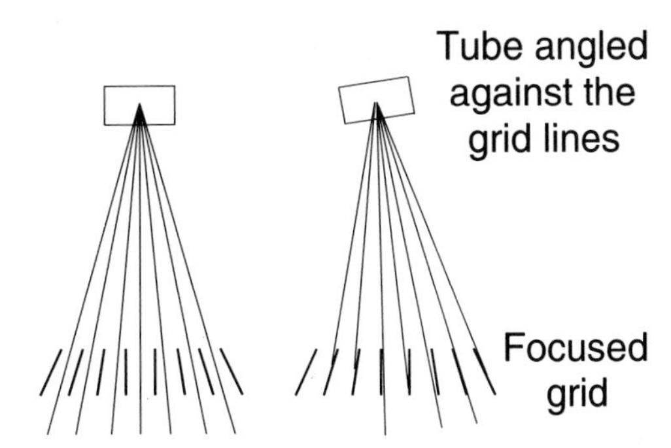

FIGURE 9–11. Grid cut-off produced by angling the x-ray beam against the grid lines.

Angle of the Grid

Grid cut-off also occurs if the x-ray tube is straight but the grid is at an angle. This causes the x-ray beam to be directed against the grid lines. This problem can occur in clinical practice during portable radiography when the patient is lying on a cassette with a grid on top of the cassette. The patient may be leaning more heavily on one side of the grid and cassette than the other. This causes the grid and cassette to be at an angle compared to the beam (Fig. 9–12).

To avoid grid cut-off the beam and grid must be perpendicular to each other.

PERFORM ACTIVITY 9.D

Centering of the X-ray Beam

Incorrect centering of the x-ray beam to the center line of the grid can cause grid cut-off on the radiograph. The x-ray tube should always be positioned so that the central ray is pointed at the center line on the grid. Grid cut-off is produced when the x-ray tube is moved across the grid lines, or perpendicular to the way the grid lines run in the grid (Fig. 9–13).

The central ray must be positioned at the center line of the grid to avoid grid cut-off.

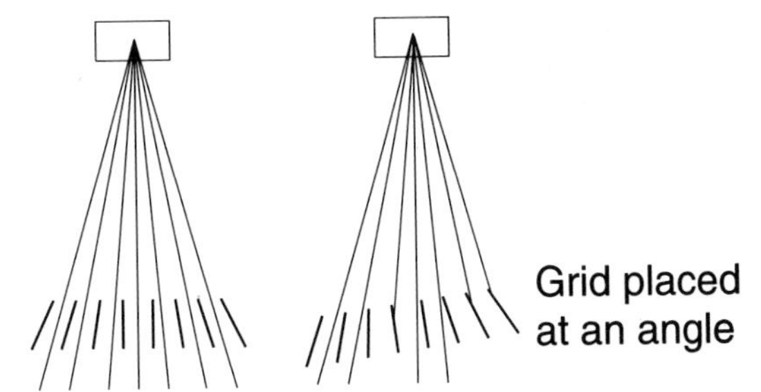

FIGURE 9–12. Grid cut-off produced by angling the grid in relation to the central ray.

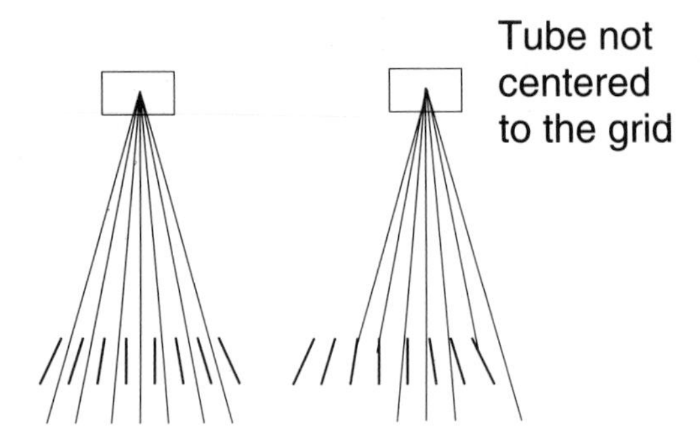

FIGURE 9–13. Grid cut-off produced because the central ray is off center to the center of the grid.

PERFORM ACTIVITY 9.E

Upside-Down Grid

Using the grid upside down can occur accidentally. The center line on the face of the grid indicates the top side of the grid. The top side should be placed toward the x-ray beam with the film underneath the grid.

If the grid is accidentally placed upside down, the center line will be pointing toward the film instead of the x-ray tube. This mistake will produce a very noticeable grid cut-off. A less dense image will be displayed in the very center of the radiograph and the sides will appear almost blank. Figure 9–14 shows what happens to x-rays passing through an upside-down grid. Figure 9–15 is a radiograph taken through an upside-down grid.

The center line of the grid must face the x-ray tube to avoid grid cut-off.

PERFORM ACTIVITY 9.F

THE BUCKY

When a radiograph is taken with a grid, it is possible to see the lines of the grid on the radiograph. In 1920, Dr. Hollis Potter invented a device called the Bucky, which

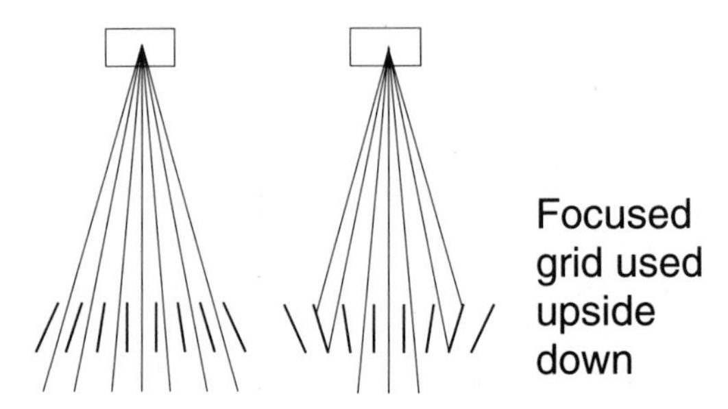

FIGURE 9–14. Grid cut-off produced by using a focused grid upside down.

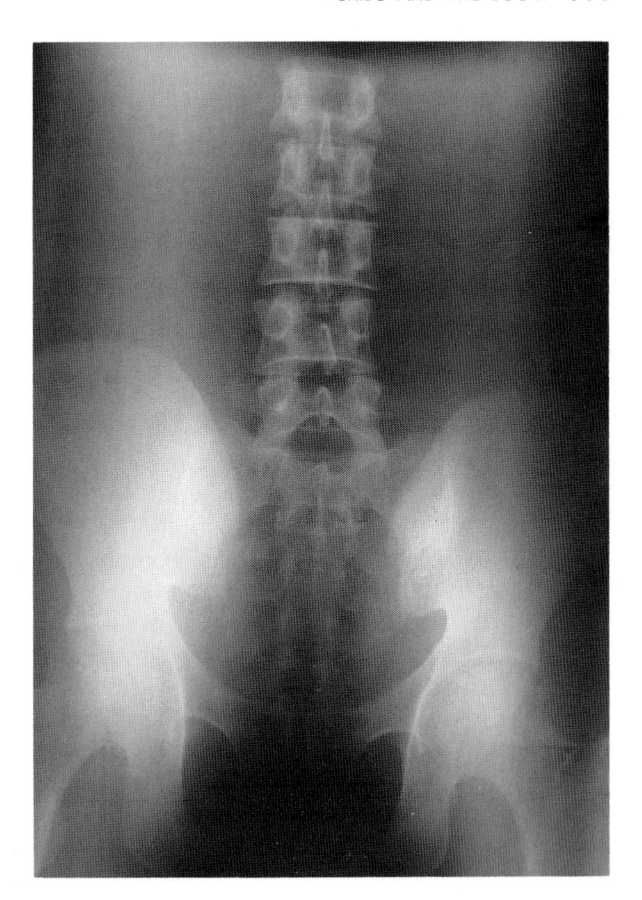

FIGURE 9–15. An example of grid cut-off caused by using a focused grid upside down.

moves the grid during the x-ray exposure. This movement blurs the grid lines so they will not be imaged on the radiograph.

The Bucky movement blurs the grid lines.

The most common type of Bucky device is a reciprocating Bucky. This moves the grid from side to side during the exposure. If the Bucky device fails to move the grid, or if it moves too slowly, the grid lines may appear on the radiograph. This is called "capturing" the grid.

A Bucky device is located directly under the x-ray table. A Bucky can also be installed in equipment used for upright radiography. The device consists of a focused grid and a motor to move the grid. The Bucky device also has a tray where the cassette is placed. The tray does not have the grid on it. The grid is positioned above the tray and cassette and usually cannot be seen.

All the precautions mentioned to avoid grid cut-off with a focused grid have to be adhered to when using the Bucky device in the x-ray table or upright equipment, because a focused grid is part of the equipment.

GRID SELECTION

How does a radiographer decide when to use a grid? And when a grid is necessary, what pattern and grid ratio should be used? In most departments there is a standard protocol for grid use. When the protocol is established, these factors should be considered: the size of the body part being examined, the kVp used, the amount of contrast required, the possibility of producing grid cut-off, and the grid pattern.

A general rule states that a grid should be used when the patient's body part measures more than 10 cm. More scattered radiation is produced when the patient's body part is large because there are more atoms for the x-ray photons to collide with.

Another general rule states that a grid should be used when the kVp has to be set above 70. More scattered radiation is produced with a high kVp.

At techniques above 90 kVp, a grid ratio of at least 8:1 is usually required. If a high grid ratio is used, the grid will be able to absorb more scattered radiation. If it is necessary to produce a radiograph with high contrast, a high ratio grid should be used.

There is a greater chance of producing grid cut-off with a higher ratio grid. During portable radiography, when problems may occur with alignment of the central ray and grid, it may be better to use a lower grid ratio.

A crossed grid will absorb the most scattered radiation, but the x-ray tube cannot be angled at all with this type of grid. The grid lines will absorb the primary radiation no matter which way the tube is angled.

PERFORM ACTIVITY 9.G

TECHNIQUE COMPENSATION WITH A GRID

The radiographer needs to increase the exposure factors whenever a grid is being used. There are two reasons for this. A radiograph taken without a grid has more scattered radiation on it than one taken with a grid. Scattered radiation puts density on the film even though it is unwanted density. The absence of the scattered radiation on a film produced with a grid makes the film less dense than one produced without a grid. Also, when a radiograph is taken with a grid, the lead in the grid will absorb some of the primary radiation, even when it is being used correctly. This causes less radiation to reach the film and produces less density on the radiograph.

Suppose a radiographer takes a good radiograph without a grid using 5 mAs and 70 kVp. If the radiograph is taken again and a grid is used for the second exposure, the exposure factors need to be increased or the second radiograph will not have enough density. If the radiographer switches from using a grid to not using a grid, the exposure factors would have to be decreased. The amount of technique compensation or the amount of exposure increase or decrease necessary depends on what grid ratio was used for the original exposure compared to the second exposure.

This book will use the "to/from" method for calculating most technique compensations. The compensation used for the grid is just one of several a radiographer uses. When using the to/from method, think of a tag on a Christmas present. The tag may say "To: Anne, From: Doug". The name of the person the present is "to" goes on top of the tag and whoever the present is "from" goes on the bottom of the tag.

Table 9–1. Grid Ratios and Multipliers for Calculating Technique Compensation

Grid Ratio	Multiplier
No grid	1
5:1	2
6:1	3
8:1	4
12:1	5
16:1	6

The first thing to do when calculating the technique compensation with a grid is to form a fraction with the grid ratio multipliers. These are listed in Table 9–1. The number beside the grid ratio is the **multiplier**. The multiplier of the grid ratio being changed ***to*** goes on the top of the fraction and becomes the numerator. The multiplier of the grid ratio being changed ***from*** goes on the bottom of the fraction and becomes the denominator. The number 5 is the multiplier for a 12:1 ratio grid, and 3 is the multiplier for a 6:1 ratio grid. So if the grid ratio is changed ***to*** a 12:1 ratio grid ***from*** a 6:1 ratio grid, the fraction would be 5/3. For another example, the fraction would be 4/1 if the change is to an 8:1 ratio grid from no grid.

After forming the fraction, multiply the original mAs by the fraction. The answer is the new mAs to be used because of the grid change.

Example 1

The original radiograph was taken with a 6:1 ratio grid at 5 mAs and 80 kVp. The repeat radiograph is taken with a 16:1 ratio grid. What new mAs is required?

To: 16:1 multiplier of 6
From: 6:1 multiplier of 3

$$\text{New mAs} = 5 \times \frac{6}{3}$$

$$\text{New mAs} = 10$$

Example 2

The original radiograph was taken without a grid at 8 mAs and 70 kVp. The repeat radiograph is taken with a 12:1 ratio grid. What new mAs is required?

To: 12:1 multiplier of 5
From: Nongrid multiplier of 1

$$\text{New mAs} = 8 \times \frac{5}{1}$$

$$\text{New mAs} = 40$$

Some radiography references suggest increasing or decreasing the kVp to compensate for grid use. Since kVp changes the amount of scattered radiation produced, this is not wise. If a grid is being used to decrease scattered radiation on the radiograph, and then the kVp is increased to compensate for the use of the grid, the increase in kVp will cause more scattered radiation to be produced. Therefore the higher contrast achieved by using a grid would be canceled by the lower contrast caused by increasing the kVp. mAs should be the factor used to compensate for grid use because mAs does not change the amount of scattered radiation produced.

PERFORM ACTIVITY 9.H

PERFORM ACTIVITY 9.I

SUMMARY

A grid is used to absorb scattered radiation and prevent it from reaching the film. A grid consists of lead strips standing on edge separated by interspaces. The focused grid is the most common pattern.

Grid cut-off is the unwanted absorption of primary radiation by the grid. Grid cut-off can be avoided by using the source-image distance within the focal range, angling the tube only in the direction of the grid lines, avoiding an angle of the grid, centering the central ray to the center of the grid, and using the grid right side up.

A Bucky device moves the grid so that the grid lines will not appear on the radiograph.

To compensate for the addition or elimination of a grid, the mAs must be increased or decreased. Form a fraction by placing the multiplier of the grid ratio being changed to in the numerator and the multiplier of the grid ratio being changed from in the denominator. To calculate the new mAs, multiply the old mAs by this fraction.

PERFORM ACTIVITY 9.J

CHAPTER 10

METHODS TO CONTROL SCATTER

CHAPTER OUTLINE

OBJECTIVES

At the end of this chapter you should be able to:

- List two advantages of restricting the x-ray beam to the size of the film being used.
- Describe the construction and function of a collimator.
- Explain the purpose of automatic collimation.
- Calculate the new mAs to be used when the collimation field size is changed.
- Describe the effect of a change in collimation field size on contrast and density.
- List the main purpose for using filtration.
- Describe the effect of filtration on contrast and density.
- Differentiate between inherent, added, and total filtration.
- Explain the purpose and clinical applications of the wedge and trough compensatory filters.
- Explain how these methods act to control scattered radiation: the air-gap technique, lead blockers, compression, and the cassette back.

Chapter 9 discussed the grid, which prevents scattered radiation from reaching the film. This chapter will present a variety of other methods to control scatter. X-ray beam restriction by using the collimator will be discussed first. This prevents the production of too much scattered radiation in the patient's body. The grid and collimator are the primary methods used to control scattered radiation.

The main purpose of the filter is to protect the patient's body from excess radiation, but a filter also changes the quantity and quality of the x-ray beam and affects both contrast and density. Several miscellaneous methods to control scatter are also discussed in this chapter. Some are more popular than others. They are the air-gap technique, lead blockers, compression, and using a cassette upside down.

X-RAY BEAM RESTRICTION

Scattered radiation is produced in the patient's body when primary photons from the x-ray tube hit matter in the patient. The photons then travel off in a changed direction and they also have less energy. Thus it is in the patient's body where the majority of scattered radiation is produced.

The amount of scatter produced depends on how much matter in the body is hit with radiation. If a large area of radiation covers the patient's body, the radiation will hit more matter and produce more scattered radiation because there are more atoms for the photons to collide with. If the size of the x-ray beam when it hits the patient's body is small, less scattered radiation will be produced. Also if the patient is large, there is more matter present in the area of radiation, and more scattered radiation will be produced than if the patient is small. The saying "more matter = more scatter" will help you remember how this works.

More matter = More scatter

The x-ray beam as it emerges from the x-ray tube takes the shape of a cone. The photons diverge, or move away from each other, as they leave the anode of the x-ray tube. Therefore as the beam travels away from the tube, it gets larger in size. If it were unrestricted when it reached the patient's body, it would be quite large and cover a large area of the body. This would not only produce a lot of scattered radiation but also radiate more of the patient's body than necessary and increase the radiation dose to the patient.

A small beam size reduces scattered radiation production and reduces the patient's radiation dose.

A beam that is larger than the x-ray film being used will not record any more information on the film than a beam that is adjusted to match the size of the film. There is never an advantage to having the x-ray beam larger than the size of the film. There are two advantages to using a small beam size: less scattered radiation production and a lower radiation dose to the patient.

The x-ray beam should never be larger than the size of the film being used.

There are several devices used to restrict the x-ray beam. Two older devices are aperture diaphragms and cones. The collimator is the most effective and used almost exclusively now, so this is the only device this book will discuss.

The Collimator

The collimator, sometimes called a variable aperture diaphragm, is a boxlike device attached at the edge of the x-ray tube, right under the window of the x-ray tube (Fig. 10-1). The x-ray tube sits right above the collimator.

The collimator box has several sets of lead shutters in it. The lead shutters absorb the edges of the beam as it emerges from the anode so that the beam will be smaller

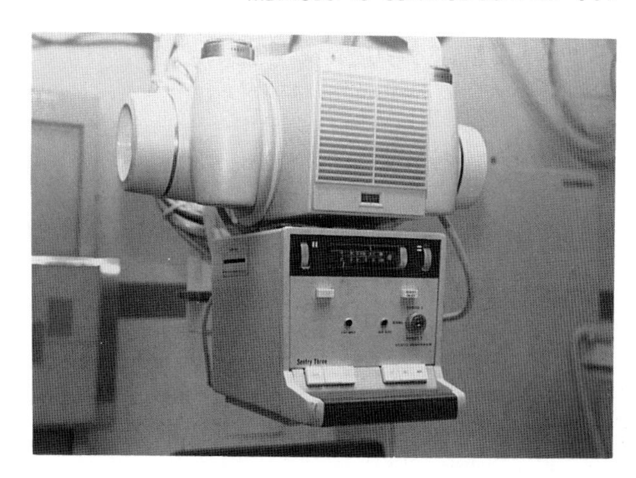

FIGURE 10–1. The x-ray tube and collimator.

when it hits the patient (Fig. 10–2). The collimators also shape the beam so that it will be rectangular to match the rectangular shape of the film being used.

The radiographer can adjust the shutters inside the collimator with dials that are on the outside of the collimator. The shutters move in and out, making the x-ray field size smaller or larger.

Modern x-ray equipment uses a device called automatic collimation or positive beam limitation. This device automatically adjusts the size of the x-ray beam to the size of the film being used. A sensor, located in the Bucky tray, detects the size of the film. This causes a motor to move the collimator shutters to adjust the beam to match the size of the film in the Bucky tray. By federal law, automatic collimation must be available on all modern x-ray equipment.

Automatic collimation only works when the Bucky tray is being used. There are many times in clinical situations when the Bucky tray is not used. Sometimes the radiographer places the cassette on the top of the x-ray table or directly under the patient's body when the patient cannot be moved from a stretcher or wheelchair. The Bucky is also not used during portable radiography. During these instances, it is the radiographer's responsibility to adjust the collimation field size to limit scatter production and limit the patient's radiation dose.

Modern collimators are always equipped with a light that indicates the size of the x-ray beam at the patient's body. The collimator light is produced from a light bulb in the collimator box. The light bulb shines on a mirror that is placed in the collimator at an angle. The mirror reflects the light from the light bulb onto the patient's body. This light image indicates the location of the x-ray beam on the patient's body. It is important that this light beam be adjusted correctly, otherwise the light on the patient's body might not coincide with where the x-ray beam is actually being directed (Fig. 10–3).

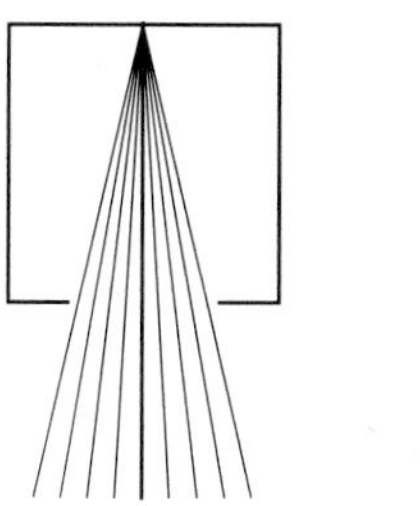

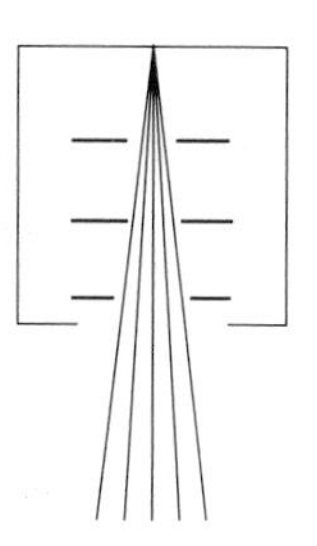

FIGURE 10–2. The collimator shutters cut off part of the beam.

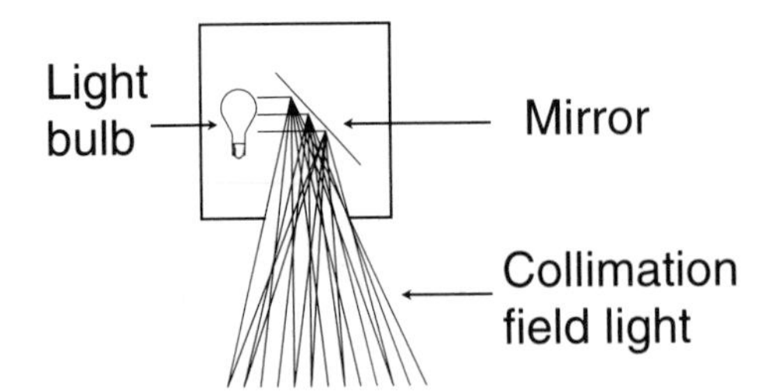

FIGURE 10–3. The field light is produced by a light bulb in the collimator box.

The collimator usually includes two centering guides. One guide placed in the collimator casts its shadow in the field light and indicates the exact center of the beam. The shadow usually shows up as a circle or "X" shadow. The other guide is a line of light that extends out the side of the collimation field. This helps the radiographer line up the center of the x-ray beam with the center of the film. Some x-ray equipment uses laser lights to show the center and edges of the collimation field.

Technique Compensation

An increase or decrease in the area of radiation at the patient's body determined by the collimator changes the amount of scattered radiation produced. Scattered radiation affects contrast and it also puts density on the film. If the area of radiation at the patient's body increases, more scattered radiation is produced. On the radiograph the density is increased and the contrast is decreased. If the area of radiation at the patient's body decreases, less scattered radiation is produced. The density is then decreased and the contrast is increased. The mAs needs to be changed to compensate for the density changes when the area of radiation or collimation field size is changed.

A change in collimation field size affects both density and contrast.

If the collimation field size is changed from a size that will cover a 14 × 17 inch film to a size that will cover a 10 × 12 inch film, the mAs should be increased by about 25%. If the change is from 14 × 17 inches to 8 × 10 inches, the mAs should be increased by about 40%. A change from a small area of radiation to a larger area of radiation will require a corresponding decrease in mAs.

In Chapter 9 the "to/from" technique compensation method was discussed. This same method can be used to calculate the new mAs when a change in collimation field size is necessary.

Table 10–1 shows the multipliers for three sizes of collimation. Form a fraction by placing the multiplier for the collimation field size that is being changed *to* in the numerator and the multiplier for the collimation field size that is being changed *from*

Table 10–1. Multipliers for Changes in Collimation Field Size

Collimation Field Size	Multiplier
14 × 17	1
10 × 12	1.25
8 × 10	1.40

in the denominator. Then multiply the original mAs by this fraction. The answer is the new mAs to be used because of the collimation change.

Example 1

A KUB radiograph is taken on a 14 × 17 inch film using 10 mAs and 70 kVp. The radiologist requests a "coned-down" (smaller field size) film of the left upper quadrant on a 10 × 12 inch film to increase radiographic contrast because of a suspected kidney stone in the left kidney. What new mAs is required?

To: 10 × 12 multiplier of 1.25
From: 14 × 17 multiplier of 1

The fraction is $\frac{1.25}{1}$

$$\text{New mAs} = 10 \times \frac{1.25}{1}$$

$$\text{New mAs} = 12.5$$

Example 2

A preliminary film of the gall bladder is taken of the right upper quadrant on an 8 × 10 inch film using 20 mAs and 70 kVp. The radiologist requests a KUB on a 14 × 17 inch film because he or she thinks the patient might have an early bowel obstruction and he or she needs to see the whole abdomen. What new mAs is required?

To: 14 × 17 multiplier of 1
From: 8 × 10 multiplier of 1.40

The fraction is $\frac{1}{1.40}$

$$\text{New mAs} = 20 \times \frac{1}{1.40}$$

$$\text{New mAs} = 14.3$$

When changing from a 10 × 12 inch film to an 8 × 10 inch film, the fraction is 1.40/1.25. When changing from an 8 × 10 inch film to a 10 × 12 inch film, the fraction is 1.25/1.40.

PERFORM ACTIVITY 10.A

PERFORM ACTIVITY 10.B

FILTRATION

A filter is a material placed between the anode of the x-ray tube and the patient's body. A filter absorbs low energy photons from the x-ray beam, and this decreases the patient's radiation dose. Filtration also affects the amount of scattered radiation on the radiograph and the amount of radiation reaching the film. Filtration has an effect on both the quantity and quality of the x-ray beam and therefore affects both contrast and density. However, filtration's primary purpose is not to affect contrast and density. The main purpose of filtration is to protect the patient's body from excess radiation.

The x-ray beam is polyenergetic. This means that the photons in the beam have many different energies. When the beam reaches the patient's body, the photons with low energy would probably hit the patient's skin and stop right in the skin or just under it, damaging the tissues there. These low energy photons don't have enough energy to go through the patient's body and put density on the film. Thus it is a good idea to put something between the anode of the x-ray tube and the patient's body to absorb these low energy photons before they ever reach the patient's body, since they won't do the radiograph any good anyhow. The device used to do this is called a filter.

A filter absorbs low energy photons and decreases the patient's radiation dose.

Filters absorb more of the low energy photons from the beam compared to the high energy photons. Because low energy photons are absorbed, what remains in the beam are high energy photons. Therefore the average energy of the whole beam is increased by filtration. This increase in beam energy will reduce radiographic contrast because the higher energy beam will be able to produce more scattered radiation.

The filter's main effect is on low energy photons, but photons of all energies can be absorbed by a filter. The reduction of photons of all energies from the beam will decrease density on the radiograph because the total quantity of radiation in the beam is decreased.

Filtration decreases density and decreases contrast.

There are two sources of filtration, inherent and added.

Inherent Filtration

Inherent filtration is present because of the design of the x-ray tube. It is a part of the tube and cannot be eliminated. The x-ray tube has a leaded glass covering or envelope around it. The glass has a thinner spot in it called the window. This window is positioned under the anode. The x-ray photons have to pass through the window after they leave the anode and are traveling through space to the patient. As the x-ray photons pass through this window, lower energy photons are absorbed by the lead glass. Thus the window of the x-ray tube removes or filters some of the photons from the beam.

Added Filtration

An added filter can be a piece of metal, usually aluminum, that is placed under the window between the x-ray tube and collimator (Fig. 10–4). It functions the same way as inherent filtration. It absorbs lower energy photons and increases the average energy of the beam.

It is called added filtration because it was removable in older equipment. It could be used for some exposures and removed for other exposures. Now by federal

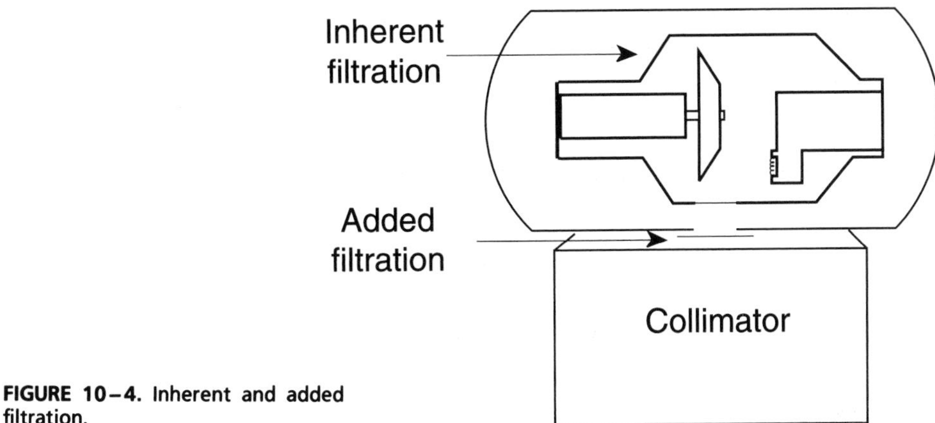

FIGURE 10–4. Inherent and added filtration.

law, the added filtration has to be included in every x-ray tube. It is not removable in modern equipment, but it is still called "added" to distinguish it from inherent.

Any material placed between the x-ray tube window and the patient acts as a filter. The mirror of the collimator also filters the beam, and contributes to the added filtration.

Total Filtration

The total filtration is the sum of both the inherent and added filtration. Since inherent and added filtration are made of different materials, they are made equal in the measurement of their effect by equating their effect to what aluminum would do. The term **aluminum equivalent** is used. The amount of inherent filtration is about .5 to 1.0 mm of aluminum equivalent. This means that the lead glass in the x-ray tube must filter the same amount of photons as .5 to 1.0 mm of aluminum.

The amount of added filtration is about 2.0 to 3.0 mm of aluminum equivalent. Other metals can be used, but they must do what 2.0 to 3.0 mm of aluminum would do.

Federal law requires at least 2.5 mm of aluminum equivalent total filtration for general-purpose x-ray tubes operated above 70 kVp. For x-ray tubes operated between 50 and 70 kVp, at least 1.5 mm of aluminum equivalent total filtration is required. A total filtration of .5 mm of aluminum equivalent is required for x-ray tubes operated below 50 kVp.

Since the amount of filtration in a modern x-ray tube must be present and cannot be removed, there is no need for technique compensation because of variable amounts of filtration. However, it is important to remember what effect filtration has on density and contrast. Any additional filtration above the usual amount would decrease density and decrease contrast.

Compensatory Filtration

Another type of filtration, but not one that is always required, is compensatory filtration. These are special filters used only during certain clinical applications. The filters are placed in a track under the collimator. Their purpose is to provide a more uniform film density across the whole film when the patient's body part varies greatly in size or tissue density. There are two commonly used shapes, the wedge and trough filters.

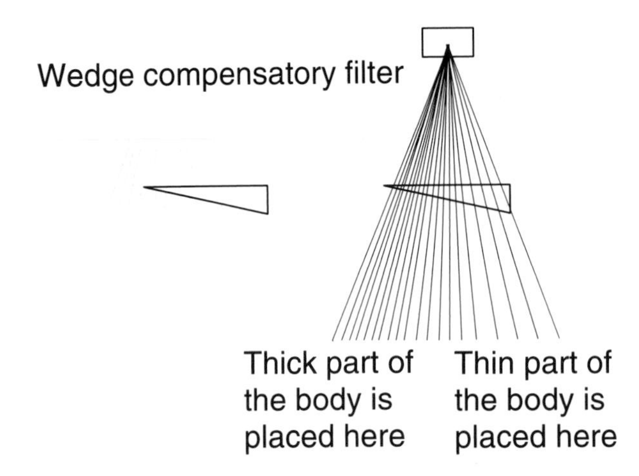

FIGURE 10–5. Wedge compensatory filter.

Wedge Compensatory Filter

A wedge compensatory filter is shaped like a wedge or triangle. The purpose of a wedge compensatory filter is to give a uniform density to the radiograph when the body part being examined is larger on one side of the radiograph than on the other side.

The filter has a thin end and a thick end and must be placed correctly under the collimator. The filter must be placed so that the thick end of the filter is over the smaller part of the patient, and the thin end of the filter is over the larger part of the patient (Fig. 10–5). More radiation will be absorbed by the thick end of the filter, which reduces the density on the radiograph at the smaller end of the patient. Less radiation will be absorbed by the thin end of the filter, which increases the density on the radiograph at the larger end of the patient compared to the smaller end. Thus, the density on the radiograph becomes more even.

The thorax is smaller at the superior end and larger at the inferior end. An anteroposterior (AP) radiograph of the thoracic spine shows an increased density at the superior end and a decreased density at the inferior end. If a wedge compensatory filter is used, this density difference evens out across the radiograph. In this instance, the thick part of the filter would have to be placed over the superior part of the thoracic spine.

Trough Compensatory Filter

The trough filter is thicker on its edges and thin in the middle. It is useful for frontal views of the chest. The mediastinum, or center part of the chest, is composed of the heart, spine, sternum, and thick blood vessels. It has more tissue density than the lungs, which are made up of lung tissue and air.

When used for an anteroposterior (AP) or posteroanterior (PA) chest radiograph, the shape of the trough filter allows more radiation through its thin center, which is placed over the mediastinum. The thicker ends of the filter, placed over the lungs, allow less radiation through (Fig. 10–6). The density of the chest radiograph should be more even across the radiograph with the trough filter.

PERFORM ACTIVITY 10.C

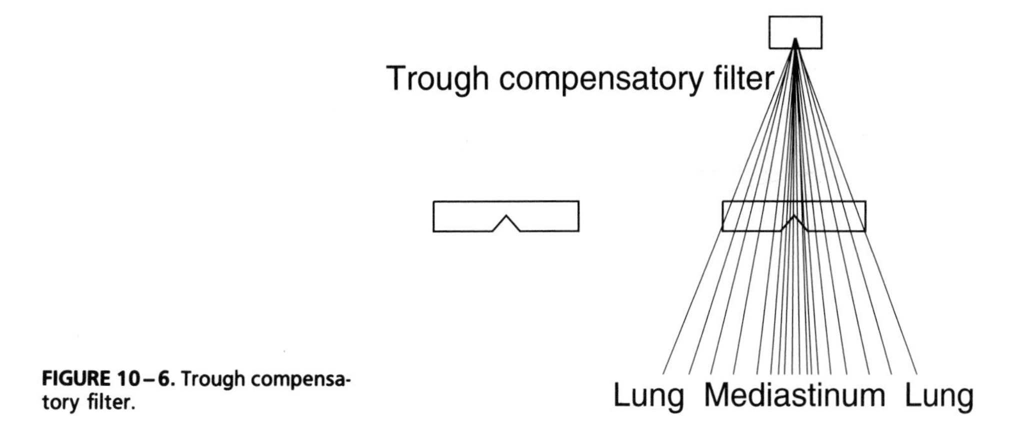

FIGURE 10–6. Trough compensatory filter.

MISCELLANEOUS METHODS TO CONTROL SCATTER

The grid and the collimator are the best methods to control scattered radiation. There are several other methods to control scattered radiation that are not widely used. A brief discussion of each follows.

The Air-Gap Technique

The air-gap technique uses a large object-image distance. By placing the body part farther away from the film, some of the scattered radiation produced in the patient's body will miss hitting the film (Fig. 10–7). This increases radiographic contrast, but reduces density. The amount of scattered radiation reduction achieved with the air-gap technique is about equivalent to the effect of using a 6:1 ratio grid.

An air-gap increases contrast but decreases density.

A large object-image distance will produce a very noticeable increase in magnification. This is compensated for by increasing the source-image distance. In clinical practice the air-gap technique is used most often for a PA chest radiograph. A 10-inch OID or air gap is usually used with a compensating 10-foot SID. The increase in SID will also require an increase in mAs using the density maintenance formula to maintain film density.

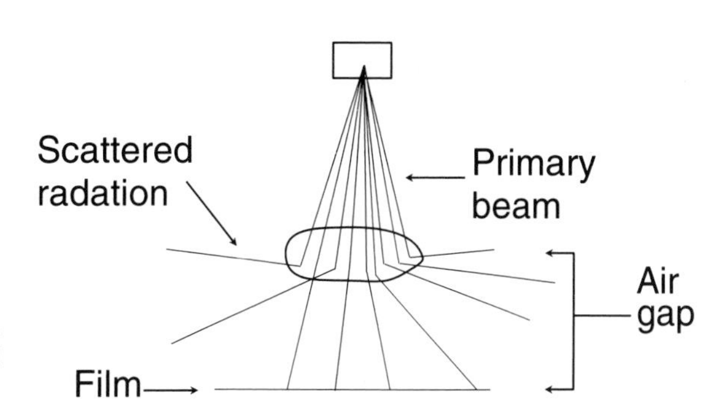

FIGURE 10–7. The air-gap technique works because some of the scattered photons miss hitting the film.

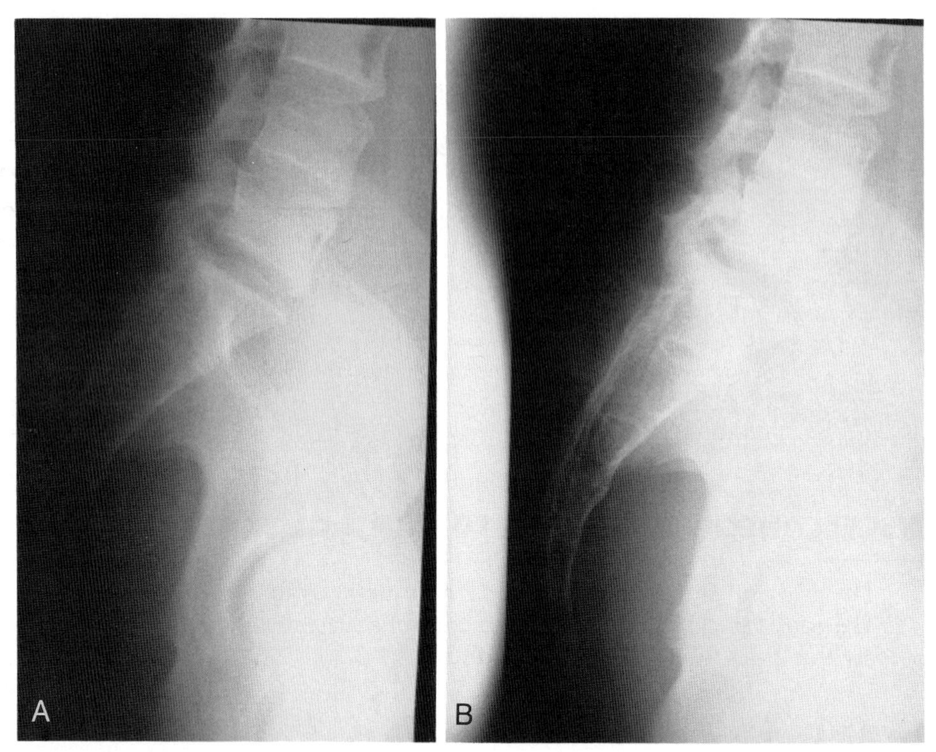

FIGURE 10–8. The lead blocker is placed in an area of unabsorbed primary radiation. (*A*) Radiograph taken without a lead blocker. (*B*) Radiograph taken with a lead blocker shows higher contrast.

PERFORM ACTIVITY 10.D

Lead Blocker

A lead blocker can be used for thick body parts on exposures where there is a large area of unabsorbed primary radiation on a radiograph (Fig. 10–8). A good example of this is with the lateral view of the sacrum. For the lateral position of the sacrum, the sacrum should be placed in the center of the film. This leaves one side of the film with no image on it. The film will be very dense in this area because there is nothing there to absorb the radiation.

Unabsorbed primary radiation produces scattered radiation when the photons hit the x-ray table top. This scatter decreases the contrast on the radiograph in the area of the sacrum. If lead blockers or a lead apron are placed on the table next to the patient's body where the unabsorbed radiation will fall, the lead will absorb this radiation. The radiograph will show higher contrast with the lead blocker than without it.

PERFORM ACTIVITY 10.E

Compression

Recall the saying "more matter = more scatter." A thick body part will produce more scattered radiation than a thin body part. If it were possible to compress a thick body part and make it thinner, less scattered radiation would be produced.

In clinical practice this is possible during abdominal radiography. An AP KUB provides no compression of the abdomen. If the patient is turned over and lies on his or her abdomen, the abdomen will be compressed. This is especially true of a patient with a large abdomen.

The PA radiograph will show more contrast because less scattered radiation will be produced due to the compression (Fig. 10–9). This effect may be seen on an intravenous pyelogram (IVP) exam. This exam usually requires several AP radiographs of the abdomen and at least one PA radiograph. Figure 10–9 shows an AP and PA radiograph taken during an IVP. The PA radiograph shows higher contrast because of the removal of some scattered radiation and also more density because the abdomen is compressed.

Cassette Back

The back of a cassette contains a thin layer of lead. This lead will absorb x-rays and can act like a filter if the cassette is used upside down. This application is limited though, because it only works on cassettes with a solid lead back. If anything else is included in the lead back, it will be imaged on the film.

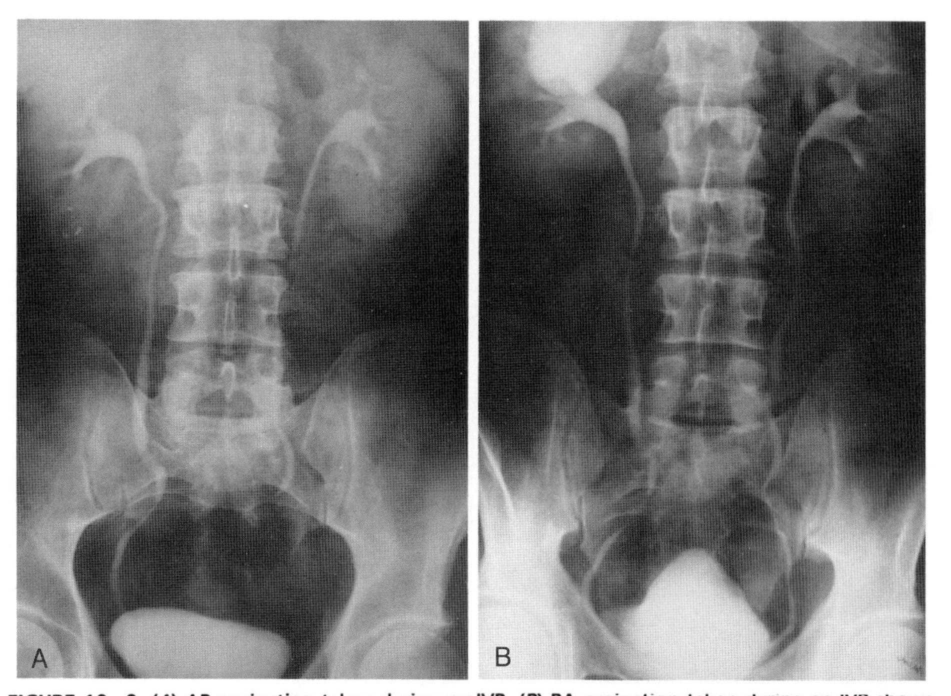

FIGURE 10–9. (*A*) AP projection taken during an IVP. (*B*) PA projection taken during an IVP shows higher contrast and also more density because the abdomen is compressed by the prone position.

SUMMARY

The collimator is used to limit the area of radiation to the size of the film being used. Collimation reduces the production of scattered radiation because less matter in the patient's body is being hit with radiation. A change in the collimation field size changes contrast and density. The mAs must then be changed to maintain film density.

A filter absorbs low energy photons from the x-ray beam before the photons can enter the patient's body, thus reducing the patient's radiation dose. Filtration increases the average energy of the beam. The decrease of photons from the beam produces less density, but the increase in beam energy produces more scattered radiation, which reduces contrast. The total amount of filtration is the sum of the inherent and the added filtration.

The air-gap technique, lead blockers, compression, and the back of the cassette can all be used to decrease the amount of scattered radiation. This increases radiographic contrast.

PERFORM ACTIVITY 10.F

Control of Scattered Radiation Section Review Activities

PERFORM ACTIVITY 10.G

PERFORM ACTIVITY 10.H

SECTION V

RECORDED DETAIL

CHAPTER 11

GEOMETRIC FACTORS AFFECTING RECORDED DETAIL

CHAPTER OUTLINE

OBJECTIVES

At the end of this chapter you should be able to:

- Define recorded detail.
- List the seven factors that affect recorded detail.
- Differentiate between recorded detail and visibility of detail.
- Describe the construction and function of the resolution grid.
- Define the terms penumbra and edge gradient.
- Explain how recorded detail is affected when unsharpness changes.
- List the geometric factors that affect recorded detail.
- Explain the effect of a change in focal spot size on unsharpness and recorded detail.
- Explain the effect of a change in object-image distance on unsharpness and recorded detail.
- Explain the effect of a change in source-image distance on unsharpness and recorded detail.
- Describe the relationship between recorded detail and size distortion.
- Given the focal spot size, the object-image distance, and either the source-object distance or the source-image distance, calculate the amount of unsharpness produced.

The four radiographic qualities introduced in Chapter 1 are density, contrast, recorded detail, and distortion. The three chapters in this section describe the quality of recorded detail.

Some factors that affect recorded detail are easily seen on the radiograph. Others are very subtle and it seems easier to just trust that they happen, because the changes are difficult to see on the radiograph. However, if several of these subtle factors are changed at the same time, a change in recorded detail can be seen easily.

The geometric factors that affect recorded detail are discussed in this chapter.

They are the focal spot size, the object-image distance, and the source-image distance. The later chapters in this section will discuss the material factors that affect recorded detail. These are film and intensifying screens that are the components of the film and screen imaging system. The contact inside the cassette between the film and intensifying screens also affects recorded detail.

Motion of the body during the exposure affects recorded detail. Immobilization of the body part so it won't move during the exposure is an affective method to control motion on the radiograph. Using a short exposure time is also effective for reducing the chance of motion on the radiograph. This was discussed in Chapter 5 with the reciprocity law, and Chapter 8 with the 15% rule.

RECORDED DETAIL

Recorded detail, formerly called definition, is the sharpness of the lines of the image. If the lines are recorded as sharp, the radiograph has good recorded detail. Poor recorded detail is seen as a fuzzy or blurry edge around the lines.

Recorded detail is the sharpness of the lines of the image.

The factors that influence recorded detail affect the whole image. All the lines that form the image are affected equally by the factors influencing recorded detail. The factors can't selectively affect one part of the image and leave the other parts unaffected unless the image has shape distortion. However, seeing the effect of poor recorded detail on the radiograph is sometimes difficult.

When thinking about the lines of the image, do not think just of the outside edges of the body part. Each image has internal lines that appear on a radiograph, and these must be sharp also. When radiographing the skull, the image of the sella turcica must be sharp, the edges of the orbits must be sharp, and the image of the bony markings in the skull must be sharp. Looking at the edges of an internal bony structure on a radiograph is the best area to detect poor recorded detail.

Figure 11 – 1 shows two radiographic images, one with good recorded detail and one with poor recorded detail.

Recorded Detail Versus Visibility of Detail

There are seven factors that affect recorded detail. These are listed in Table 11 – 1 along with a mnemonic to help remember the factors. These are the only factors that affect recorded detail and it is important to remember them.

There are many factors that affect the visibility of detail. **Visibility of detail** is a term used by radiographers and radiologists to describe how well they can see the image. Visibility of detail is the overall quality of the finished radiograph. It is affected by everything that went into producing the image.

Visibility of detail is the overall quality of the finished radiograph.

When a radiologist says that the detail on the image is not good, it could mean that the image has too much density, not enough density, does not have enough

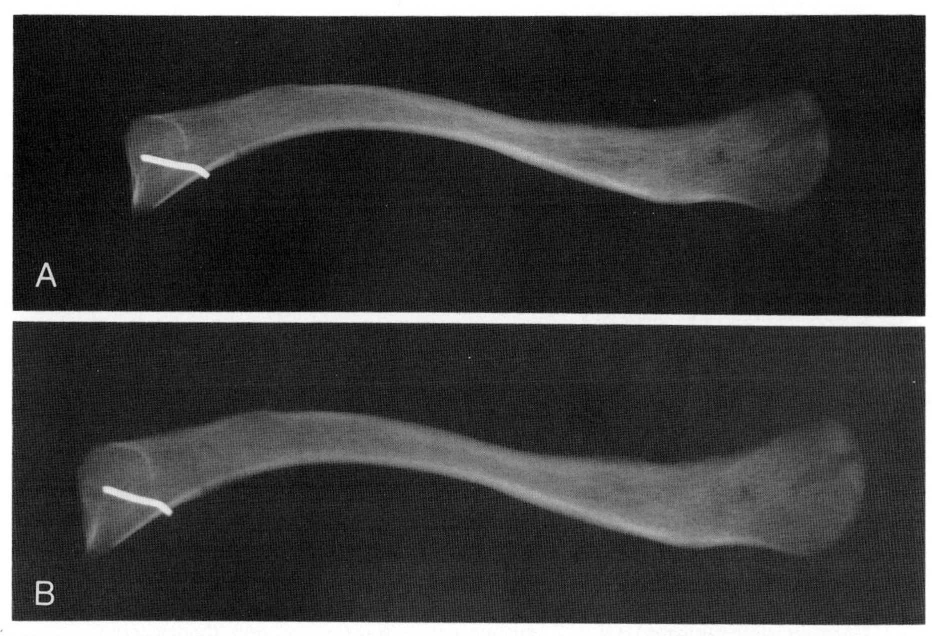

FIGURE 11–1. (*A*) Radiograph demonstrates good recorded detail. (*B*) Radiograph demonstrates poor recorded detail.

contrast, or even that the recorded detail is poor. Visibility of detail and recorded detail are two distinct qualities and cannot be confused by students.

MEASUREMENT OF RECORDED DETAIL

Resolution is defined as the ability of an imaging system to record two adjacent structures as separate structures. The term imaging system means the equipment that was used to form the image. If two very small adjacent structures are seen as two separate individual images on the radiograph, the radiograph has good resolution. It will also have good recorded detail.

Resolution is defined as the ability of an imaging system to record two adjacent structures as separate structures.

Since it is sometimes difficult to see poor recorded detail on a radiograph unless it is obvious, a special device called a **resolution grid** (Fig. 11–2) is used to measure

Table 11–1. Factors That Affect Recorded Detail

Factor	Mnemonic
SID	*S*TAT
OID	*O*rders
Focal Spot Size	*F*rom
Screen Speed	*S*urgery
Film Speed	*F*ollow
Contact of Screen and Film	*C*utting
Motion	*M*istakes

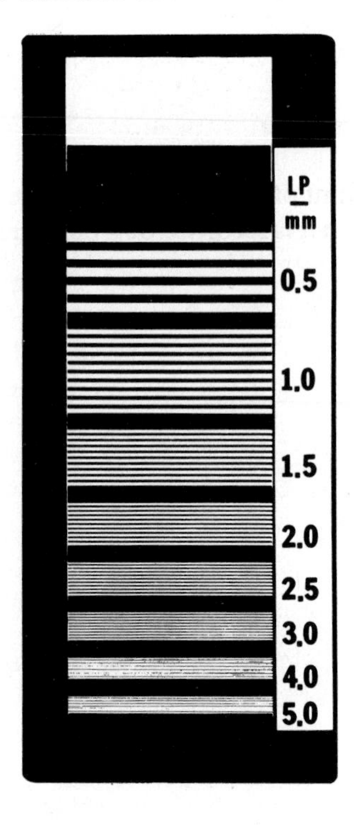

FIGURE 11–2. A resolution grid. (Photo courtesy of Nuclear Associates, 100 Voice Road, Carle Place, NY 11514.)

recorded detail. A radiograph is taken of the resolution grid using the same conditions used for a radiograph. Poor recorded detail can be seen more easily on the image of the resolution grid than on an image of a patient.

A resolution grid is a flat piece of metal with slits cut into it. The slits, called spaces, are interlaced with the metal lines of the grid. One metal line and the slit or space next to it is called a **line pair**. The resolution grid is constructed to have a variety of sets of line pairs, each having different sizes. A number is usually written on the resolution grid next to each set of line pairs, indicating how many line pairs in that set will fit into a millimeter. An area indicating five line pairs per millimeter would have smaller lines and spaces than an area indicating three line pairs per millimeter. The smaller line pairs are more difficult to render sharp or resolved on the radiograph.

The radiograph of the resolution grid is examined with the eye to see the maximum number of line pairs per millimeter that are resolved or seen as separate and sharp. An imaging system that produces good resolution will show a large number of line pairs as sharp or definite. This system will be able to display good recorded detail.

Resolution and recorded detail are good when a large number of line pairs per millimeter are resolved.

UNSHARPNESS TERMS

All radiographs have some amount of unsharpness. When it can be seen with the eye, the radiograph has poor recorded detail. If a radiograph has poor recorded detail, the lines in the image will have an area of unsharpness or a blurry area around them. There are several terms that describe unsharpness and recorded detail.

The area of unsharpness can be called the **penumbra**. If the penumbra increases, the recorded detail decreases.

Edge gradient is a term that describes the amount of recorded detail. Edge gradient refers to how sharp the edge of an object is when it is recorded on a radiograph. As the edge gradient increases, the recorded detail increases.

This book will use the term **unsharpness**. As unsharpness increases, recorded detail decreases.

As unsharpness increases, recorded detail decreases. As unsharpness decreases, recorded detail increases.

GEOMETRY AND RECORDED DETAIL

In geometry class, you learned about similar triangles (Fig. 11–3). With similar triangles, each corresponding angle has exactly the same degree, but the length of the lines in each triangle can be smaller or larger, making the size of the two triangles different.

The geometric factors that affect recorded detail are the size of the focal spot, the object-image distance, and the source-image distance. These factors can be arranged in a diagram to form similar triangles (Fig. 11–4). Because the triangles are similar, if one of the geometric factors in the top triangle changes, the length of the line on the bottom triangle of the diagram that represents unsharpness will also change. If the unsharpness changes, the recorded detail on the radiograph changes. If the line representing the area of unsharpness increases, the recorded detail decreases. If the line representing the area of unsharpness decreases, the recorded detail increases.

Focal Spot Size

Try this experiment. Hold a finger up about one foot from your eyes. Cover one of your eyes with your other hand. Focus on an object beyond your finger and take particular notice of where your finger is in space compared to the object. Now cover your other eye with your hand. You should see a change in the relationship of your finger and the object you were focusing on. This happens because each eye forms its own image of the finger and object. The human brain merges these two images and

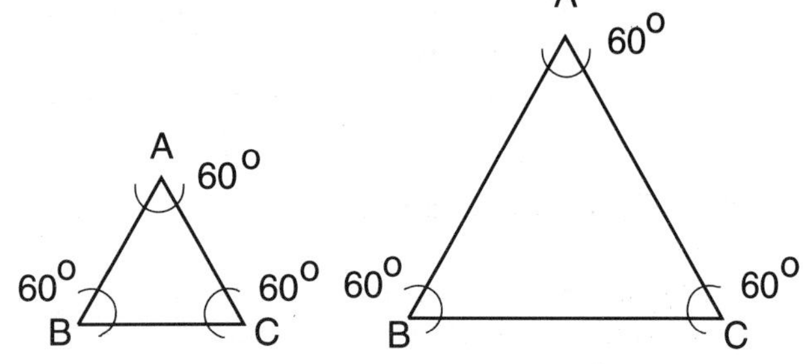

FIGURE 11–3. Two similar triangles. The size of the lines can change, but the degrees in each angle must remain the same.

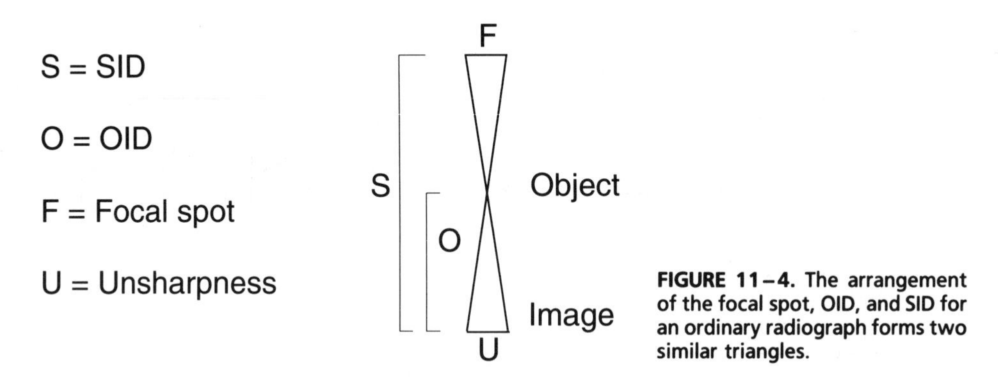

FIGURE 11–4. The arrangement of the focal spot, OID, and SID for an ordinary radiograph forms two similar triangles.

only sees one. A similar effect occurs on a radiograph, but the x-ray tube cannot merge the images and more than one image of the object is formed on the film.

X-rays are produced at the focal spot. The focal spot is the area on the anode of the x-ray tube that is hit with electrons from the filament. All x-ray photons in a beam originate from the focal spot. Because the photons come from an area instead of from one single point, each photon in the beam forms its own image of the object.

Look at Figure 11–5. Photons 1, 2, and 3 all originate from the focal spot, but the image of the object formed by each of the photons falls in a different spot on the film. The image is spread out over this area on the film and all the separate images can make the whole image appear unsharp.

If the focal spot area is smaller, the image will be spread out less and will appear sharper on the radiograph. An image formed with a small focal spot will display better recorded detail because the photons originate from a smaller area. Figure 11–6 shows a diagram of the similar triangles formed with several sizes of focal spots. As the focal spot size increases, the area of unsharpness increases.

A small focal spot produces better recorded detail.

PERFORM ACTIVITY 11.A

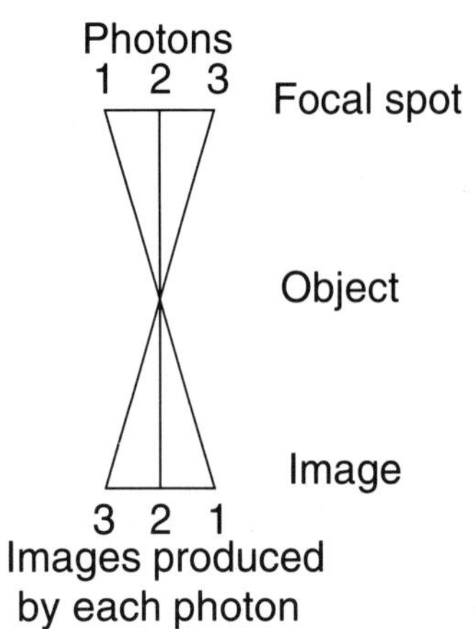

FIGURE 11–5. Each photon forms its own image of the object. Each of these separate images is projected to a different spot on the film. This spreads the image over an area on the film and can make the image appear unsharp.

FIGURE 11–6. A change in the size of the focal spot changes the area of unsharpness. If the focal spot increases, the unsharpness increases and the recorded detail decreases. If the focal spot decreases, the unsharpness decreases and the recorded detail increases.

Object-Image Distance

The object-image distance (OID) is the distance from the object being radiographed to the film or spot where the image is being formed. The radiographer controls this distance when positioning the patient.

If the object-image distance is increased, the area of unsharpness on the radiograph increases, and the image will display less recorded detail. If the object-image distance is decreased, the area of unsharpness decreases, and the image will display more recorded detail. This effect can be seen on Figure 11–7, which shows a diagram of the similar triangles formed with different object-image distances. As the OID on the diagram is increased, the area of unsharpness increases.

A small object-image distance produces better recorded detail.

PERFORM ACTIVITY 11.B

Source-Image Distance

The source-image distance (SID) is the distance from the source of x-rays, which is the x-ray tube, to where the image is formed, which is usually at the film. Most of the time in clinical practice, standard source-image distances of 40 or 72 inches are used. There are times, though, when these standard distances are varied.

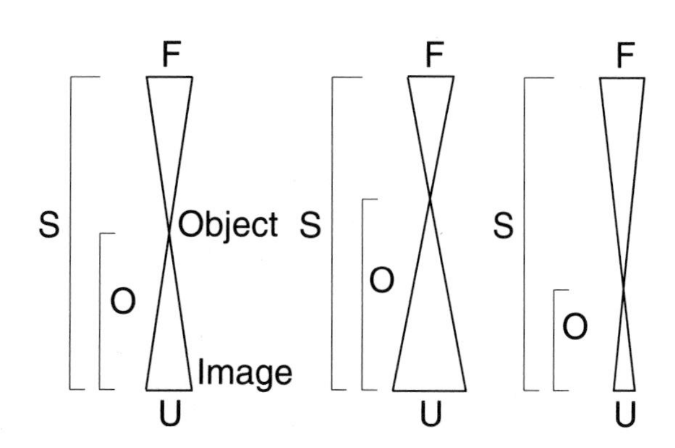

FIGURE 11–7. A change in the OID changes the area of unsharpness. If the OID increases, the unsharpness increases and the recorded detail decreases. If the OID decreases, the unsharpness decreases and the recorded detail increases.

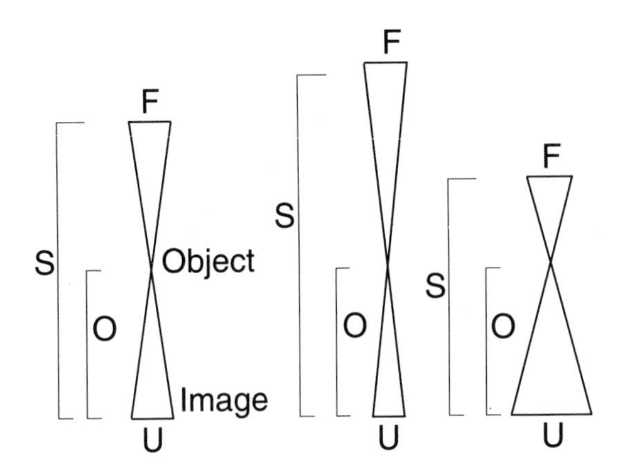

FIGURE 11–8. A change in the SID changes the area of unsharpness. If the SID increases, the unsharpness decreases and the recorded detail increases. If the SID decreases, the unsharpness increases and the recorded detail decreases.

If the source-image distance is increased, the area of unsharpness on the radiograph decreases, and the recorded detail improves. If the source-image distance is decreased, the area of unsharpness increases, and the recorded detail decreases. Figure 11–8 shows a diagram of the similar triangles formed with different source-image distances. As the SID on the diagram is increased, the area of unsharpness decreases.

A large source-image distance produces better recorded detail.

PERFORM ACTIVITY 11.C

RECORDED DETAIL AND DISTORTION

Chapter 3 discussed size distortion, which is also called magnification, and Chapter 4 discussed shape distortion. There is a relationship between distortion and recorded detail.

Size distortion and recorded detail are both affected by the source-image distance and the object-image distance. If the object-image distance increases, the image on the radiograph becomes more magnified. An increase in object-image distance also causes a decrease in recorded detail. If the source-image distance increases, the image on the radiograph becomes less magnified. An increase in source-image distance also causes an increase in recorded detail.

As magnification increases, recorded detail decreases. As magnification decreases, recorded detail increases.

An image with shape distortion is produced because the parts within the object lie at different object-image distances. One part of the image will have more magnification than another part. In this case, the amount of recorded detail will be different for each part which lies at a different object-image distance.

CALCULATION OF UNSHARPNESS

The geometric factors affecting recorded detail can be formed into an equation that is used to calculate the amount of unsharpness that will appear on the radiograph.

$$\text{Unsharpness} = \frac{\text{Focal spot size} \times \text{Object-image distance}}{\text{Source-object distance}}$$

The following conditions will be used to calculate the amount of unsharpness when each geometric factor is changed:

Focal spot size = .6 mm
Object-image distance = 2 inches
Source-object distance = 38 inches

$$\text{Unsharpness} = \frac{.6 \times 2}{38}$$

$$\text{Unsharpness} = .03$$

Focal Spot Size

If the focal spot size is increased, the amount of unsharpness increases. If the focal spot size changes from .6 to 2.0 mm, the amount of unsharpness changes to .11.

$$\text{Unsharpness} = \frac{2 \times 2}{38}$$

$$\text{Unsharpness} = .11 \quad \text{(an increase compared to .03)}$$

Object-Image Distance

If the object-image distance is increased, the amount of unsharpness increases. Referring back to the original factors, if the object-image distance changes from 2 inches to 8 inches, the amount of unsharpness changes to .13.

$$\text{Unsharpness} = \frac{.6 \times 8}{38}$$

$$\text{Unsharpness} = .13 \quad \text{(an increase compared to .03)}$$

Source-Image Distance

If the source-image distance is increased, the amount of unsharpness decreases. Remember that the source-image distance is the sum of the object-image distance and the source-object distance. Thus if the object-image distance stays the same and the source-image distance is increased, the source-object distance also is increased. The source-object distance may have to be calculated before using it in the unsharpness formula. Referring back to the original factors, if the source-object distance changes from 38 inches to 70 inches, the amount of unsharpness changes to .02. In this instance the SID is increased from 40 inches (38 + 2) to 72 inches (70 + 2).

$$\text{Unsharpness} = \frac{.6 \times 2}{70}$$

$$\text{Unsharpness} = .02 \quad \text{(a decrease compared to .03)}$$

PERFORM ACTIVITY 11.D

PERFORM ACTIVITY 11.E

SUMMARY

Recorded detail is affected by seven factors: the source-image distance, the object-image distance, the focal spot size, the speed of the intensifying screen, the speed of the film, the contact between the film and intensifying screen, and motion.

The focal spot size, the object-image distance, and the source-image distance are the geometric factors that affect recorded detail.

Recorded detail improves and the radiograph will show less unsharpness with a small focal spot size, a short object-image distance, and a long source-image distance. Recorded detail decreases and the radiograph will show more unsharpness with a large focal spot size, a long object-image distance, and a short source-image distance.

PERFORM ACTIVITY 11.F

CHAPTER 12

RADIOGRAPHIC FILM AND DEVELOPMENT

CHAPTER OUTLINE

OBJECTIVES

At the end of this chapter you should be able to:

- Describe the construction and characteristics of the film base and emulsion.
- List the layers of a single- and double-emulsion film in order from top to bottom.
- Describe the use of these types of film: single and double emulsion, screen, non-screen, roll, and special purpose.
- List the sections the film goes through in the automatic processor in order from beginning to end.
- Explain the purpose of each section of the processor.
- Name the agents and chemicals in the developer and fixer and state the purpose of each.
- Explain why it is important to monitor developer temperature.
- Describe how a film travels through the processor.
- Describe the special function of the entrance, turnaround, and crossover rollers.
- Explain how the processor chemicals become contaminated.
- Describe how the developer and fixer are replenished.
- Describe three ways to produce a characteristic curve.
- Draw a characteristic curve and label its parts.
- Define the term average gradient.
- Compare the film speed, contrast, and exposure latitude of two characteristic curves of different films drawn on the same graph.
- State the effect of film speed on recorded detail.
- Explain how the information from the characteristic curve is used for quality control of the processor.

The geometric factors that affect recorded detail are the focal spot size, the object-image distance, and the source-image distance. These were discussed in Chapter 11. This chapter discusses one of the material factors that affects recorded detail, radiographic film. Film is usually used with intensifying screens, which are discussed in Chapter 13.

The relationship between the exposure a film receives and the amount of density it is able to record is called film speed. Film speed affects recorded detail.

Film speed can be represented on a graph called the characteristic curve. This graph is used to show the speed, contrast scale, and exposure latitude that can be expected of a film. The information from this curve allows the radiographer to describe the characteristics of a type of film and also to monitor the processing conditions used on the film.

In addition to film and the characteristic curve, this chapter will include a discussion of film development. Film development affects the radiographic qualities of density and contrast.

RADIOGRAPHIC FILM CONSTRUCTION

Radiographic film is composed of two main parts, the base and the emulsion. The base and emulsion have several important characteristics.

Film is composed of a base and an emulsion.

The Base

The base of an x-ray film is a sheet of plastic made of **polyester** that is about .007 inch thick, depending on the type of film and the manufacturer. The polyester base is called a **safety base**. This means that it will not burn easily. It melts when ignited. This is a good feature since one type of film base formerly used was unstable and caused fires in several hospitals.

The base has a characteristic called **dimensional stability**. This means that it keeps its size and shape under all processing conditions, which can include subjecting the film to temperature variations and pH scale variations.

Most film has a **blue tint** added to the base when the base is manufactured. When a film is placed on a view box, the blue tint absorbs about 15% of the light from the view box. The blue tint makes the film more pleasing to the eye and reduces eye strain on radiologists who look into view boxes all day. The tint also helps to enhance radiographic contrast.

The Emulsion

The emulsion is a gelatin substance that is spread on the base like peanut butter on a piece of bread. If the emulsion is spread on just one side of the base, the film is *single-emulsion film*. If the emulsion is spread on both sides of the base, the film is *double-emulsion film*. One layer of emulsion is about.0005 inch thick, depending on the type of film and the manufacturer.

The emulsion consists of microscopic crystals of **silver bromide** suspended in a **gelatin**, kind of like the fruit suspended in a Jell-o salad. The image is formed in the silver bromide crystals.

The emulsion consists of silver bromide crystals suspended in a gelatin.

The gelatin has several important characteristics. It is a **colloid**, which means it is capable of suspending the silver bromide crystals. It forms a coating around each crystal separating it from the others. The gelatin is also **amphoteric**, which means it can be used with either an acid or alkali. This is important since one of the chemicals used in the automatic processor, the developer, is an alkali solution and another chemical, the fixer, is an acid solution.

Film Layers

When the film is put together at the factory, the base is first coated with an **adhesive**, which is sometimes called a substratum layer. When the emulsion is applied to the base it sticks well because of the adhesive. A protective coating called a **supercoating** is applied on top of the emulsion to protect it from scratching. Figure 12–1 shows a diagram of the layers of a double-emulsion and a single-emulsion film.

PERFORM ACTIVITY 12.A

PERFORM ACTIVITY 12.B

TYPES OF FILM

A wide variety of film types is used in radiology. The most common type is screen film, but radiology departments also use non-screen film and roll film. There are also many special-purpose films used.

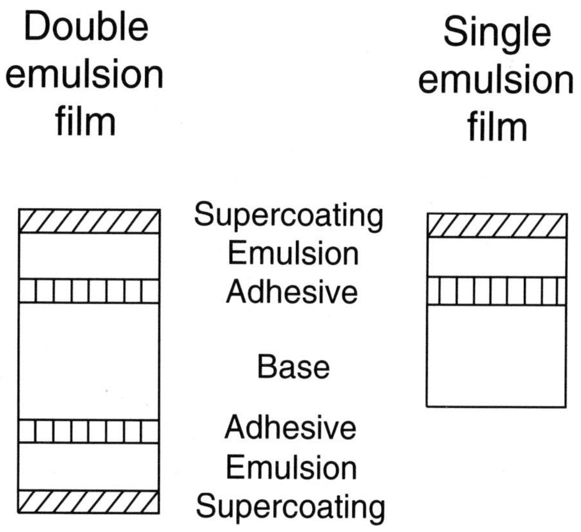

FIGURE 12–1. Layers of a double and single emulsion film.

Table 12–1. Common Film Sizes

Film Sizes
8 × 10
9 ½ × 9 ½
10 × 12
11 × 14
7 × 17
14 × 17

Screen Film

The single- and double-emulsion film described above are usually used in a cassette that contains intensifying screens. Intensifying screens give off light, which exposes the film. They will be described in Chapter 13. The type of film used with intensifying screens is called **screen film**. It is manufactured to be sensitive to both light and x-rays. Screen film comes in a variety of sizes. Table 12–1 lists the most commonly used sizes of film.

Non-Screen Film

A type of film called **non-screen film** is designed to be used without intensifying screens. It is manufactured to be sensitive to x-rays more than to light. Instead of being placed in a cassette with intensifying screens, it is encased in a light-tight cardboard or plastic holder. The emulsion of a non-screen film is thicker than screen film and it contains more silver. Non-screen film requires much more radiation than screen film to produce an adequate density. This causes the patient's radiation dose to be much higher. The use of non-screen film has been eliminated from most departments except for a few special-purpose films.

Periapical film is a very small non-screen film used to produce radiographs of teeth. An **occlusal** film is just like periapical film but it is a little bit larger. Occlusal film is used for a few special intraoral radiographs.

Roll Film

There are several types of film that are packaged in a roll, somewhat like a roll of tape. They are used in special devices that unroll the unexposed film as it is being used, and roll up the exposed film into a light-tight container sometimes called a magazine. The magazine can be detached and taken to the darkroom without exposing the film inside to light. Then one end of the roll of film must be taped onto a larger film called a **leader**. The leader film is fed into the automatic processor and the roll film follows it. This procedure keeps the roll film from jamming in the processor.

The **105-mm camera** uses roll film. The 105-mm camera is used as a spot film device during fluoroscopy when rapid exposures are required. A **Franklin** rapid film changer also uses roll film. This device is used during a procedure called an angiogram. **Cinefluorography** roll film is used during some special procedures and also in the cardiac catheterization lab. Cinefluorography film requires a different type of developer from the automatic processor.

Special-Purpose Film

Mammography film is a single-emulsion film used during a mammogram. It is able to display a high contrast and very good recorded detail, which are necessary to see early breast cancer.

Duplicating or copy film is single-emulsion film used to make a copy of a radiograph.

Subtraction film is used after an angiogram during a photographic technique designed to subtract the superimposing bone away from the angiographic image. This enables the arteries to be seen better.

Nuclear medicine, ultrasound, magnetic resonance imaging, and computed tomography equipment all use a computer to form the image. The image appears on a computer screen. **Laser** film, **video** film, or **electronic imaging** film are used to record these computer-generated images.

PERFORM ACTIVITY 12.C

RADIOGRAPHIC FILM DEVELOPMENT

The automatic processor (Fig. 12–2) develops or processes radiographic film. After the film is processed it will have the radiographic image on it and will be ready for the radiologist to read. Automatic processors usually develop the film in 45 to 90 seconds depending on the type of processor. Processors that develop the film in 45 seconds use a higher temperature for the processor chemicals, and a film that has a very thin emulsion compared with a processor that develops the film in 90 seconds.

Inside the processor the film is transported by a series of rollers. The film passes through a **developer** chemical, a **fixer** chemical, water called the **wash**, and a **dryer**.

In the processor the film goes through the developer, fixer, wash, and dryer.

The radiographer is expected to have a basic knowledge of how the processor works. Sometimes the processor jams, the films may be developed too light or too

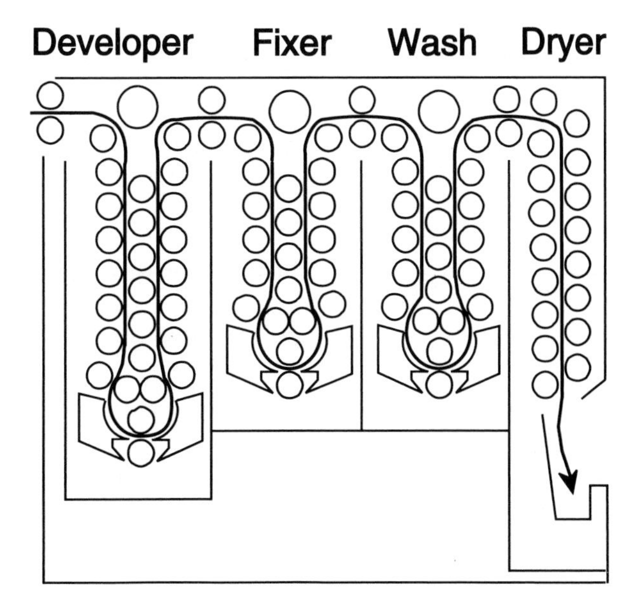

FIGURE 12–2. The inside of an automatic processor.

dark, or the film may have a gray fog over it. The radiographer should be able to recognize these problems, know the most likely reason for the problem, and fix minor difficulties.

SECTIONS OF THE PROCESSOR

The Developer

The first section the film goes through is the developer, which is an alkaline solution. When the film is exposed inside the cassette, the silver bromide crystals in the film emulsion are changed by the light and radiation that hit the film. The changes produce a **latent image** in the film. The latent image is the invisible image in the film after it is exposed to radiation or light and before it is put into the processor. When the film is placed in the processor, the developer chemical reduces the silver bromide crystals that were exposed to light or radiation to metallic silver. This produces a **visible** or **manifest** image on the film.

Developer reduces the exposed silver bromide crystals to metallic silver.

The developer has five agents in it. Each agent has its specific purpose. An agent consists of one or more chemicals and sometimes each chemical has its own purpose. Table 12–2 lists the agents and chemicals used in the developer and the purposes for each.

The temperature of the developer is important for film quality. Developer temperature is usually between 93 and 98°F, depending on the speed of the processor. If the temperature is too high, the film will be overdeveloped, have excess density, and will appear too dark. This excess density is called **fog**, and it reduces radiographic contrast just as the increased density from scattered radiation does. If the developer temperature is too low, the film will be underdeveloped and will appear too light.

Table 12–2. Developer Agents and Chemicals

Agent	Purpose	Chemical	Purpose
Developing, reducing	Reduces the exposed silver bromide to metallic silver	Phenidone	Develops the gray areas; fast acting
		Hydroquinone	Develops the black areas; slow acting
Accelerator, activator, alkali	Swells the emulsion; maintains the alkaline pH level	Sodium carbonate	
Restrainer	Prevents the developer from reducing unexposed silver bromide; controls fog	Potassium bromide	
Preservative	Prolongs the life of the developer	Sodium sulfite	
Hardener	Keeps the emulsion from becoming too soft	Glutaraldehyde	

Table 12–3. Fixer Agents and Chemicals

Agent	Purpose	Chemical
Fixing, clearing	Removes the unexposed and undeveloped silver bromide crystals; clears the film	Ammonium thiosulfate (hypo)
Activator, acid	Stops the action of the developer; maintains the acid pH level	Acetic acid
Preservative	Prolongs the life of the fixer	Sodium sulfite
Hardener	Hardens the emulsion	Potassium alum

There is usually a temperature gauge on the outside of the processor so that the developer temperature can be monitored.

Developer temperature affects density and contrast.

The Fixer

After the developer the film goes into the fixer tank. The fixer is an acid solution. Its purpose is to remove the unexposed and undeveloped silver bromide crystals from the film. This is called clearing the film. The fixer also hardens and preserves the image. A list of the agents and chemicals in the fixer is in Table 12–3.

Fixer removes the unexposed and undeveloped silver bromide crystals.

Since silver bromide is removed in the fixer, used fixer contains silver. This silver can be recovered, so used fixer is ordinarily saved until the silver is removed from it.

The Wash

When the film comes out of the fixer it goes into the wash. This is a tank of constantly recirculating water. The water washes away any chemicals that remain on the film.

The Dryer

The last section of the processor is the dryer. Here, hot air is blown onto both sides of the film to dry it before it comes out of the processor.

PERFORM ACTIVITY 12.D

SYSTEMS OF THE PROCESSOR

The roller transport and replenishment systems of the processor are the ones that are usually involved if something malfunctions in the processor. The roller transport system can cause the film to jam, and a poorly functioning replenishment system can cause variations in film development.

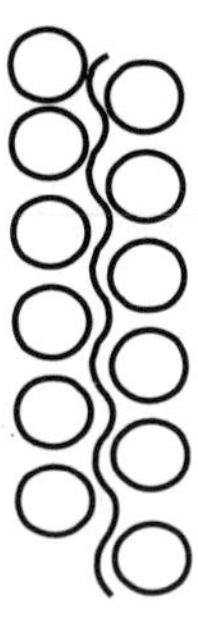

FIGURE 12–3. The rollers in the processor are offset, which makes the film flex and bend as it travels through the processor.

Roller Transport

The roller transport system consists of the rollers, gears, chains, crossovers, and turnarounds that transport the film from the feeding tray through the four sections of the processor and out.

The film travels between two sets of rollers. The rollers are not parallel to each other but are **offset**, causing the film to flex and bend as it is moved along (Fig. 12–3). This **agitates** the film in each chemical, which helps keep the chemicals mixed and ensures even development of the film.

The film travels down in each section, turns around at the bottom, and travels back up. The film must then cross over into the next section. Special devices help the film with these motions (Fig. 12–4). **Turnaround** rollers are at the bottom of each section, and **crossover** rollers are at the top of each section. These rollers have metal guides called **guide shoes**, which help the film make the turns. The guide shoes have ridges in them, and if they are adjusted too tight, the ridges can scratch the film emulsion.

The crossover rollers squeeze off some of the chemical from the previous section before the film goes on to the next section. If the alkaline developer is carried over and mixes with the acid fixer, the acid would gradually be neutralized.

The ends of the rollers are connected to gears that are turned by a chain. If a roller, a gear, or a section of the chain is not working as it should, the processor may jam. A jam means that the films all stop at about the same place inside the processor. A jam is not usually discovered until the processor starts making a knocking noise or somebody realizes that a film has not come out of the processor for a while. By that time several films are usually ruined, especially the films jammed in the developer or fixer tanks where they are not finished developing.

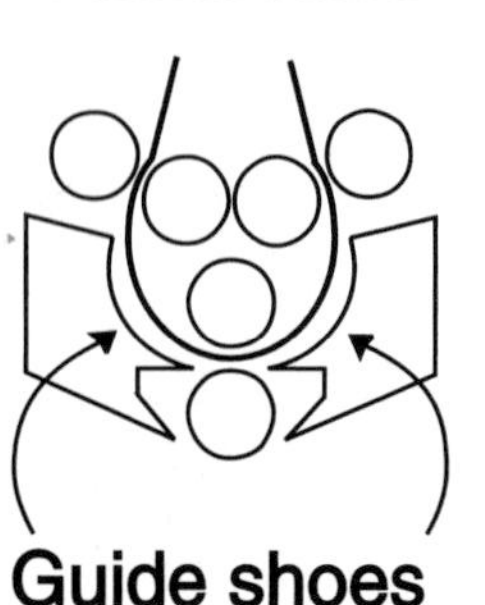

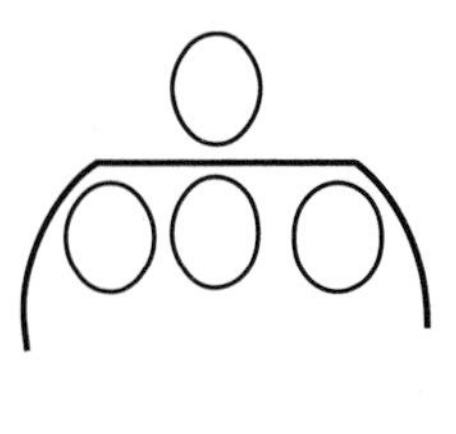

FIGURE 12–4. Turnaround rollers are at the bottom of each section. Crossover rollers are at the top of each section.

To clear a jam, the lid of the processor must be removed. This exposes the films inside of the processor to light. The roller sections in the area of the jam need to be taken out of the processor and all the jammed films removed. When the jam is cleared and the problem fixed, the rollers have to be replaced carefully or the processor chemicals may be contaminated.

Contamination of the chemicals occurs when fixer is accidentally splashed into the developer. It only takes a small amount of fixer in the developer to cause contamination. If the developer becomes contaminated, it cannot be used again until the developer tank has been drained and the chemicals completely replaced. A contaminated developer chemical usually smells like ammonia.

The first two rollers of the transport system are called **entrance** rollers. As the film is passing through these rollers a switch is triggered. This switch turns off the safelight right above the feeding tray so the light won't fog the film. After the film is completely through the first two rollers, a bell rings or a buzzer sounds, telling the person in the darkroom that it is all right to feed another film into the processor. This prevents the films from jamming by being placed too close to each other. The entrance rollers also control the replenishment rate.

The entrance rollers control the film feeding rate and the replenishment rate.

Replenishment

When the film goes through the entrance rollers, the replenishment system is triggered. As the developer and fixer are used to process films, the chemicals gradually lose their strength. The chemicals must be replenished to bring them back to their original strength. So as each film is developed, some of the used developer and fixer are removed from the processor and new developer and fixer are added to the processor.

The developer and fixer replenishment tanks usually sit alongside the processor. Tubes come out of the bottom of each replenishment tank and enter the respective sections of the processor. The replenishment chemicals travel into the processor through these tubes.

PERFORM ACTIVITY 12.E

THE CHARACTERISTIC CURVE

It is important that the processor be monitored with a quality control system to assure that it is working properly. Then the radiographer can depend on the processor to develop films consistently. The characteristic curve is a graph that is used for quality control of the processor. The information from the curve tells the radiographer about a film's speed, contrast, and exposure latitude, and enables monitoring of the function of the automatic processor.

The characteristic curve is also called the *H* and *D* curve, the *D* log *E* curve, and the sensitometric curve. The characteristic curve is a graph showing how a film responds to a series of gradually increasing exposures. It can be produced in three ways.

A characteristic curve could be produced by first exposing a section of a film to a

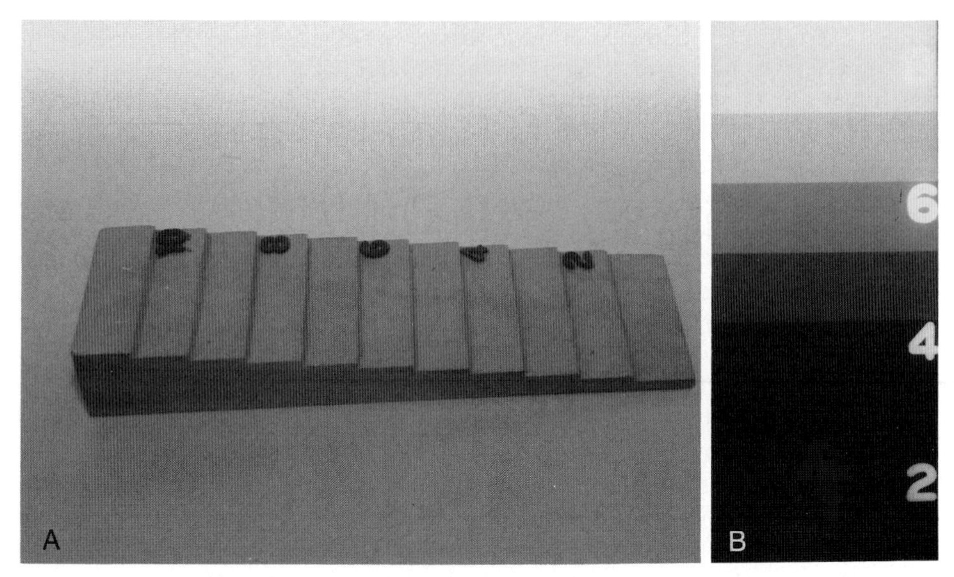

FIGURE 12–5. (*A*) A step wedge. (*B*) A step wedge radiograph.

very light exposure. Then as the exposure is doubled for the next section of the film, the density would also double. This pattern of doubling the exposure factors each time a new section of film is exposed continues until the exposure becomes very heavy and the section of film is very black.

A characteristic curve can also be produced by taking one radiograph of a step wedge, which is also called a **penetrometer**. A step wedge is constructed of solid aluminum or tissue-equivalent plastic shaped into small sections or steps that each have a gradually increasing thickness. A radiograph taken of the step wedge will show a gray scale that looks like blocks of gradually decreasing densities (Fig. 12–5). The thicker steps of the penetrometer will produce less radiographic density and the thinner steps will produce more radiographic density.

On an 11-step penetrometer each different density corresponds to doubling the film density with exposure factors. To produce a characteristic curve, each density step on the radiograph is measured with a densitometer. The reading is then plotted on a graph, and a characteristic curve is produced.

The third way to produce a characteristic curve is with a **sensitometer**. A sensitometer exposes a film with light and produces an image that looks like a step wedge image (Fig. 12–6). This is the best system, since the image is not produced in an x-ray room that can cause some variations in the image from day to day.

The characteristic curve (Fig. 12–7) is plotted with density on the vertical axis and the log of the exposure on the horizontal axis. The **toe** of the characteristic curve is the area of underexposure. This is where the exposure a film receives is too small to record any density on the film. The toe never drops to zero on the curve because the film usually has a blue tint in the base that will measure about .15 on the densitometer. In addition to the tint, the film may have some fog on it, which is also a measurable density. The toe area takes into account the **base-plus-fog** measurement.

The **threshold** is the area where the curve begins to turn upward. This happens when the film begins to record density. The **shoulder** is at the top of the curve and it is the area of overexposure. This is where the film would be black from receiving a high exposure. **D-max** is the maximum density the film can record.

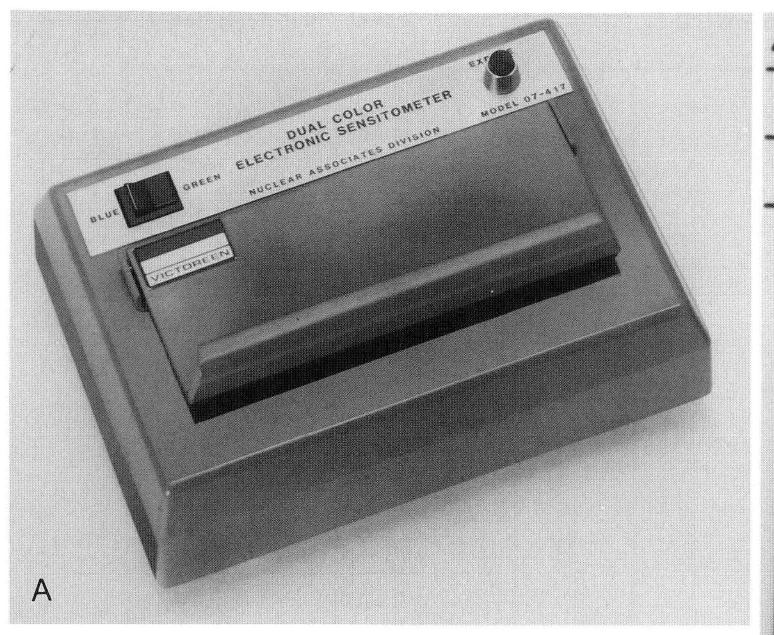

FIGURE 12–6. A radiograph produced with a sensitometer looks like a step wedge radiograph. It is used for processor quality control. (Photo courtesy of Nuclear Associates, 100 Voice Road, Carle Place, NY 11514.)

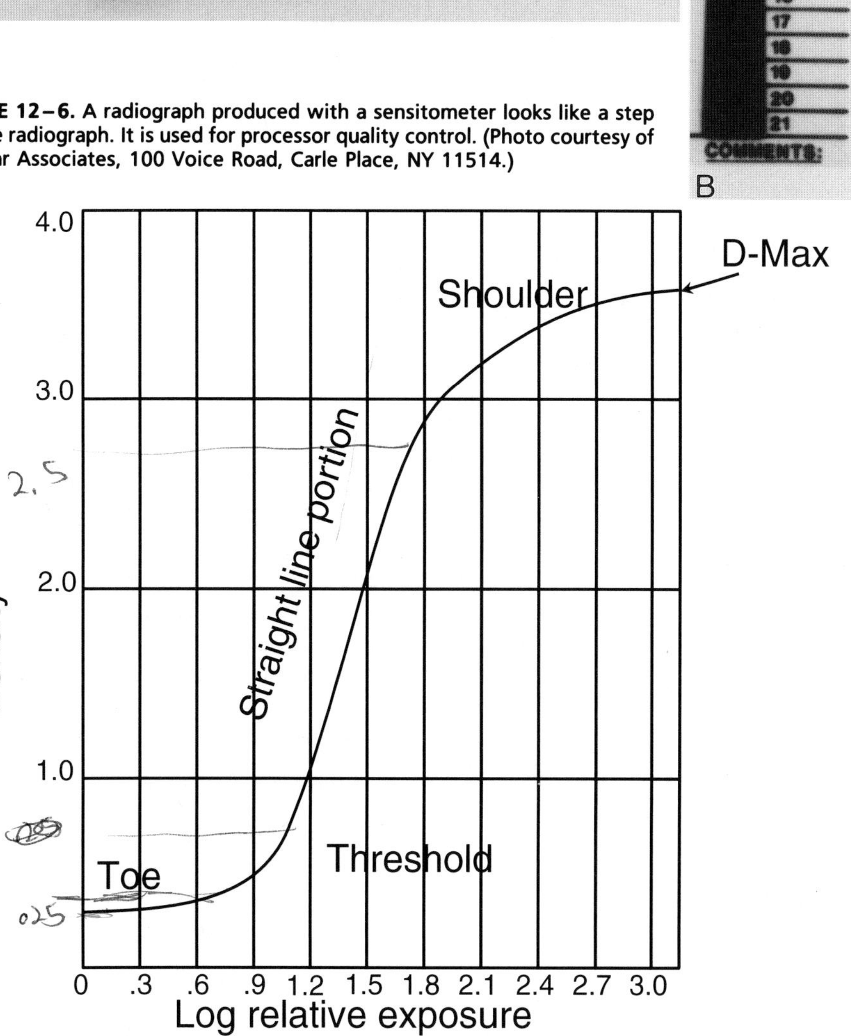

FIGURE 12–7. The characteristic curve.

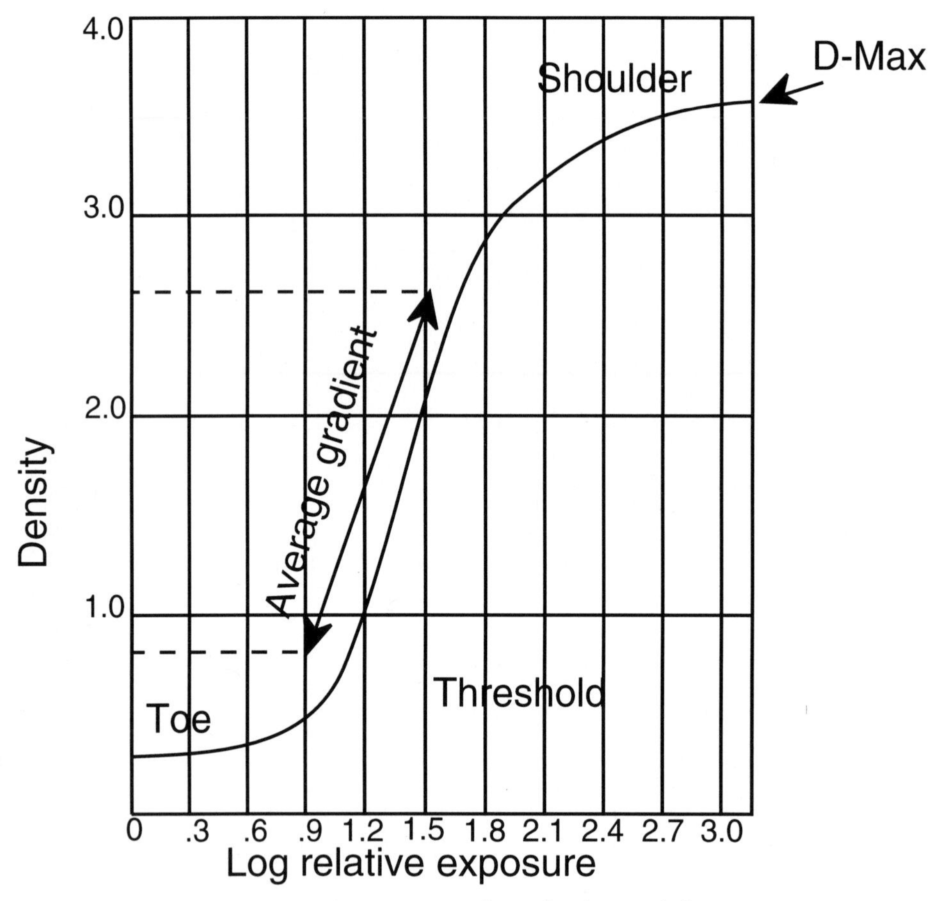

FIGURE 12–8. The average gradient of a characteristic curve.

The area between the threshold and shoulder is called the **straight-line** portion of the curve. It can also be called the **slope** or the **gamma**. A line drawn on the slope representing the densities within the image is called the **average gradient** (Fig. 12–8). In an ordinary radiographic image, this range of densities will measure on a densitometer between .25 and 2.0 above the base-plug-fog measurement. Therefore if the base-plus-fog measures .17, the range of densities for the average gradient for that film will measure between .42 (.25 + .17) and 2.17 (2.0 + .17). Other areas on the radiograph surrounding the image will measure above or below this average gradient range. These areas are not within the image but may be on the edges of the film. The average gradient shows the slope of the curve within the image.

The average gradient shows the slope of the characteristic curve within the image.

The position of the slope on the graph and the steepness of the slope give the radiographer information about a film's **speed, contrast**, and **exposure latitude**.

Film Speed

Film speed or **sensitivity** is a measure of a film's ability to respond to radiation or light. If two different types of film (film A and B) are given the same exposure conditions, and film A records more density than film B, film A has a higher speed because it is more sensitive to the exposure. To make the films equal in density, less radiation exposure is required on film A. The characteristic curve of film A would lie closer to the vertical axis than film B because film A has a higher speed (Fig. 12–9).

The curve of a high speed film lies close to the vertical axis.

The speed of a film is a characteristic of the film that is determined during the manufacture of the film. X-ray departments usually select only one speed of film for routine radiography exams, so that the radiographer does not need to compensate for different film speeds.

Film speed affects **recorded detail**, although it is not a major factor. As film speed increases, recorded detail decreases.

A high speed film decreases recorded detail.

Film is ordinarily used in a cassette with an intensifying screen. Intensifying screens also have a speed so that the speed of the film and the intensifying screen the

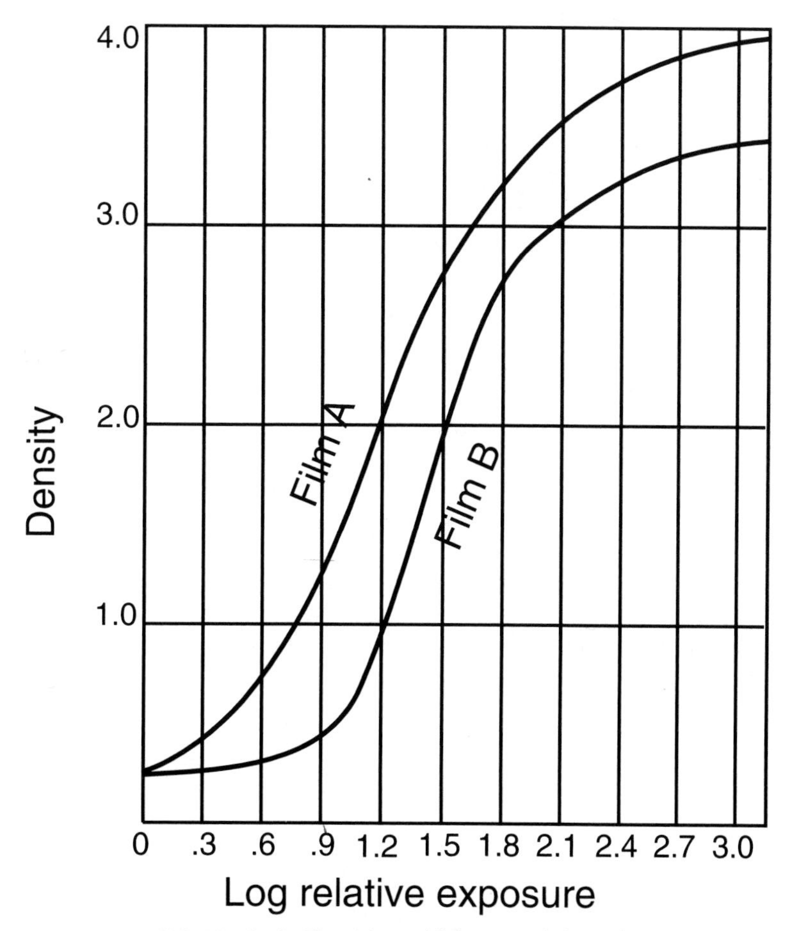

FIGURE 12–9. Film A has a higher speed than Film B.

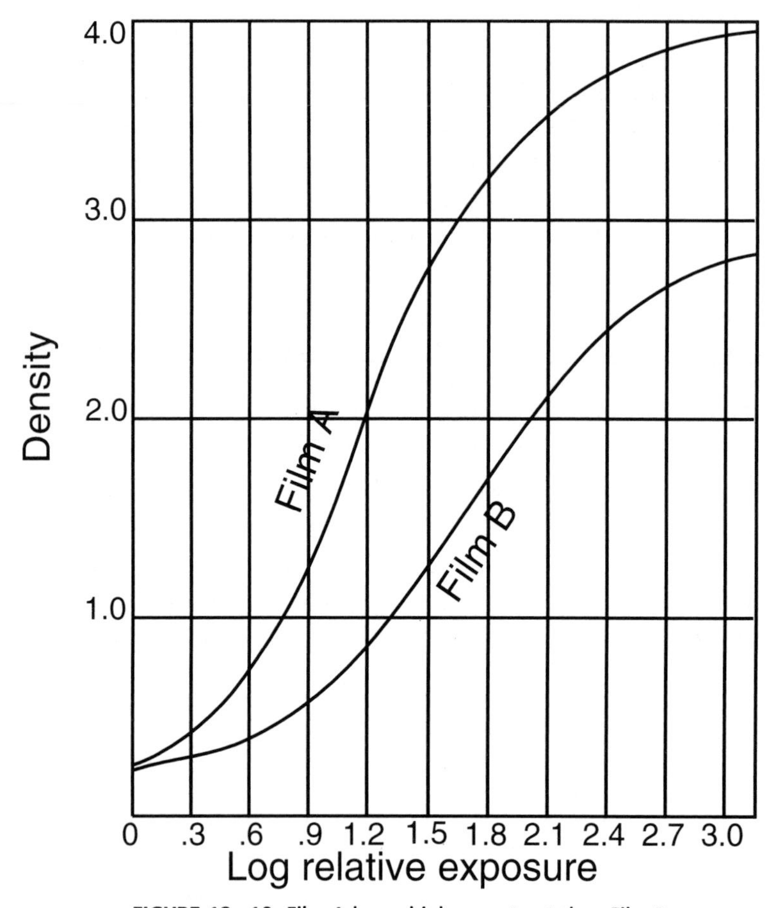

FIGURE 12–10. Film A has a higher contrast than Film B.

film is used with, the film-screen system, is what ultimately determines the amount of recorded detail.

Film Contrast

The steepness of the slope of the characteristic curve shows the amount of contrast a film is capable of displaying. A film with a steep slope will produce high contrast or short scale contrast, which is a mostly black-and-white image. A film with a flat slope will produce low contrast or long scale contrast, which is an image with many gray tones. In Figure 12–10, film A will display a higher contrast than film B.

A film with a steep slope produces high contrast.

Film contrast, like speed, is also determined during the manufacture of the film. Film contrast affects radiographic contrast in addition to the other factors affecting radiographic contrast like kVp and scattered radiation.

Exposure Latitude

Exposure latitude gives the radiographer some room for error. If a fantastic radiograph is produced using the perfect exposure factors, the same radiograph could be made with some variation in the exposure factors and the film would still be acceptable. How far the exposure factors can be varied from perfection is exposure latitude.

Exposure latitude allows room for error.

There is a relationship between film contrast and exposure latitude. A film that would display long scale contrast will also give the radiographer a wide exposure latitude (Fig. 12–11). A film with a wide exposure latitude gives more room for error than a film with a narrow exposure latitude.

PROCESSOR QUALITY CONTROL

The characteristic curve tells about the film's speed and contrast, and this information can be used to monitor processor conditions. If the processor is always working

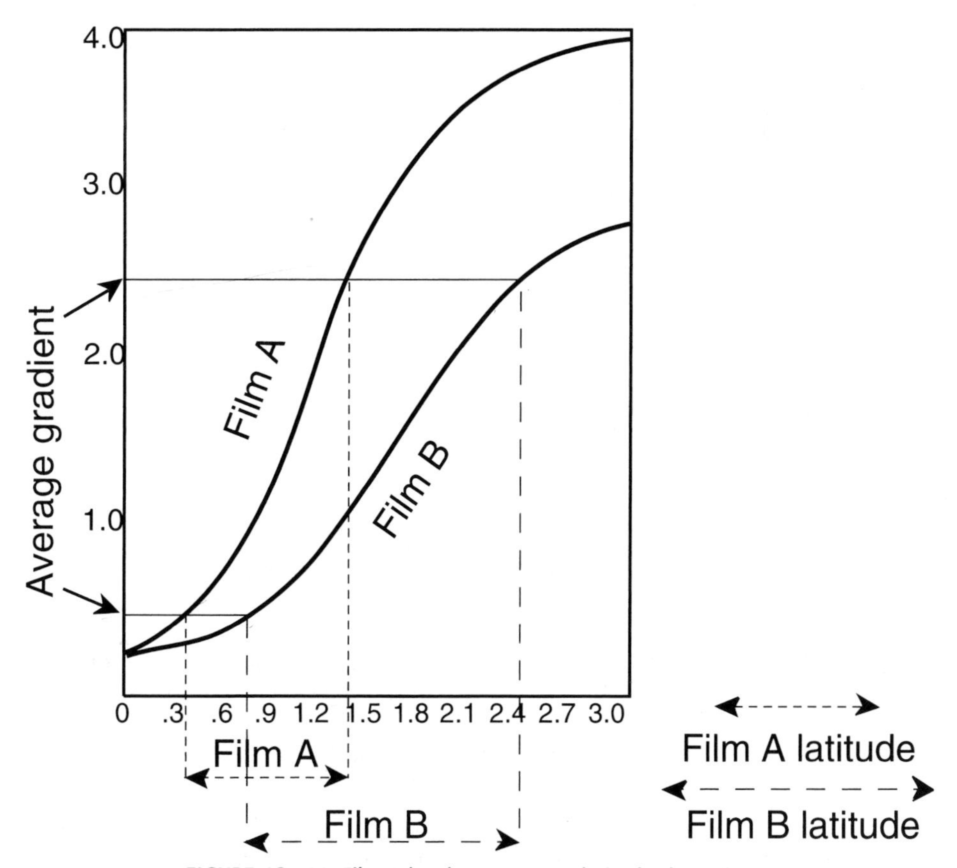

FIGURE 12–11. Film A has less exposure latitude than Film B.

well, the characteristic curve of a film should show about the same speed and contrast from day to day. So if the film speed and contrast are checked every day, a large variation indicates that something is wrong with the processor.

A quality control system usually uses a film produced with a sensitometer (see Fig. 12–6). Measurements are made with a densitometer on the sensitometry radiograph and the readings indicate the film's speed and contrast.

A medium density area is measured and this reading is called **speed**. A high density area is also measured. Then the speed or medium density reading is subtracted from the high density reading. This value is called **contrast**. Remember that contrast is the difference between adjacent densities, so by subtracting one density reading from another, the answer measures contrast or the difference between two densities.

A blank area of the film is also measured and this value is called **base-plus-fog**. This measures the density resulting from the tint in the base, plus any fog that might be on the film. The three values—speed, contrast, and base-plus-fog—are plotted on a chart, which is analyzed for proper processor function (Fig. 12–12).

Table 12–4 shows some possible reasons for variations in the speed, contrast, or base-plus-fog readings.

PERFORM ACTIVITY 12.F

SUMMARY

Radiographic film consists of a polyester base and an emulsion of silver bromide crystals suspended in gelatin. Some types of film in use are double and single emulsion, screen and non-screen, periapical, occlusal, 105-mm, cinefluorography, mammography, duplicating, subtraction, laser, video, and electronic imaging.

In the automatic processor the film goes through the developer, which changes the exposed silver bromide to metallic silver; then through the fixer, which removes

Table 12–4. Reasons for Speed, Contrast, and Base-Plus-Fog Variations From Normal

Increased speed	Developer temperature too high
	Overreplenishment
	Densitometer not set to zero
	Film fog
	Safelight fog
Decreased speed	Developer temperature too low
	Underreplenishment
Contrast variations	Developer temperature too high
	Developer temperature too low
	Film fog
	Safelight fog
	Contamination of chemicals
	Overreplenishment
	Underreplenishment
Base-plus-fog variations	Developer temperature too high
	Developer temperature too low
	Underreplenishment
	Film fog
	Safelight fog
	Contamination of chemicals

Processing Control Chart

Location: ______ Processor No. M6 AW

Month: July Prepared by ______

Replenishment Rate	Developer	
	Fixer	

Date: 1 2 | 5 6 7 8 9 | 12 13 14 15 16 | 19 20 21 22 23 | 26 27 28 29 30

Day: M T W T F | M T W T F | M T W T F | M T W T F | M T W T F

Processor Tank: Fresh Developer; Fresh Fixer

Replenisher Tank: Fresh Developer; Fresh Fixer

Base + Fog: 0.3; 0.2; .17; 0.1; 0.0

Speed Index: Upper Limit +0.15; Standard 1.3; Lower Limit -0.15

Contrast Index: Upper Limit +0.15; Standard .75; Lower Limit -0.15

Agfa Division of Miles, Inc.

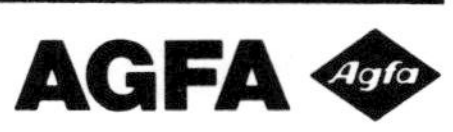

FIGURE 12–12. A quality control chart. (Courtesy of AGFA Division, Miles Inc.)

the unexposed silver bromide from the film; then through the wash, which removes any chemicals left on the film; and finally through the dryer, which dries the film.

The roller transport system moves the film through the processor with a series of rollers. Malfunctions of this system can cause the films to jam.

The developer and fixer get replenished as each film is developed. This keeps the chemicals at their correct strength. The temperature of the developer must be monitored because changes can affect density and contrast.

The characteristic curve of a film tells the radiographer about a film's speed, contrast, and exposure latitude. Variations in speed, contrast, and base-plus-fog are monitored as part of a quality control system because a variation can indicate a malfunction of the processor.

Film speed affects recorded detail, but it is not a major factor. An increase in film speed or sensitivity will cause a decrease in recorded detail.

PERFORM ACTIVITY 12.G

CHAPTER 13

INTENSIFYING SCREENS

CHAPTER OUTLINE

OBJECTIVES

At the end of this chapter you should be able to:

- List the two parts of an intensifying screen.
- Describe the construction of the base and active layer.
- Describe the action of a phosphor and correlate the amount of radiation hitting the phosphor with the intensity of its action.
- Define fluorescence and phosphorescence.
- Describe the phenomenon of light diffusion.
- Explain how light diffusion reduces recorded detail.
- Relate screen speed to the amount of density produced on a radiograph.
- Explain how fast screens reduce recorded detail.
- Describe the problem of poor screen contact and explain how it reduces recorded detail.
- Perform a wire mesh test for poor screen contact.
- List the phosphors used and color of light emitted for the calcium tungstate and rare earth intensifying screen systems.
- Define the term conversion efficiency and explain how it relates to recorded detail.
- Given a relative screen speed, calculate the multiplication factor for the screen.
- Calculate the new mAs required to maintain film density when the intensifying screen speed changes.
- Describe the difference between a direct exposure and an exposure made with an intensifying screen.
- Briefly explain how a computed radiography image is produced.
- Relate the computed radiography terms of brightness, gray scale, and resolution to density, contrast, and recorded detail.
- Explain how a computed radiography image can be manipulated to alter brightness, gray scale, and resolution.

The subject of the last chapter in this section dealing with recorded detail is intensifying screens. Film and intensifying screens are the material factors affecting recorded detail. Source-image distance, object-image distance, and the focal spot are the geometric factors that affect recorded detail.

There are two types of intensifying screen systems and a variety of speeds to choose from in each system. Density, recorded detail, and the exposure to the patient change with each choice.

Intensifying screen construction will be discussed first. Phosphors that are in the intensifying screens give off light when x-ray photons hit them. Light diffusion is a problem with intensifying screens and causes a loss of recorded detail. Poor screen contact can also be a problem.

Relative speed value is a way to equate the speed of different intensifying screens. When a radiographer changes to a different intensifying screen speed, a new mAs must be calculated because each relative speed value produces a different density.

Radiographs can also be produced without intensifying screens. This system, called direct exposure, requires a very large exposure to the patient, so many x-ray facilities only use intensifying screens.

Computed radiography is a new system of producing radiographic images in which a computer forms the image. The image will appear on a TV screen (cathode-ray tube), and while it is on this screen density, contrast, and recorded detail can be changed to enhance the image. In some systems the image from the cathode-ray tube is then transferred to a film. In other systems, the image is only on the screen, and the film is eliminated.

INTENSIFYING SCREEN CONSTRUCTION

Intensifying screens are composed of two parts, a base and an active layer. The screens are mounted inside a cassette, usually in pairs with one in the front and one in the back of the cassette. The x-ray film is placed inside the cassette between the two screens.

The Base

The base of an intensifying screen is made of a piece of cardboard or plastic. It needs to be flexible, rugged, moisture resistant, and chemically inert. The base has a **white reflecting surface** that directs the light given off by the intensifying screens back to the film.

The Active Layer

The active layer consists of microscopic crystals of a **phosphor** suspended in a matrix. The active layer is spread on the base. The active layer of the screens is then coated with a protective coating to keep the active layer from being scratched. The basic construction of an intensifying screen is similar to the construction of a film that has a base, an emulsion coating, and a protective layer. Figure 13–1 shows the layers of an intensifying screen.

Active layer
Reflecting layer
Base

FIGURE 13–1. The layers of an intensifying screen.

PHOSPHOR ACTION

Luminescence is the ability of a material to emit light. A **phosphor** is a material that emits light when it is struck by x-ray photons.

A phosphor gives off light when struck by x-ray photons.

The amount of light emitted by the phosphor after it is hit by x-ray photons corresponds to how much radiation got through the patient's body and into the phosphor. In places where a lot of radiation got through the patient's body, the light from the phosphors will be very bright. In areas where not much radiation got through the patient, such as areas under bone, the light from the phosphors will not be very bright.

When an x-ray exposure is made, the pattern of light emitted by the intensifying screen phosphors contains the image of the patient's body in the form of a light and dark pattern on the intensifying screen. This pattern is then transferred to the film.

When the film is hit with a bright light from the intensifying screen, that area of the film will be developed as black. In areas that are exposed by only a little light, the film will develop a light gray tone or maybe even white.

When the film is placed into a cassette and the cassette is closed, the intensifying screens and the film are in very close contact with each other. There is usually a compression pad in the front and back of the cassette so that the film and screens remain in good contact with each other.

The light emitted by the phosphors is given off isotropically, which means in all directions, like a sphere of light (Fig. 13–2). The phosphors are supposed to begin the emission of light promptly when hit by x-ray photons and stop emitting light promptly when the photons stop hitting them. This property is called **fluorescence**. Fluorescence is defined as the ability of a material to give off light when struck by x-rays.

Fluorescence is the ability of a material to give off light when struck by x-rays.

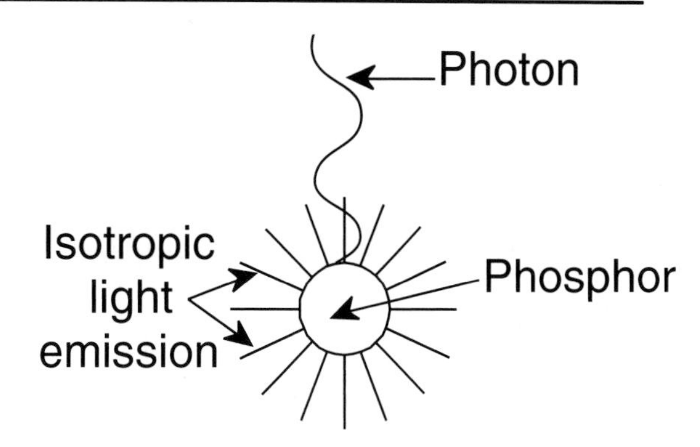

FIGURE 13–2. Isotropic light emission of a phosphor after being struck by x-ray photons.

In older intensifying screens a problem called **phosphorescence** can occur. Phosphorescence causes the phosphors to continue to emit light after the x-ray photons have stopped hitting them. This can cause an increased density on the film because the film is exposed to the light for too long. Phosphorescence is also called **afterglow** or **screen lag**.

Phosphorescence is continued light emission after the x-rays have been turned off.

Light Diffusion

Light diffusion is the phenomenon that causes a lack of recorded detail on a radiograph produced with intensifying screens. Even though the phosphors in the active layer of a screen are in good contact with the film when the cassette is closed, there is still a minute space between the phosphor and film. Since the light from the phosphor is emitted isotropically, by the time the light travels to the film it has spread out a little bit (Fig. 13–3). This spreading of light is called **light diffusion**.

The light from the intensifying screen is what exposes the film and produces the image on the film. Since it has spread out at the film surface, the image produced loses some of its distinctness. The image shows less recorded detail because of light diffusion. Every film taken with an intensifying screen has this problem. The problem becomes more acute when the intensifying screen speed is increased.

Light diffusion reduces recorded detail.

Screen Speed

Intensifying screen speed is the ability of a screen to respond to radiation. Increasing the speed of an intensifying screen enables the screen to respond more intensely and give off more light with the same amount of radiation. If a screen gives off more light, the radiograph displays more density. Suppose identical exposures are made on film A and film B. Film A is produced with a slow screen and film B is produced with a faster screen. Film B would display more density. If film A is a good film, the exposure for film B should be reduced because the screen is faster (Fig. 13–4).

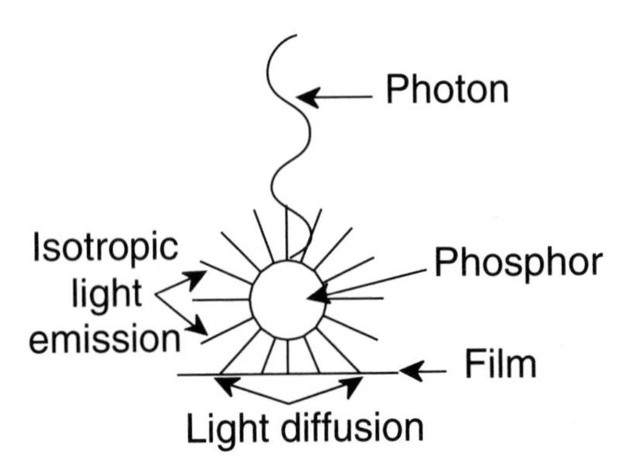

FIGURE 13–3. Light diffusion is caused by the slight distance between the phosphor and film inside the cassette. Light diffusion decreases recorded detail.

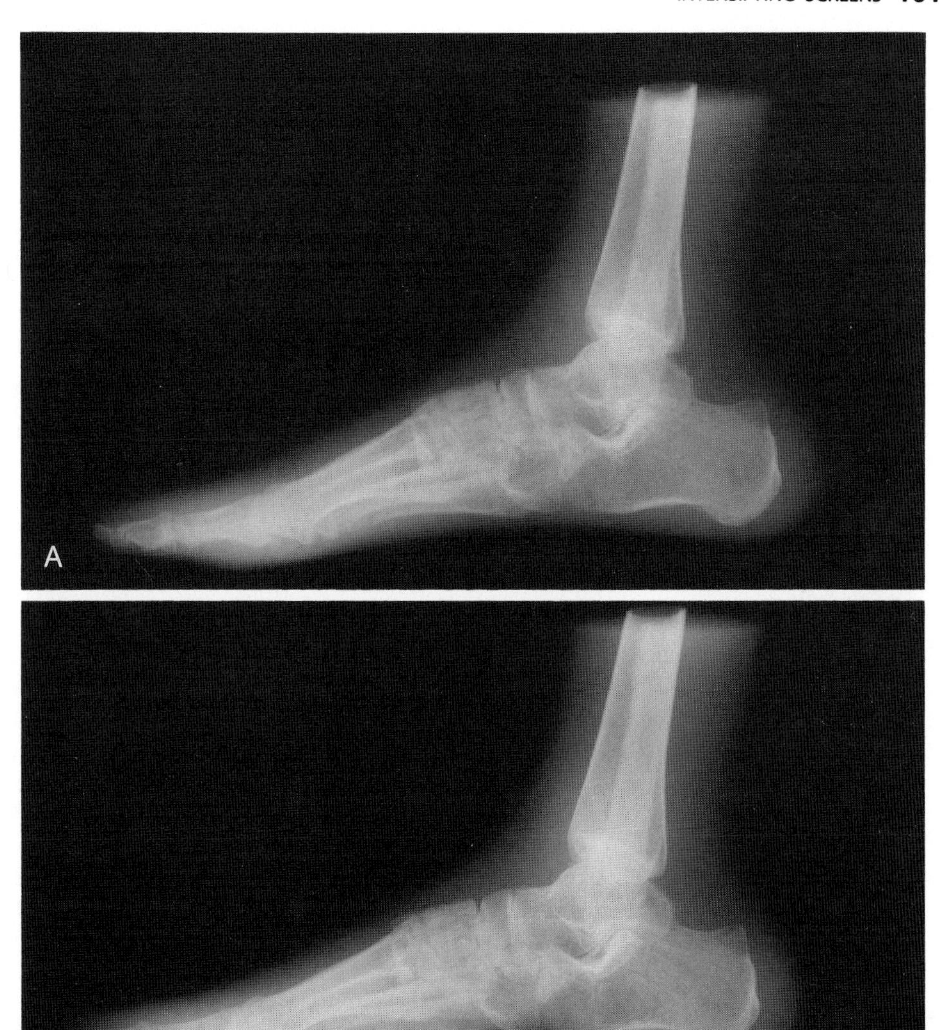

FIGURE 13–4. (*A*) Radiograph taken on a slow speed screen using 6 mAs and 60 kVp. (*B*) Radiograph taken on a fast screen with an adjustment of the mAs to 1.25 to produce an adequate density.

Fast screens emit more light than slower screens.

Screen speed is a major factor in reducing the radiation dose to the patient. By changing to a faster screen that requires less radiation to produce the image, the radiographer can cut the patient's radiation dose. That's the good news! The bad news is that there are two methods used to make a screen faster and both methods produce an increase in light diffusion and therefore a decrease in recorded detail.

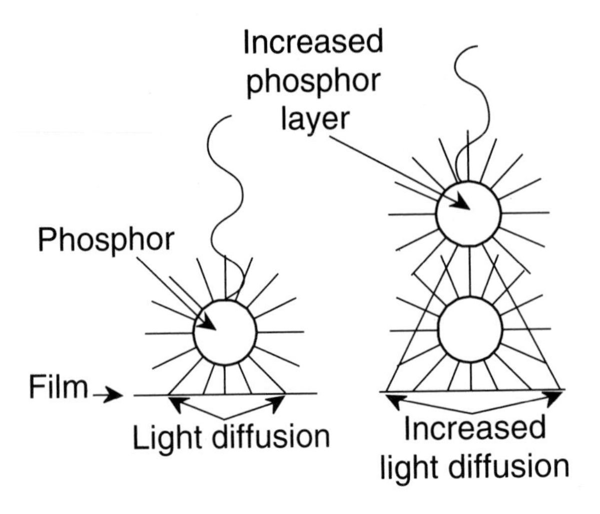

FIGURE 13–5. Increased light diffusion caused by increasing the phosphor layers. This increases the intensifying screen speed but reduces recorded detail.

Fast screens produce less recorded detail than slower screens.

One way to increase screen speed is to put more layers of phosphor in the active layer of the screen. This causes the screen to give off more light, but it moves some of the phosphors farther away from the film. The light from these phosphors will spread out more by the time the light reaches the film because the phosphor is placed farther away from the film (Fig. 13–5). This increases light diffusion and reduces recorded detail.

Another way to increase screen speed is to increase the size of the phosphor crystals. This method also increases light diffusion because the light from a large crystal has to travel farther to reach the film than the light from a smaller crystal (Fig. 13–6).

Poor Screen Contact

It is important for the film and screen to be in good contact with each other when the cassette is closed. If there is an area that is not in good contact, there will be an increased distance between the phosphors and the film. This increases the light diffusion of those phosphors and produces less recorded detail in the area of poor contact (Fig. 13–7).

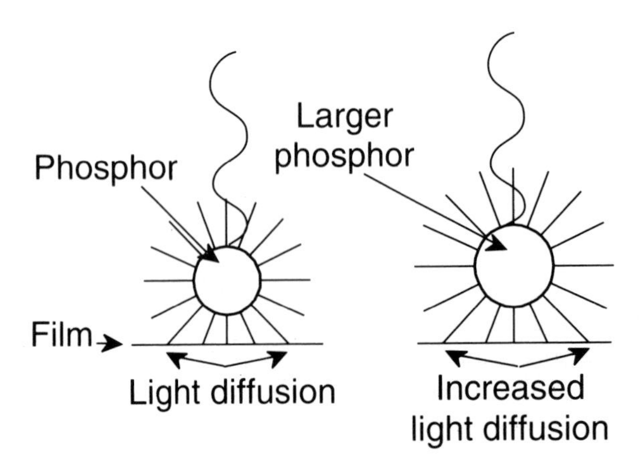

FIGURE 13–6. Increased light diffusion caused by using larger phosphor crystals. This increases the intensifying screen speed but reduces recorded detail.

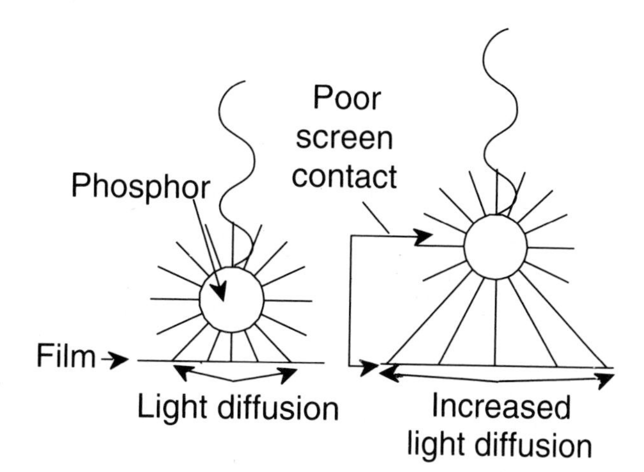

FIGURE 13–7. Increased light diffusion caused by poor screen contact, which reduces recorded detail.

Poor screen contact reduces recorded detail.

Poor screen contact is caused by dropping cassettes and by bending them. This can warp the screens. Poor screen contact is produced more often on larger cassettes.

A test can be performed on a cassette to see if it has poor screen contact. The device used is a wire mesh, which looks like a window screen. The wire mesh is encased in plastic. The cassette that is suspected to have poor screen contact is placed on the x-ray tabletop, and the wire mesh is placed directly on top of it. An exposure is made of the wire mesh using about the same technique used for a radiograph of a foot. It is easier to see poor recorded detail of the wires than it is to see poor recorded detail on an image of the body.

After the film is developed, the recorded detail of the wires is analyzed. An area of poor recorded detail caused by poor screen contact will produce a blurry image around the edges of the wires. Figure 13–8 shows a radiograph with an area of poor screen contact and the wire mesh test performed on that cassette.

PERFORM ACTIVITY 13.A

INTENSIFYING SCREEN SYSTEMS

There are two different intensifying screen systems in use today, calcium tungstate and rare earth. There are several speeds to choose from in each system, and the recorded detail and exposure to the patient changes with the use of the different systems and speeds.

Calcium Tungstate Intensifying Screens

Calcium tungstate intensifying screens were used exclusively until the 1970s when rare earth screens were developed. The phosphor used in this system is **calcium tungstate**. This type of phosphor emits a **blue-violet** light when struck by x-ray photons.

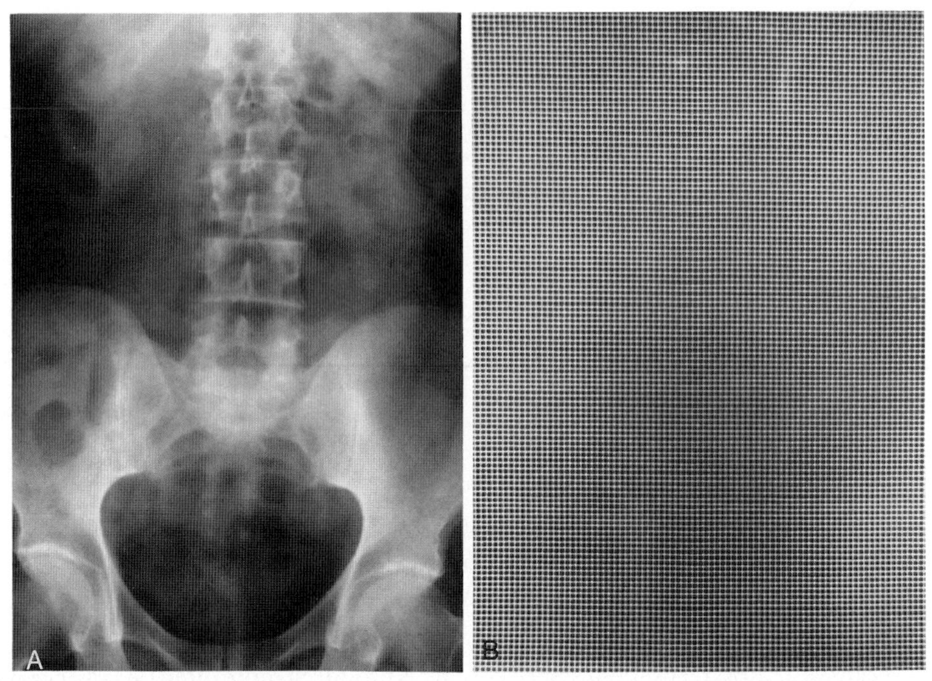

FIGURE 13–8. (*A*) Radiograph has probable poor screen contact in the lower center of the screen. (*B*) The wire mesh test performed on the cassette demonstrates the area of poor screen contact.

Rare Earth Intensifying Screens

The phosphors used for rare earth intensifying screens are the rare earth elements of **gadolinium, lanthanum,** or **yttrium**. These phosphors usually emit a **yellow-green** light.

PERFORM ACTIVITY 13.B

The rare earth system is generally faster than the calcium tungstate system. Rare earth screens are able to produce about the same recorded detail as high speed calcium tungstate screens but with a reduced radiation dose to the patient. They can do this because rare earth phosphors have better **conversion efficiency**.

Rare earth phosphors have better conversion efficiency.

Conversion efficiency is the ability to convert x-ray energy to light. With the same amount of x-ray energy rare earth phosphors emit more light than calcium tungstate phosphors. This causes rare earth screens to have an increased speed. The increased speed of rare earth screens is achieved without sacrificing recorded detail. The rare earth system produces increased light without layering more phosphors or increasing the phosphor size, which increases light diffusion and reduces recorded detail.

The film used with either intensifying screen system must be sensitive to the color of light emitted by the screen. The safelights in the darkroom must also be matched to the calcium tungstate or rare earth screens so that they will subtract out the color of light given off by the screens. This is called **spectral matching**.

TECHNIQUE COMPENSATION

If the same exposure conditions were used on the same radiograph with all the different intensifying screen speeds, each speed would produce a different density on the radiograph. The slow speed screens would produce less density than the higher speed screens. So when the radiographer has to change from one screen speed to another, the exposure factors must be changed or the film will be too dark or too light.

Relative Speed Value

Three descriptive names were traditionally used for the different screen speeds: **slow**, which is also called **detail**; **medium** or **par**; and **fast** or **high** speed. This got confusing when two intensifying screen systems were developed. Since there are now several speeds in each system and a variety of manufacturers, the relative speed value was developed as a way of equating the speed of the different screens.

When the relative speed value (RSV) was established, a value of 100 was chosen for the medium or par speed screen. Every other speed value was then made relative to 100. Slow speed screens have a relative speed value of less than 100 and high speed screens have a relative speed value of more than 100. Rare earth screens usually have relative speed values between 200 and 1200.

Multiplication Factors

In order to calculate the new mAs to be used when changing screen speeds, each screen speed needs a multiplication factor. This multiplication factor is then used in the "to/from" system to calculate the new mAs. The multiplication factor is calculated by forming a fraction with 100 in the numerator and the relative speed value of the other screen in the denominator. Then divide the numerator by the denominator and the decimal produced is the multiplication factor.

A slow speed screen with a relative speed value of 50 would have a multiplication factor of 2, while a high speed screen of 200 would have a multiplication factor of .5, and a rare earth screen at a 400 relative speed value would have a multiplication factor of .25.

$$\frac{100}{50} = 2 \quad \frac{100}{200} = .5 \quad \frac{100}{400} = .25$$

With this system a multiplication factor can be figured for any screen speed. Table 13–1 lists the multiplication factors for some common screen speeds.

Calculating the New mAs

When calculating the new mAs to be used to maintain film density when changing screen speeds, form a fraction with the multiplication factors by placing the multiplication factor of the screen speed being changed *to* in the numerator and the multiplication factor of the screen speed being changed *from* in the denominator. Multiply

Table 13–1. Multiplication Factors for Common Intensifying Screen Speeds

Screen Speed	Multiplication Factor
50	2
100	1
200	.5
300	.33
400	.25
500	.2
600	.17
700	.14
800	.125

the mAs used before the change (the old mAs) by this fraction and the answer is the new mAs to be used because of the change in screen speeds.

Example 1

An exposure of 10 mAs and 80 kVp is used on a slow speed screen (RSV = 50). A change is made to a high speed screen (RSV = 200). What new mAs should be used because of the change?

To: High speed (RSV = 200) multiplication factor = .5
From: Slow speed (RSV = 50) multiplication factor = 2

$$10 \text{ mAs} \times \frac{.5}{2} = 2.5 \text{ mAs (the new mAs)}$$

Example 2

An exposure of 15 mAs and 70 kVp is used on a medium speed screen (RSV = 100). A change is made to a rare earth screen (RSV = 400). What new mAs should be used because of the change?

To: Rare earth (RSV = 400) multiplication factor = .25
From: Par speed (RSV = 100) multiplication factor = 1

$$15 \text{ mAs} \times \frac{.25}{1} = 3.75 \text{ mAs (the new mAs)}$$

Another way to calculate the new mAs required when changing RSV is to place the RSV of the intensifying screen being changed *from* in the *numerator* of a fraction and the RSV of the intensifying screen being changed *to* in the *denominator*. Then the from/to fraction is multiplied by the old mAs and the answer is the new mAs to be used because of the change in intensifying screen speed.

These examples use the same factors as above and the identical answer is produced.

Example 1

From: Slow speed (RSV = 50)
To: High speed (RSV = 200)

$$10 \text{ mAs} \times \frac{50}{200} = 2.5 \text{ mAs} \quad \text{(the new mAs)}$$

Example 2

From: Par speed (RSV = 100)
To: Rare earth (RSV = 400)

$$15 \text{ mAs} \times \frac{100}{400} = 3.75 \text{ mAs} \quad \text{(the new mAs)}$$

This second method eliminates the calculation of the multiplication factor. However, the second method requires the radiographer to remember that this is the only from/to calculation. By using the first method requiring calculation of the multiplication factor, all the calculations of the new mAs required when exposure conditions change are to/from calculations. So it may be easier to calculate the multiplication factor first and then insert the multiplication factor in a to/from fraction rather than eliminating the calculation of the multiplication factor and then having to remember that this is the only from/to calculation.

PERFORM ACTIVITY 13.C

PERFORM ACTIVITY 13.D

OTHER IMAGING SYSTEMS

Direct Exposure

Direct exposure refers to producing radiographs without intensifying screens. This is an old system that was used only on small body parts. It has been almost eliminated except for a few special applications because of the large exposure required to produce the image. In this system, the film is placed in a cardboard or plastic holder. It cannot be used with a Bucky device. When the exposure is made, 100% of the density recorded on the film is produced with radiation. With intensifying screens about 95% of the density is due to exposing the film with light. So the exposure required with direct exposure is a lot more than with intensifying screens. For example, a direct exposure of a foot requires about 300 mAs and 60 kVp, while the same radiograph produced with intensifying screens would only require about 5 mAs and 60 kVp.

The big advantage of direct exposure is the better recorded detail produced. Whenever more radiation and less light is used to expose a film, the recorded detail improves. Light diffusion is what causes the loss of recorded detail when using an intensifying screen. Direct exposure uses no light so there is no light diffusion problem.

Radiographic contrast is also different between radiographs produced with direct exposure and intensifying screens. Direct exposure produces an image with long scale contrast, which has many gray tones. A radiograph made with an intensifying screen produces an image with short scale contrast, which is a mostly black-and-white image. Figure 13–9 shows radiographs taken with direct exposure and an intensifying screen.

Computed Radiography

Computed radiography, sometimes called digital radiography, is a newer system of producing a radiographic image. All the principles of radiographic exposure are still

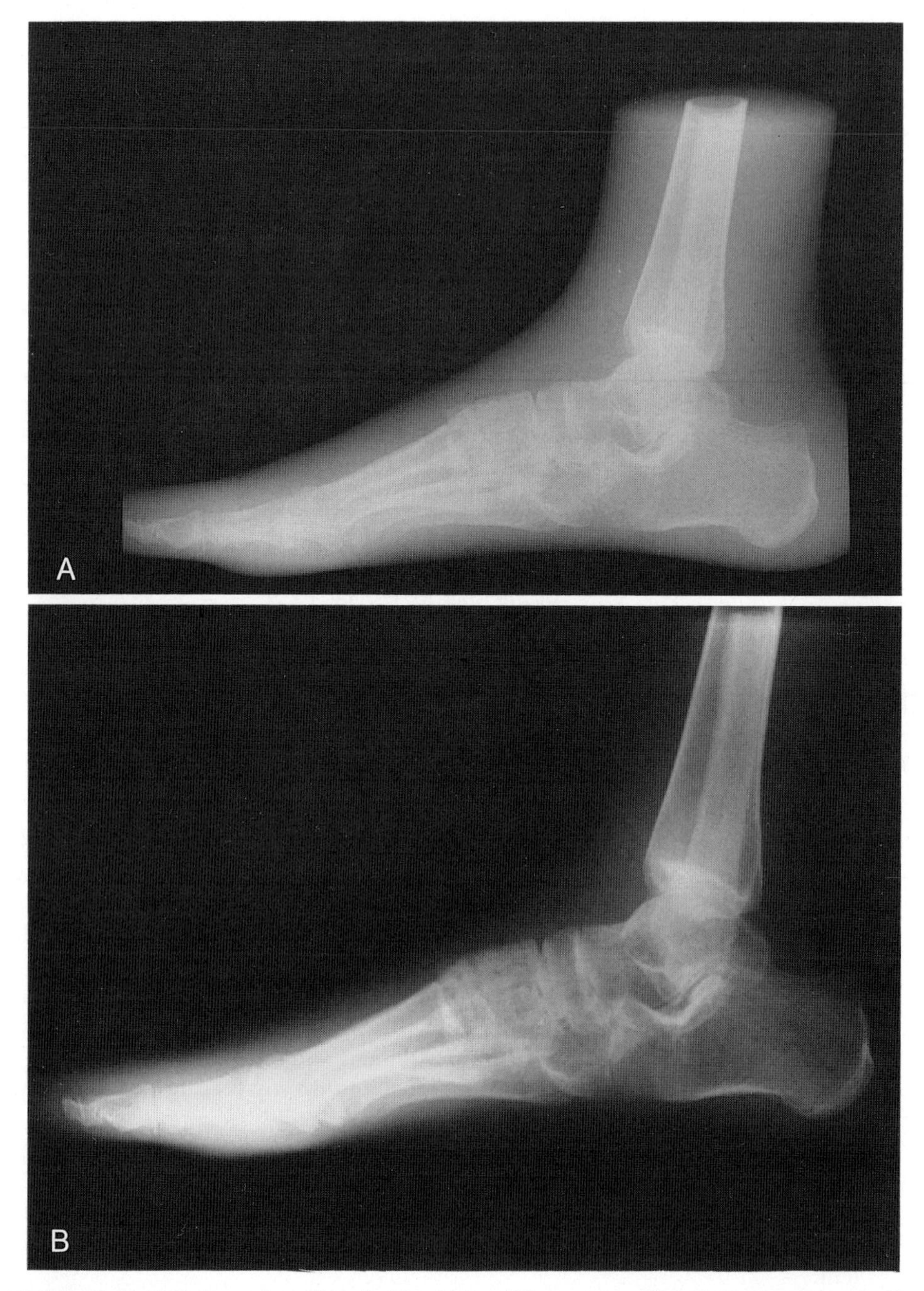

FIGURE 13–9. (*A*) Radiograph produced without intensifying screens. (*B*) Radiograph produced with intensifying screens.

used with this system, but this is not a film and screen system, and in some computed radiography systems film is eliminated. Computed radiography uses an imaging plate in the place of a cassette. The patient, imaging plate, and x-ray tube are positioned in the same manner as if a cassette were being used, and an ordinary x-ray exposure is made.

The imaging plate is then scanned by a computer and the image appears on a screen that looks like a TV screen. The screen is a cathode-ray tube (CRT). When the radiographic image is on the CRT, the image can be changed to enhance its appearance without taking the exposure over and radiating the patient again (Fig. 13–10).

Some systems eliminate the use of the imaging plate and send the image data produced during the exposure directly to the computer. The image will then appear on a CRT. The image from the CRT can be recorded on a film with either system.

The density, contrast, and recorded detail of the image can all be changed while the image is on the CRT. One problem with learning about computed radiography is that the terminology is different. Density is called brightness, contrast is called gray scale, and recorded detail is called resolution. The terminology is changed because the image is produced in a different manner. In order to understand the new terms, it is helpful to understand how a computer forms a radiology image on a CRT.

Density = brightness
Contrast = gray scale
Recorded detail = resolution

A computer cannot analyze an entire image the way the human brain can, so the first thing a computer must do when forming a radiography image is to break the

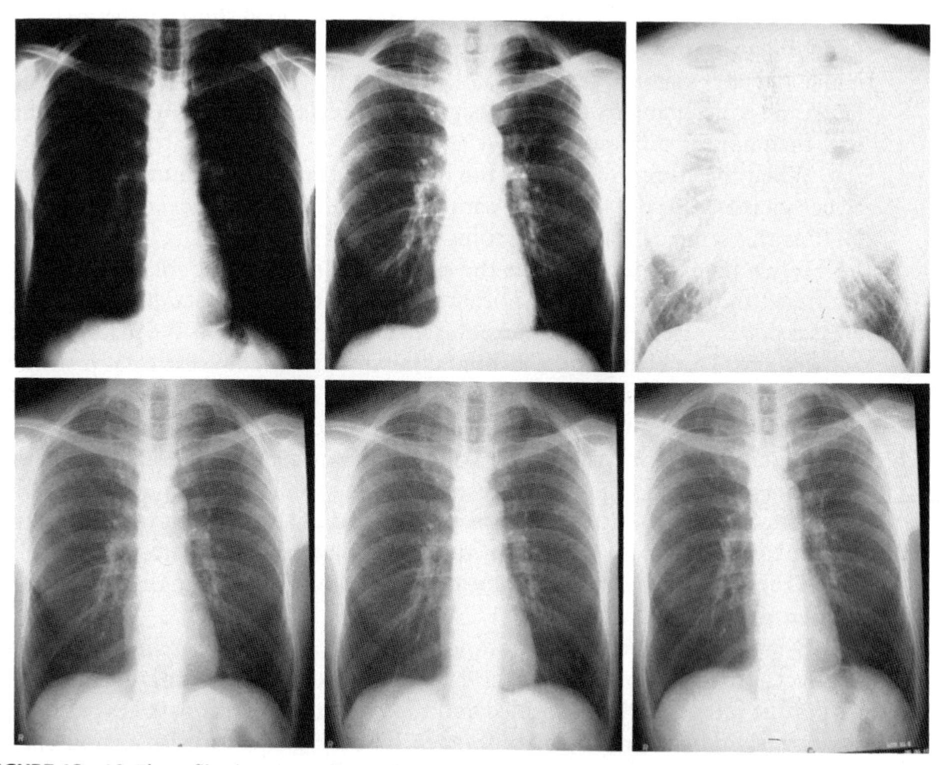

FIGURE 13–10. Three film/screen radiographs that vary in quality. Below each radiograph is the image after it was enhanced using computed radiography. (Courtesy of Fuji Medical Systems.)

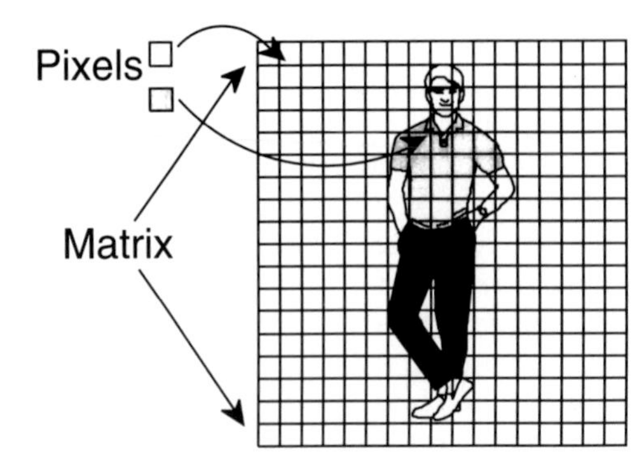

FIGURE 13–11. A computer matrix superimposed over an image.

image down into very small pieces. The way the computer breaks down the image is to superimpose a **matrix** over the image information it receives. Each small part of the matrix is called a **pixel** (Fig. 13–11).

The computer then assigns a number to each pixel, because computers can quickly perform functions with numbers. The number assigned to the pixel corresponds to the amount of radiation that got through the patient's body when the exposure was made. Each pixel is then made into a shade of gray by the computer. The darkness of this shade of gray is determined by the number the computer assigned to the pixel.

Once this process is finished, the computer displays the gray shades in the form of an image on the CRT. The radiographer only needs to turn a dial to adjust or enhance the appearance of the image. When the image is being enhanced or manipulated, the computer very quickly assigns the pixels a different number and the image will then appear different.

When the computer adjusts the image **brightness**, the number for all pixels is either increased or decreased the same amount. The brightness of the image on the CRT is the same as the radiographic quality of **density**.

When the computer adjusts the **gray scale**, the number for one pixel might be increased and the number for another pixel might be decreased. As the computer increases or decreases pixel numbers, the shade of gray it makes the pixels in the image will change. This changes the radiographic quality of **contrast** by adjusting the degree of difference between the various densities in the image. Short scale contrast produces an image that is mostly black and white and the computer will only use a few gray shades to form the image. Long scale contrast produces an image with many gray tones, so the computer will use more gray shades to form this type of image.

When the computer adjusts the **resolution** of the image it forms a matrix with more pixels to increase the resolution of an image and one with fewer pixels to decrease the resolution. Image resolution is the same as the radiographic quality of **recorded detail**.

One additional feature of computed radiography is the ability of the computer to select a small part of the image and enhance just that part of the image. The smaller part of the image can be magnified and this sometimes demonstrates pathology that can be missed on a film and screen image. The computer can also change the brightness and contrast of this smaller part of the image.

SUMMARY

Intensifying screens are composed of a base and an active layer. The active layer contains phosphors that give off light when struck by x-rays. The light exposes the film and produces an image. The phosphor light diffuses by the time it reaches the film because of the slight distance between the phosphor and film. Light diffusion causes a loss of recorded detail. This loss is very noticeable if the film and screens are not in good contact with each other inside the cassette.

Increasing the amount of light given off by an intensifying screen increases its speed and reduces the amount of radiation needed to produce an image. When the speed is increased, the recorded detail is reduced if light diffusion increases.

The two intensifying screen systems are calcium tungstate and rare earth. There are several screen speeds in each system. When changing screen speeds, the radiographer must calculate a new mAs because each screen speed produces a different density.

Direct exposure radiographs are produced without intensifying screens. These radiographs display better recorded detail than intensifying screen radiographs because they do not require light to form the image. Direct exposure has been almost eliminated because it requires a very large exposure to the patient.

Computed radiography is a new system that uses a computer to help form the image. The radiography image appears on a cathode-ray tube (CRT) and this image can be transferred to film. While the image is on the CRT the qualities of density (brightness), contrast (gray scale), and recorded detail (resolution) can be adjusted by the computer without radiating the patient again.

PERFORM ACTIVITY 13.E

Recorded Detail Section Review Activities

PERFORM ACTIVITY 13.F

PERFORM ACTIVITY 13.G

PERFORM ACTIVITY 13.H

SECTION VI

RADIOGRAPHIC TECHNIQUES

CHAPTER 14

THE RELATIONSHIP OF THE FOUR RADIOGRAPHIC QUALITIES

CHAPTER OUTLINE

DENSITY
CONTRAST
RECORDED DETAIL
DISTORTION
RELATIONSHIPS
SUMMARY

OBJECTIVES

At the end of this chapter you should be able to:

- Explain the effect on density, contrast, recorded detail, and distortion with either an increase or decrease in the following factors:
  mA
  Exposure time
  mAs
  kVp
  SID
  OID
  Focal spot
  Grid ratio
  Collimation field size
  Filtration
  Intensifying screen speed
  Developer temperature

This last section of the book deals with radiographic techniques. In this chapter you will learn to analyze the effect of any change in exposure conditions on the four radiographic qualities of density, contrast, recorded detail, and distortion. In Chapters 15 and 16 you will learn how to make changes in exposure factors when one or several exposure conditions change.

This section will include a chapter on the two types of technique charts, fixed and variable kVp charts. The last chapter describes the use of automatic exposure control or phototiming.

Throughout this book, you have learned how various factors affect the radiographic qualities of density, contrast, recorded detail, and distortion. You have learned the concepts in bits and pieces. This chapter helps you put it all together so that you can see the relationship among the four radiographic qualities. A good radiographer must be able to anticipate the effect of any changes in exposure conditions on the quality of the radiograph.

Some of the factors described in this book have an effect on one radiographic quality and some have an effect on more than one quality. Table 1–2 in Chapter 1 lists the four qualities and the factors that control and affect each quality. Depending on the way the factors are changed, some changes cause an increase and some cause a decrease in the quality. Some other factors don't affect the quality at all. A good way to summarize this is to develop a table for each quality in which a plus (+) sign indicates an increase, a minus (−) sign indicates a decrease, and a zero (0) indicates no change.

DENSITY

Table 14–1 lists the most important factors that affect any of the radiographic qualities. In this table all of the factors are first ***increased*** and then all the factors are ***decreased***. The + for an increase, − for a decrease, and 0 for no change indicate the factor's effect on density after the factor is either increased or decreased. For example, as the mA is increased, density is increased, and as the mA is decreased, density is decreased. As the grid ratio is increased, density is decreased, and as the grid ratio is decreased, density is increased. A short explanation of why the change affects density is included in the table.

Table 14–1. Evaluation of Density

Factor	All Factors Increased	All Factors Decreased	Explanation
mA	+	−	mA and density are directly proportional
Time	+	−	Time and density are directly proportional
mAs	+	−	mAs controls density; mAs and density are directly proportional
kVp	+	−	kVp affects density
SID	−	+	SID and density are inversely proportional
OID	−	+	OID and density are inversely proportional because of the air-gap
Focal spot size	0	0	Focal spot size only affects recorded detail
Grid ratio	−	+	A grid with a higher ratio contains more lead and reduces density
Collimation field size	+	−	A larger collimation field size produces more scatter and therefore more density
Filtration	−	+	An increase in filtration reduces the amount of radiation in the beam
Screen speed	+	−	A higher speed screen will produce more light and more density
Developer temperature	+	−	Developer temperature and density are directly proportional

Table 14–2. Density Factors in a Clinical Situation

A good radiograph was produced using the factors listed. Each change is made independently, and the effect on density after the change is indicated as + for increase, − for decrease, and 0 for no change.
Good radiograph:

300 mA	80 kVp	.6-mm focal spot	2.5-mm filtration
.05 sec	72″ SID	8:1 grid ratio	100 speed screen
15 mAs	2″ OID	14 × 17 collimation field size	94° developer temperature

Factors Changed	Effect on Density
400 mA	+
.02 sec	−
30 mAs	+
70 kVp	−
40″ SID	+
8″ OID	−
2.0 mm focal spot	0
12:1 grid ratio	−
10 × 12 collimation field size	−
3.0 mm filtration	−
200 speed screen	+
88° developer temperature	−

Any factor that affects the amount of radiation reaching the film has to affect density. mA, time, mAs, kVp, and SID all determine the amount of radiation reaching the film. Using any method that controls the amount of scattered radiation that reaches the film also affects density. These methods include using a large OID in the air-gap technique, and the use of grids, collimation, and filtration. The speed of the intensifying screen also determines the amount of density produced. Any time the developer temperature is increased or decreased, density will usually be affected.

Table 14–2 lists specific factors that might be used in a clinical situation. The first factors listed were used to produce a good quality radiograph. In the table these factors are either increased or decreased, and the effect on density is indicated by a +, −, or 0.

PERFORM ACTIVITY 14.A

PERFORM ACTIVITY 14.B

PERFORM ACTIVITY 14.C

CONTRAST

Contrast will be analyzed in the same way as density, by developing a table in which all factors are first increased and then decreased (Table 14–3). Any factor that

Table 14–3. Evaluation of Contrast

Factor	All Factors Increased	All Factors Decreased	Explanation
mA	0	0	mA does not affect contrast
Time	0	0	Time does not affect contrast
mAs	0	0	mAs controls density; mAs does not affect contrast
kVp	−	+	kVp controls contrast; kVp and contrast are inversely proportional
SID	0	0	SID does not affect contrast
OID	+	−	OID and contrast are directly proportional because of the air gap
Focal spot size	0	0	Focal spot size only affects recorded detail
Grid ratio	+	−	A grid with a higher ratio reduces more scatter
Collimation field size	−	+	A larger collimation field size produces more scatter
Filtration	−	+	An increase in filtration produces a beam with more energy, which produces more scatter
Screen speed	0	0	A change in screen speed usually does not affect contrast
Developer temperature	−	−	Developer temperature changes usually reduce contrast

changes the amount of scattered radiation produced or the amount of scattered radiation that reaches the film has to change contrast. These factors include using a large OID in the air-gap technique, using a grid, and collimation. Also, any factor that changes the penetrating quality of the beam will change contrast. These factors are kVp and filtration. When the developer temperature is increased or decreased, contrast will usually be affected.

Table 14–4 lists factors that might be used in a clinical situation to produce a good quality radiograph. Then these factors are changed, and the effect of the changes on contrast are indicated by a +, −, or 0.

PERFORM ACTIVITY 14.D

PERFORM ACTIVITY 14.E

PERFORM ACTIVITY 14.F

RECORDED DETAIL

It's easy to get confused with the factors that affect recorded detail, because the terms recorded detail and visibility of detail are often used to mean the same thing when they are not the same. The term visibility of detail takes into account all of the factors that make the image visible on the radiograph, whereas only seven factors affect re-

Table 14–4. Contrast Factors in a Clinical Situation

A good radiograph was produced using the factors listed. Each change is made independently, and the effect on contrast after the change is indicated as + for increase, − for decrease, and 0 for no change.

Good radiograph:

400 mA	80 kVp	1.5-mm focal spot	2.5-mm filtration
⅓ sec	56″ SID	8:1 grid ratio	400 speed screen
133 mAs	2″ OID	14 × 17 collimation field size	90° developer temperature

Factors Changed	Effect on Contrast
200 mA	0
½ sec	0
50 mAs	0
70 kVp	+
50″ SID	0
8″ OID	+
1.2 mm focal spot	0
6:1 grid ratio	−
10 × 12 collimation field size	+
2.0 mm filtration	+
200 speed screen	0
96° developer temperature	−

corded detail. These seven factors are SID, OID, focal spot, screen speed, film speed, the contact between the screen and film, and motion.

Table 14–5 lists the effects on recorded detail when all the factors on the table are first increased and then decreased. Table 14–6 shows the factors used to produce a good quality radiograph. Recorded detail is affected only when the seven factors listed above are changed.

PERFORM ACTIVITY 14.G

PERFORM ACTIVITY 14.H

PERFORM ACTIVITY 14.I

DISTORTION

Of the factors listed on the tables for density, contrast, and recorded detail, not many affect distortion. Distance changes always produce more or less magnification, which affects size distortion. When magnification decreases, size distortion decreases. A decrease in distortion improves radiographic quality. The factors that affect shape distortion are situational and are difficult to use on a table, so these factors are not included on the tables. These factors are the alignment of the central ray, object, and film.

Table 14–5. Evaluation of Recorded Detail

Factor	All Factors Increased	All Factors Decreased	Explanation
mA	0	0	mA does not affect recorded detail
Time	0	0	Time does not affect recorded detail
mAs	0	0	mAs controls density; mAs does not affect recorded detail
kVp	0	0	kVp controls contrast; kVp does not affect recorded detail
SID	+	–	SID and recorded detail are directly proportional
OID	–	+	OID and recorded detail are inversely proportional
Focal spot size	–	+	Focal spot size and recorded detail are inversely proportional
Grid ratio	0	0	Grid ratio does not affect recorded detail
Collimation field size	0	0	Collimation does not affect recorded detail
Filtration	0	0	Filtration does not affect recorded detail
Screen speed	–	+	Screen speed and recorded detail are inversely proportional
Developer temperature	0	0	Developer temperature does not affect recorded detail

Table 14–6. Recorded Detail Factors in a Clinical Situation

A good radiograph was produced using the factors listed. Each change is made independently, and the effect on recorded detail after the change is indicated as + for increase, – for decrease, and 0 for no change.

Good radiograph:

100 mA	80 kVp	1.5-mm focal spot	2.5-mm filtration
.2 sec	72″ SID	6:1 grid ratio	200 speed screen
20 mAs	2″ OID	10 × 12 collimation field size	94° developer temperature

Factors Changed	Effect on Recorded Detail
300 mA	0
.5 sec	0
10 mAs	0
70 kVp	0
50″ SID	–
6″ OID	–
.6-mm focal spot	+
8:1 grid ratio	0
14 × 17 collimation field size	0
2.0-mm filtration	0
100 speed screen	+
92° developer temperature	0

Table 14–7 lists the effects on distortion when all the factors are first increased and then decreased. Table 14–8 shows the factors used to produce a good quality radiograph. Size distortion is only affected when SID and OID change.

PERFORM ACTIVITY 14.J

PERFORM ACTIVITY 14.K

RELATIONSHIPS

In order to see how the four radiographic qualities are related, Table 14–9 lists the effects on all the qualities as the factors are increased. Table 14–10 lists the effects on all the qualities as the factors are decreased.

PERFORM ACTIVITY 14.L

PERFORM ACTIVITY 14.M

PERFORM ACTIVITY 14.N

PERFORM ACTIVITY 14.O

Table 14–7. Evaluation of Distortion

Factor	All Factors Increased	All Factors Decreased	Explanation
mA	0	0	mA does not affect distortion
Time	0	0	Time does not affect distortion
mAs	0	0	mAs controls density; mAs does not affect distortion
kVp	0	0	kVp controls contrast; kVp does not affect distortion
SID	–	+	As SID changes, magnification is changed, which changes distortion
OID	+	–	As OID changes, magnification is changed, which changes distortion
Focal spot size	0	0	Focal spot size does not affect distortion
Grid ratio	0	0	Grid ratio does not affect distortion
Collimation field size	0	0	Collimation does not affect distortion
Filtration	0	0	Filtration does not affect distortion
Screen speed	0	0	Screen speed does not affect distortion
Developer temperature	0	0	Developer temperature does not affect distortion

Table 14–8. Distortion Factors in a Clinical Situation

A good radiograph was produced using the factors listed. Each change is made independently, and the effect on distortion after the change is indicated as + for increase, − for decrease, and 0 for no change.

Good radiograph:

200 mA	75 kVp	2.0-mm focal spot	3.0-mm filtration
20 msec	48″ SID	16:1 grid ratio	100 speed screen
4 mAs	2″ OID	14 × 17 collimation field size	94° developer temperature

Factors Changed	Effect on Distortion
100 mA	0
30 msec	0
2 mAs	0
85 kVp	0
60″ SID	−
6″ OID	+
.3-mm focal spot	0
No grid	0
8 × 10 collimation field size	0
2.0-mm filtration	0
400 speed screen	0
98° developer temperature	0

Table 14–9. Effect on Radiographic Quality if All Factors Are Increased

Factors	Density	Contrast	Recorded Detail	Distortion
mA	+	0	0	0
Time	+	0	0	0
mAs	+	0	0	0
kVp	+	−	0	0
SID	−	0	+	−
OID	−	+	−	+
Focal spot size	0	0	−	0
Grid ratio	−	+	0	0
Collimation field size	+	−	0	0
Filtration	−	−	0	0
Screen speed	+	0	−	0
Developer temperature	+	−	0	0

Table 14–10. Effect on Radiographic Quality if All Factors Are Decreased

Factors	Density	Contrast	Recorded Detail	Distortion
mA	−	0	0	0
Time	−	0	0	0
mAs	−	0	0	0
kVp	−	+	0	0
SID	+	0	−	+
OID	+	−	+	−
Focal spot size	0	0	+	0
Grid ratio	+	−	0	0
Collimation field size	−	+	0	0
Filtration	+	+	0	0
Screen speed	−	0	+	0
Developer temperature	−	−	0	0

SUMMARY

When an exposure condition changes, one or more of the four radiographic qualities may be affected. Density is always affected by a change in the amount of radiation reaching the film. Contrast is always affected by changes in the amount of scattered radiation and changes in the beam quality. Recorded detail is affected by only seven factors. Size distortion is affected by distance changes. A summary of these effects is shown in Tables 14–9 and 14–10.

CHAPTER 15

EXPOSURE COMPENSATION

CHAPTER OUTLINE

OBJECTIVES

At the end of this chapter you should be able to:

- Calculate mAs, mA, or time.
- Calculate the new mA and time to be used to control motion, select the small focal spot, and use the breathing technique.
- Calculate the new mAs required to compensate for a change in the:
  SID
  kVp
  Grid ratio
  Collimation field size
  Intensifying screen speed
  X-ray generation

This chapter reviews the technique calculations that were each presented separately in other chapters. The math that will be reviewed involves the factors the radiographer uses most often in clinical situations. Whenever a change is made in an exposure condition, the density on the radiograph is usually affected. The mAs then needs to be changed to compensate for the effect on density. This compensation brings the density of the radiograph back to being satisfactory. Of course this assumes that the original density was satisfactory. The calculations reviewed include: mAs, reciprocity, the density maintenance formula, the 15% rule, grid ratio, collimation field size, and intensifying screen speed.

One other technical factor will be introduced in this chapter. X-rays can be generated using single-phase equipment or three-phase equipment. X-ray facilities often have both types of equipment. Radiographers must use a different mAs on single-phase equipment than on three-phase equipment to produce the same density.

All of the calculations that involve determining a new mAs because of a change in an exposure condition use the "to/from" system except for the 15% rule and reciprocity law calculations. In the to/from system, a fraction is formed by placing the multiplier of the factor being changed *to* in the numerator and the multiplier of the factor being changed *from* in the denominator. Then the old mAs is multiplied by

Table 15–1. The Multipliers Used in To/From Calculations

Grid Ratio	Collimation Field Size	Intensifying Screen Speeds	X-Ray Generation
No grid = 1	14 × 17 = 1	50 RSV = 2	single phase = 2
5:1 = 2	10 × 12 = 1.25	100 RSV = 1	three phase = 1
6:1 = 3	8 × 10 = 1.40	200 RSV = .5	
8:1 = 4		300 RSV = .33	
12:1 = 5		400 RSV = .25	
16:1 = 6		500 RSV = .20	
		600 RSV = .17	
		700 RSV = .14	
		800 RSV = .125	

this fraction and the answer is the new mAs required to maintain density after the change in the exposure condition. Table 15–1 shows the multipliers used for to/from calculations.

mAs

Milliampere-seconds, or mAs, the product of mA and exposure time, determines the quantity of x-rays produced in a beam. mAs, mA, and time affect only the radiographic quality of density. An increase in mAs, mA, or time causes an increase in density, and a decrease in mAs, mA, or time causes a decrease in density. Exposure time can be stated in fractions, decimals, or milliseconds. Milliseconds must be converted to a fraction or decimal before mAs can be calculated.

To Calculate mAs

$$\text{mA} \times \text{time} = \text{mAs}$$
$$300 \text{ mA} \times .05 \text{ sec} = 15 \text{ mAs}$$
$$500 \text{ mA} \times \tfrac{2}{5} \text{ sec} = 200 \text{ mAs}$$
$$600 \text{ mA} \times 20 \text{ msec} = 12 \text{ mAs } (20 \text{ msec} = .02 \text{ sec})$$

To Calculate mA

$$\text{mA} = \frac{\text{mAs}}{\text{time}}$$
$$300 \text{ mA} = \frac{15}{.05}$$
$$500 \text{ mA} = \frac{200}{\frac{2}{5}}$$
$$600 \text{ mA} = \frac{12}{.02}$$

To Calculate Time

$$\text{Time} = \frac{\text{mAs}}{\text{mA}}$$

$$.05 = \frac{15}{300}$$

$$\frac{2}{5} = \frac{200}{500}$$

$$.02 = \frac{12}{600}$$

RECIPROCITY

Several combinations of mA and time can equal the same mAs.

100 mA × .2 sec = 20 mAs
50 mA × $\frac{2}{5}$ sec = 20 mAs
400 mA × 50 msec = 20 mAs

This is the reciprocity law. The radiographer uses this law to control motion by using a short time and therefore a high mA, to select the small focal spot by using a low mA and therefore a long time, and to use a breathing technique by using a long time and therefore a low mA.

Motion Control

100 mA × .06 sec = 6 mAs
600 mA × .01 sec = 6 mAs (shorter time to control motion)

Focal Spot Selection

500 mA × .03 sec = 15 mAs
50 mA × .3 sec = 15 mAs (small focal spot range)

Breathing Technique

500 mA × .10 sec = 50 mAs
25 mA × 2 sec = 50 mAs (a breathing technique)

THE DENSITY MAINTENANCE FORMULA

If the source-image distance (SID) is increased, the intensity of radiation at the film decreases and the density of the radiograph will also decrease. And if the SID is decreased, the intensity of radiation at the film increases and the density of the radiograph will increase. The density maintenance formula is used to calculate the new mAs to be used when the SID is changed, so that the density on the radiograph will remain the same.

To Calculate the New mAs

$$\text{New mAs} = \frac{\text{old mAs} \times \text{new distance}^2}{\text{old distance}^2}$$

If a radiographer were using 10 mAs at a 40-inch SID and had to change to a 72-inch SID

$$\text{New mAs} = \frac{10 \times 72^2}{40^2}$$

$$\text{New mAs} = \frac{10 \times 5184}{1600}$$

$$\text{New mAs} = \frac{51{,}840}{1600}$$

$$\text{New mAs} = 32.4 \quad \text{(increased because the SID increased)}$$

The density maintenance formula is a to/from calculation because the old mAs is multiplied by the new distance (the distance being changed to) and divided by the old distance (the distance being changed from).

THE 15% RULE

mAs is the controlling factor for density. kVp is the controlling factor for contrast. mAs does not affect contrast; however, kVp does affect density. If the kVp is increased, more scattered radiation is produced and contrast decreases, causing the radiograph to appear grayer (long scale contrast). An increase in kVp will also increase density. If the kVp is decreased, less scattered radiation is produced and contrast increases, causing the radiograph to appear mostly black and white (short scale contrast). A decrease in kVp will also decrease density. An increase or decrease in the kVp of 15% will cause the same density change as doubling or halving the mAs.

To calculate the new mAs to be used in order to maintain film density when the kVp is changed, the 15% rule is used. If the kVp is increased by 15%, the mAs must be cut in half to maintain density. If the kVp is decreased by 15%, the mAs must be doubled to maintain density. Radiographs produced with the changed kVp and mAs will have the same density but a different contrast. Within the 60 to 90 kVp range, a change of 10 kVp is considered equal to a 15% change in kVp.

Increase in the kVp

The original factors are 15 mAs and 70 kVp.

$$70 \text{ kVp} + 10 = 80 \text{ kVp}$$

$$15 \frac{\text{mAs}}{2} = 7.5 \text{ mAs}$$

The new factors are 7.5 mAs and 80 kVp. The radiograph will have the same density as the original but lower contrast because of the increase in kVp.

Decrease in the kVp

The original factors are 12 mAs and 80 kVp.

$$80 \text{ kVp} - 10 = 70 \text{ kVp}$$

$$12 \text{ mAs} \times 2 = 24 \text{ mAs}$$

The new factors are 24 mAs and 70 kVp. The radiograph will have the same density as the original but higher contrast because of the decrease in kVp.

GRID RATIO

When a grid is used or the grid ratio is changed the goal is to change the amount of scattered radiation on the radiograph and this changes radiographic contrast. Scattered radiation also puts density on the radiograph. So if the density was adequate before a grid change, the mAs must be changed after a grid change. The change in mAs brings the density back to the original satisfactory density before the grid change was made.

Each grid ratio has a multiplier that is used to form a fraction. The multiplier of the grid ratio being changed *to* becomes the numerator of the fraction and the multiplier of the grid ratio being changed *from* becomes the denominator. The fraction formed is multiplied by the old mAs to obtain the new mAs to be used because of the grid change.

To Calculate the New mAs With a Grid Ratio Change

The original factors are 10 mAs, 75 kVp, with a 6:1 ratio grid. A change is made to a 12:1 ratio grid.

$$\text{Fraction} = \frac{5 \text{ (the multiplier for a 12:1 grid ratio)}}{3 \text{ (the multiplier for a 6:1 grid ratio)}}$$

$$\text{New mAs} = 10 \times \frac{5}{3}$$

$$\text{New mAs} = 16.7 \text{ mAs}$$

COLLIMATION FIELD SIZE

The collimation field size affects the amount of scattered radiation that is produced. A large collimation field size will produce more scattered radiation than a small collimation field size. Since scattered radiation affects density, a change in the collimation field size will require a compensating change in mAs. The three commonly used collimation field sizes each have a multiplier, and the multiplier is used to form a to/from fraction as in the grid ratio change. Then this fraction is multiplied by the old mAs to obtain the new mAs to be used because of the change in collimation field size.

To Calculate the New mAs with a Change in Collimation Field Size

The original factors are 5 mAs, 80 kVp, with a 14 × 17 size collimation. A change is made to a 10 × 12 size collimation.

$$\text{Fraction} = \frac{1.25 \text{ (the multiplier for } 10 \times 12)}{1 \text{ (the multiplier for } 14 \times 17)}$$

$$\text{New mAs} = 5 \times \frac{1.25}{1}$$

$$\text{New mAs} = 6.25 \text{ mAs}$$

INTENSIFYING SCREEN SPEED

The speed of an intensifying screen affects density. If the intensifying screen speed is increased, the density will increase, and if the intensifying screen speed is decreased, the density will decrease. To compensate for the change with mAs, the relative speed values of each intensifying screen must be known. The multiplier for the screen speed is calculated by placing 100 in the numerator and the relative speed value for the screen in the denominator. This fraction is then changed to a decimal by dividing the numerator by the denominator and this forms the screen speed multiplier.

A to/from fraction then is formed by placing the multiplier of the screen speed being changed *to* in the numerator and the multiplier of the screen speed being changed *from* in the denominator. This fraction is multiplied by the old mAs and the answer is the new mAs to be used because of the screen speed change.

The original factors are 8 mAs and 76 kVp with a 500-speed screen. A change is made to a 300-speed screen.

To Calculate the Screen Speed Multiplier

$$\frac{100}{500} \quad \begin{array}{l}\text{(always placed in the numerator)}\\ \text{(the given relative speed value of the screen)}\end{array}$$

$$\frac{100}{500} = .2 \quad \text{(the multiplier for a screen speed of 500)}$$

$$\frac{100}{300} = .33 \quad \text{(the multiplier for a screen speed of 300; the one being changed from)}$$

To Calculate the New mAs with a Change in Screen Speed

$$\text{New mAs} = 8 \times \frac{.33}{.2}$$

$$\text{New mAs} = 13.2 \quad \text{(a higher mAs is required because the new screen speed is slower)}$$

X-RAY GENERATION

Two different types of equipment are often used in the same x-ray facility. The two types, single-phase and three-phase generators, are different because they generate x-rays in a different manner. The beam produced with three-phase equipment is about two times more intense than the beam produced with single-phase equipment. If the same exposure factors are used, a radiograph produced with three-phase equipment would have about two times more density than a radiograph produced with single-phase equipment. Therefore, different exposure factors must be used on the two different types of equipment.

To calculate the new technique when changing from one type of equipment to the other, a to/from fraction is formed by placing the multiplier for the type of equipment being changed to in the numerator and the multiplier for the type of equipment being changed from in the denominator. Then this fraction is multiplied by the old mAs and the answer is the new mAs to be used because of the equipment change.

The multiplier for single phase is 2.
The multiplier for three phase is 1.

Example 1

Suppose a radiographer produced a good radiograph of a shoulder in x-ray room 4, which has single-phase equipment. The technique used was 300 mA, .05 sec, and 70 kVp. The film jammed in the processor and was ruined. The exposure needs to be repeated, but the only available x-ray room is room 5, which has three-phase equipment. The radiographer must adjust the technique or the radiograph will have too much density.

$$\text{mAs} = 300 \times .05$$
$$\text{mAs} = 15 \quad \text{(the old mAs)}$$
$$\text{New mAs} = 15 \times \frac{1 \text{ (the multiplier for 3 phase)}}{2 \text{ (the multiplier for single phase)}}$$
$$\text{New mAs} = 7.5$$

The new mAs of 7.5 used with three-phase equipment will produce the same density as 15 mAs used with single-phase equipment.

Example 2

It is Monday and you are assigned to room 6, which has a single-phase generator. The first patient, an average size patient, is in for a KUB radiograph. The radiographer you are working with asks you to set the technique factors on the control panel while she positions the patient for the exposure. Last week you were working in room 2, which has three-phase equipment. You remember that you used 20 mAs at 70 kVp for most of the KUBs on patients of average size.

$$\text{New mAs} = 20 \times \frac{2 \text{ (the multiplier for single phase)}}{1 \text{ (the multiplier for three phase)}}$$
$$\text{New mAs} = 40$$

The new mAs of 40 used with single-phase equipment will produce the same density as 20 mAs used with three-phase equipment.

PERFORM ACTIVITY 15.A

PERFORM ACTIVITY 15.B

PERFORM ACTIVITY 15.C

SUMMARY

Many changes in exposure conditions require a compensating change in mAs. This brings the density back to the original density, before the change was made assuming the original density was good. A change in mAs is required to compensate for a source-image distance change, a change in kVp, a grid ratio change, a change in the collimation field size, a change in the speed of the intensifying screen, and a change in the type of x-ray generator.

CHAPTER 16

TECHNIQUE CONVERSION AND COMPARISON

CHAPTER OUTLINE

TECHNIQUE CONVERSIONS
COMPARISON PROBLEMS
SUMMARY

OBJECTIVES

At the end of this chapter you will be able to:

- Calculate the new mAs to be used when several exposure conditions change at the same time.
- Compare several exposure conditions to see which would produce the greatest and least density.

Chapter 15 reviewed the math involved in exposure compensation when one exposure condition is changed. After the exposure compensation is calculated, the answer is the new mAs to be used because of the change in one exposure condition.

There are times in clinical situations when the radiographer is confronted with several changes in exposure conditions at the same time. This chapter will show you how to calculate the new mAs when more than one change in exposure conditions occurs at the same time.

Another math activity presented in this chapter involves evaluating several sets of exposure conditions to determine which set will produce the greatest or least density. This will give you additional practice with technique calculations.

TECHNIQUE CONVERSIONS

When several exposure conditions change at one time, it can be difficult to determine the technique factors. One change in exposure conditions might require the mAs to be increased, whereas another change might require the mAs to be decreased and neither of the changes is equal to the other. For instance, one exposure condition change might require the mAs to be doubled, while another change might require the mAs to be cut by 5 times, and still another change might require a 15% increase in the kVp.

It sounds confusing, but if the problem is approached in steps, it becomes less overwhelming. Multiple technique conversions are best approached by breaking the problem down into several single exposure compensations. The answer calculated for each part of the problem is used as the old mAs in the next part of the problem. At the end of all the calculations, the final answer is the new mAs to be used because of all the simultaneous exposure condition changes.

Example 1

Suppose the ordinary technique in the x-ray department for a posteroanterior (PA) chest radiograph on a patient of average size is 2 mAs at 110 kVp. This exposure is done at a 72-inch SID with a 12 : 1 grid. A portable chest radiograph is required on a patient who is also of average size. Since it may be difficult to get the x-ray beam and grid aligned on an exam done with a portable machine, the grid is not used. A kVp of 110 is always used on chest radiographs performed with a grid in order to penetrate the mediastinum. Without the grid, 110 kVp will generate too much scattered radiation, so the kVp must be reduced to the optimum kVp range for non-grid chest radiographs, which is 80 kVp. Also because of the arrangement in the patient's room, the maximum SID that can be achieved is only 60 inches.

To begin the calculations, arrange all the exposure conditions in columns with column A being the ordinary conditions used in the department and column B being the exposure conditions required on the portable exam. List the similar conditions across from each other. Any conditions that are not similar should be listed last. In this first example, all conditions are similar.

A		B	
2	mAs	____	mAs
110	kVp	80	kVp
72″	SID	60″	SID
12:1	Grid		No grid

The problem requires a change *from* column A conditions *to* column B conditions. Any of the changes can be calculated first, but it is easiest to work down the column one by one to make sure all changes have been accounted for.

kVp Change

A change from 110 kVp to 80 kVp is accomplished by using the 15% rule. This example requires a two-step process because the answer from the first step is not the 80 kVp required in column B.

Step 1. Reduce the kVp by 15% and double the mAs:

$$110 \times .15 = 16 \text{ kVp} \qquad 2 \times 2 = 4 \text{ mAs}$$
$$110 - 16 = 94$$

Step 2. 94 kVp is not the optimum kVp for a non-grid chest. The optimum kVp is 80. Use the answers from step 1 as the original technique in step 2.

$$94 \times .15 = 14 \text{ kvp} \qquad 4 \times 2 = 8 \text{ mAs}$$
$$94 - 14 = 80 \text{ kVp}$$

The technique after the kVp change is

8 mAs 80 kVp

SID Change

The technique factors of 8 mAs and 80 kVp are used in the next change, which is the SID change from 72 to 60 inches. This change requires a calculation with the density maintenance formula.

$$\text{New mAs} = \frac{\text{Old mAs} \times \text{New distance}^2}{\text{Old distance}^2}$$

$$\text{New mAs} = \frac{8 \times 60^2}{72^2}$$

$$\text{New mAs} = \frac{8 \times 3600}{5184}$$

$$\text{New mAs} = 5.6$$

The technique after the kVp and SID change is

5.6 mAs   80 kVp

Grid Change

The technique factors of 5.6 mAs and 80 kVp are used in the next change, which is the grid change from 12:1 to no grid. This change requires a calculation with the grid ratio multipliers. Form a fraction by placing the multiplier for the grid ratio being changed to in the numerator and the multiplier for the grid ratio being changed from in the denominator. Then multiply this fraction by the old mAs to get the new mAs to be used because of the change in grid ratio.

$$\text{New mAs} = 5.6 \times \frac{1}{5} \quad \begin{array}{l}\text{(the multiplier for no grid)}\\ \text{(the multiplier for a 12:1 grid)}\end{array}$$

$$\text{New mAs} = 1.1$$

The final technique factors after all the changes are accounted for (kVp, SID, grid) are

1.1 mAs   80 kVp

Figure 16–1 shows the two radiographs.

Example 2

Let's say you took a KUB radiograph on a 14 × 17 inch film using 20 mAs and 70 kVp. You used a 40-inch SID and took the film on a 400-speed intensifying screen. The radiologist suspects that the patient has a bony lesion on the fourth lumbar vertebra. He needs a film of that area with very good recorded detail. You decide to switch to a 200-speed screen, an 8 × 10 inch film, and a 72-inch SID.

A		B	
20	mAs	____	mAs
70	kVp	70	kVp
40″	SID	72″	SID
400	RSV	200	RSV
14 × 17	film	8 × 10	film

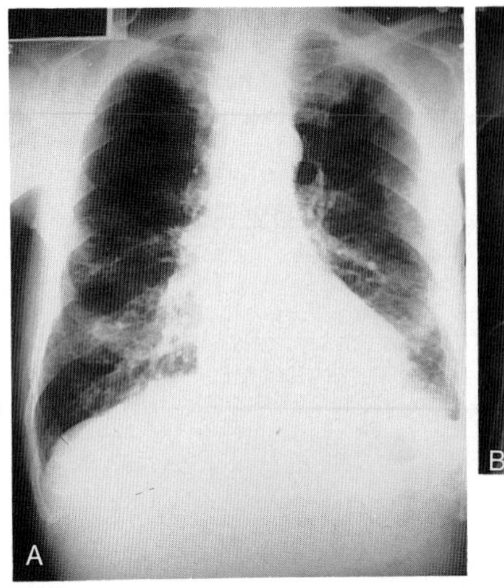

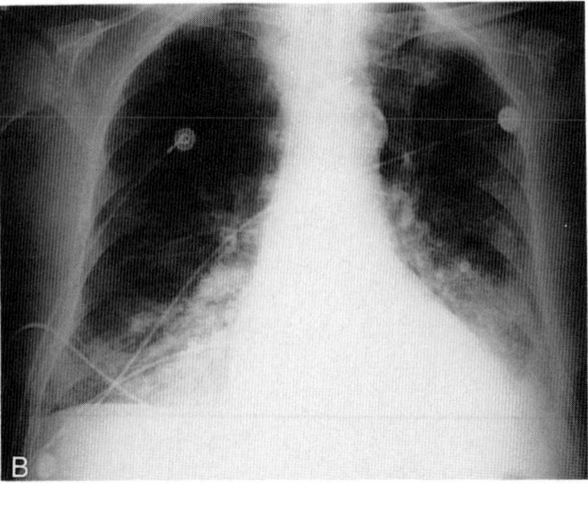

FIGURE 16–1. *(A)* A PA chest radiograph taken in the x-ray department using 2 mAs, 110 kVp, 72-inch SID, and a 12 : 1 grid. *(B)* A portable chest radiograph taken on the same patient a few days later using 1.1 mAs, 80 kVp, 60-inch SID, and no grid.

SID Change

Use the density maintenance formula:

$$\text{New mAs} = \frac{20 \times 72^2}{40^2}$$

$$\text{New mAs} = \frac{20 \times 5184}{1600}$$

$$\text{New mAs} = 64.8$$

The technique after the SID change is

64.8 mAs   70 kVp

Intensifying Screen Speed Change

First calculate the multipliers for the relative speed value (RSV) for each intensifying screen. Form a fraction by placing 100 in the numerator and the RSV of the other screen in the denominator. Then change this fraction to a decimal.

400 speed:	100 speed:
$\text{Multiplier} = \frac{100}{400}$	$\text{Multiplier} = \frac{100}{200}$
$\text{Multiplier} = .25$	$\text{Multiplier} = .5$

Now form another fraction by placing the multiplier of the speed being changed to in the numerator and the multiplier of the speed being changed from in the denominator. Multiply this fraction by the old mAs and the answer is the new mAs to be used because of the screen speed change. The old mAs is the mAs calculated after the SID change, which is 64.8.

$$\text{New mAs} = 64.8 \times \frac{.5}{.25} \quad \begin{matrix}\text{(the 200 screen multiplier} \\ \text{(the 400 screen multiplier)}\end{matrix}$$

$$\text{New mAs} = 129.6$$

The new technique after the SID and screen change is

129.6 mAs 70 kVp

Film Size Change

Assuming that you are collimating to the size of the film being used, this part of the problem is a collimation field size change. Form a fraction by placing the multiplier of the collimation field size being changed to in the numerator and the multiplier of the collimation field size being changed from in the denominator. Then multiply this fraction by the old mAs. The answer is the new mAs to be used because of the collimation field size change. The old mAs is the mAs calculated after the screen speed change, which is 129.6.

$$\text{New mAs} = 129.6 = \frac{1.40}{1} \quad \begin{matrix}\text{(the multiplier for } 8 \times 10 \text{ inch)} \\ \text{(the multiplier for } 14 \times 17 \text{ inch)}\end{matrix}$$

$$\text{New mAs} = 181.4$$

The final technique factors after all the changes are accounted for (SID, RSV, film size) are

181.4 mAs 70 kVp

Example 3

Assume that the ordinary technique you would use in the department for a patient of average size for a lateral cervical spine radiograph is 10 mAs at 80 kVp. This is ordinarily exposed at a 72-inch SID using a 12:1 grid. A trauma patient who has a neck like a pro football player needs a cross-table lateral cervical spine. You can only get a 56-inch SID because of the tight room arrangement in the ER. The stationary grids used for portable x-ray exams are 8:1 ratio. Also the technique used in the department is for three-phase equipment and the portable machine you are using is single phase equipment.

A	B
10 mAs	___ mAs
80 kVp	80 kVp
72″ SID	56″ SID
12:1 grid	8:1 grid
Three phase	Single phase
	Large patient

SID Change

$$\text{New mAs} = \frac{10 \times 56^2}{72^2}$$

$$\text{New mAs} = \frac{10 \times 3136}{5184}$$

$$\text{New mAs} = 6 \text{ mAs}$$

The technique after the SID change is

6 mAs 80 kVp

Grid Ratio Change

$$\text{mAs} = 6 \times \frac{4}{5} \quad \begin{matrix}\text{(the multiplier for an 8:1 ratio grid)} \\ \text{(the multiplier for a 12:1 ratio grid)}\end{matrix}$$

$$\text{mAs} = 4.8$$

The technique after the SID and grid ratio change is

4.8 mAs 80 kVp

X-Ray Generation

Form a fraction by placing the multiplier of the x-ray generation being changed to in the numerator and the x-ray generation being changed from in the denominator. Multiply the old mAs by this fraction

$$\text{mAs} = 4.8 \times \frac{2}{1} \quad \begin{matrix}\text{(the multiplier for single phase)} \\ \text{(the multiplier for three phase)}\end{matrix}$$

$$\text{mAs} = 9.6$$

The technique after compensating for the SID, grid ratio, and x-ray generation changes is

9.6 mAs 80 kVp

Size of the Patient

The one condition that is not similar between the two techniques is the size of the patient. You decide to double the mAs because of the patient's large size.

$$9.6 \times 2 = 19.2$$

The new technique factors after all the changes have been accounted for are

19.2 mAs 80 kVp

Suppose the highest mA station on the portable machine is 200 mA. With this mA setting the time is .096 second (19.2/200 = .096). Suppose the closest time station on the portable is .10 second. Then the new mA is 200 and the new time is .10 second for a mAs of 20, which is as close to 19.2 as possible. Figure 16–2 shows the two radiographs.

PERFORM ACTIVITY 16.A

PERFORM ACTIVITY 16.B

COMPARISON PROBLEMS

In a comparison problem, several exposure conditions are compared to assess their different densities. The best way to approach these problems is to arrange the factors in columns with all the similar factors in the same row.

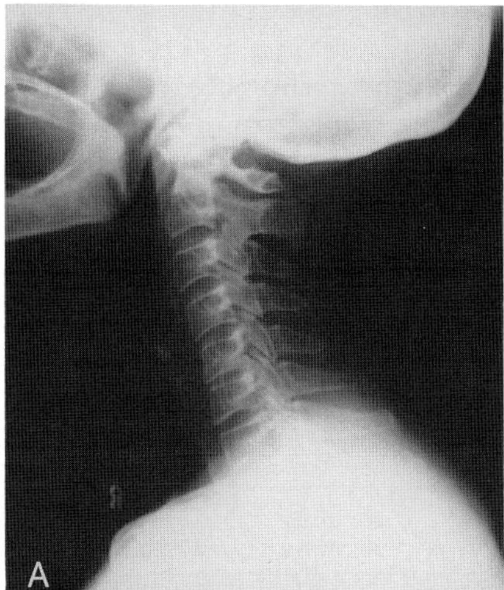

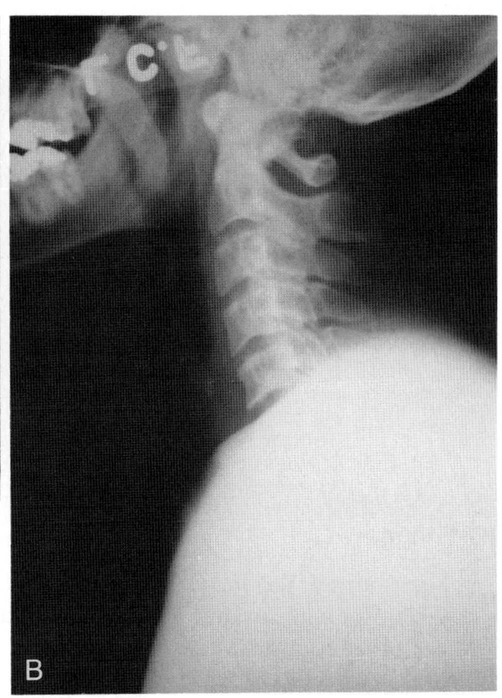

FIGURE 16–2. (*A*) A lateral cervical spine radiograph taken in the x-ray department on 3-phase equipment using 10 mAs, 80 kVp, 72-inch SID, and a 12:1 ratio grid. (*B*) A cervical spine radiograph taken on single phase portable equipment using 20 mAs, 80 kVp, 56-inch SID, and an 8:1 ratio grid on a very large patient.

Example 1

The problem in this example is to find out which set of exposure conditions will produce the greatest density.

A	B	C	D
300 mA	400 mA	100 mA	500 mA
$\frac{2}{15}$ sec	.02 sec	.20 sec	30 msec
70 kVp	80 kVp	70 kVp	80 kVp
40″ SID	56″ SID	72″ SID	44″ SID

The first thing to do is to figure out the mAs for each column.

	A	B	C	D
	300 mA	400 mA	100 mA	500 mA
	$\frac{2}{15}$ sec	.02 sec	.20 sec	30 msec
	70 kVp	80 kVp	70 kVp	80 kVp
	40″ SID	56″ SID	72″ SID	44″ SID
mAs	40 mAs	8 mAs	20 mAs	15 mAs

One of the factors in each row must be chosen as the factor that all the other columns are being changed *to*. If there are several factors in a row that match, the matching factor should be chosen. This will reduce the number of calculations necessary. If no factors match, the factor in column A should be chosen. Any of the factors in a row can be chosen, but by always choosing column A the choice becomes routine and more consistent.

kVp Change

Pick one of the kVp values to change all the other techniques *to*. Either 70 or 80 could be chosen. Let's choose 70 since there are two factors of 70 and 70 is also in column A. This change is made by using the 15% rule. In this case all the 80-kVp techniques will be changed to 70, and therefore the mAs from that column must be doubled.

	A	B	C	D
	300 mA $\frac{2}{15}$ sec 70 kVp 40″ SID	400 mA .02 sec 80 kVp 56″ SID	100 mA .20 sec 70 kVp 72″ SID	500 mA 30 msec 80 kVp 44″ SID
mAs	40 mAs	8 mAs	20 mAs	15 mAs
70 kVp	40 mAs	16 mAs	20 mAs	30 mAs

SID Change

Since none of the SID factors match, the 40-inch SID from column A is chosen. This will be the new distance in the density maintenance formula for all the calculations in the other columns. The old distance is the SID listed in each column.

Column B

$$\text{New mAs} = \frac{16 \times 40^2}{56^2}$$

$$\text{New mAs} = \frac{16 \times 1600}{3136}$$

$$\text{New mAs} = 8 \text{ mAs}$$

Column C

$$\text{New mAs} = \frac{20 \times 40^2}{72^2}$$

$$\text{New mAs} = \frac{20 \times 1600}{5184}$$

$$\text{New mAs} = 6 \text{ mAs}$$

Column D

$$\text{New mAs} = \frac{30 \times 40^2}{44^2}$$

$$\text{New mAs} = \frac{30 \times 1600}{1936}$$

$$\text{New mAs} = 25 \text{ mAs}$$

	A	B	C	D
	300 mA $\frac{2}{15}$ sec 70 kVp 40″ SID	400 mA .02 sec 80 kVp 56″ SID	100 mA .20 sec 70 kVp 72″ SID	500 mA 30 msec 80 kVp 44″ SID
mAs	40 mAs	8 mAs	20 mAs	15 mAs
kVp	40 mAs	16 mAs	20 mAs	30 mAs
SID	40 mAs	8 mAs	6 mAs	25 mAs

Column A, with the highest mAs, will produce the greatest density. Column C, with the least mAs will produce the least density.

Example 2

A	B	C	D
100 mA	300 mA	500 mA	200 mA
.35 sec	25 msec	.15 sec	$\frac{1}{10}$ sec
6:1 grid	8:1 grid	16:1 grid	12:1 grid
100 RSV	400 RSV	200 RSV	600 RSV
Single phase	Three phase	Single phase	Three phase

First calculate the mAs for each column.

	A	B	C	D
	100 mA	300 mA	500 mA	200 mA
	.35 sec	25 msec	.15 sec	$\frac{1}{10}$ sec
	6:1 grid	8:1 grid	16:1 grid	12:1 grid
	100 RSV	400 RSV	200 RSV	600 RSV
	Single phase	Three phase	Single phase	Three phase
mAs	35 mAs	7.5 mAs	75 mAs	20 mAs

Grid Change

No grid ratios match, so you must convert the values from the other columns to the 6:1 grid ratio in column A. The multiplier for the 6:1 ratio grid is the numerator and the multiplier for the grid ratio in the other columns is the denominator. Multiply this fraction by the old mAs to get the new mAs. The old mAs is the mAs already calculated in each column.

Column B

$$\text{New mAs} = 7.5 \times \frac{3}{4} \quad \begin{array}{l}\text{(multiplier for a 6:1 ratio grid)}\\ \text{(multiplier for an 8:1 ratio grid)}\end{array}$$

$$\text{New mAs} = 5.6$$

Column C

$$\text{New mAs} = 75 \times \frac{3}{6} \quad \begin{array}{l}\text{(multiplier for a 6:1 ratio grid)}\\ \text{(multiplier for a 16:1 ratio grid)}\end{array}$$

$$\text{New mAs} = 37.5$$

Column D

$$\text{New mAs} = 20 \times \frac{3}{5} \quad \begin{array}{l}\text{(multiplier for a 6:1 ratio grid)}\\ \text{(multiplier for a 12:1 ratio grid)}\end{array}$$

$$\text{New mAs} = 12$$

	A	B	C	D
	100 mA	300 mA	500 mA	200 mA
	.35 sec	25 msec	.15 sec	$\frac{1}{10}$ sec
	6:1 grid	8:1 grid	16:1 grid	12:1 grid
	100 RSV	400 RSV	200 RSV	600 RSV
	Single phase	Three phase	Single phase	Three phase
mAs	35 mAs	7.5 mAs	75 mAs	20 mAs
Grid	35 mAs	5.6 mAs	37.5 mAs	12 mAs

Screen Speed Change

To calculate the change for the intensifying screen speed, first calculate the multipliers for the screen speed values. Place 100 in the numerator of the fraction and the new screen speed in the denominator. Then change this fraction to a decimal.

Multipliers

Column A	Column B	Column C	Column D
$\frac{100}{100} = 1$	$\frac{100}{400} = .25$	$\frac{100}{200} = .5$	$\frac{100}{600} = .17$

Now insert the multipliers in a new fraction by placing the multiplier of the screen speed being changed to in the numerator and the multiplier of the screen speed being changed from in the denominator. Multiply this fraction by the old mAs and the answer is the new mAs. All the columns will be changed to a 100 RSV, which has a multiplier of 1.

Column B

$$\text{New mAs} = 5.6 \times \frac{1}{.25} \quad \begin{matrix}\text{(a 100-speed multiplier)} \\ \text{(a 400-speed multiplier)}\end{matrix}$$

$$\text{New mAs} = 22.4$$

Column C

$$\text{New mAs} = 37.5 \times \frac{1}{.5} \quad \begin{matrix}\text{(a 100-speed multiplier)} \\ \text{(a 200-speed multiplier)}\end{matrix}$$

$$\text{New mAs} = 75$$

Column D

$$\text{New mAs} = 12 \times \frac{1}{.17} \quad \begin{matrix}\text{(a 100-speed multiplier)} \\ \text{(a 600-speed multiplier)}\end{matrix}$$

$$\text{New mAs} = 70.6$$

	A	B	C	D
	100 mA .35 sec 6:1 grid 100 RSV Single phase	300 mA 25 msec 8:1 grid 400 RSV Three phase	500 mA .15 sec 16:1 grid 200 RSV Single phase	200 mA $\frac{1}{10}$ sec 12:1 grid 600 RSV Three phase
mAs	35 mAs	7.5 mAs	75 mAs	20 mAs
Grid	35 mAs	5.6 mAs	37.5 mAs	12 mAs
Screen	35 mAs	22.4 mAs	75 mAs	70.6 mAs

X-Ray Generation Change

Pick column A and change all the columns with three phase to single phase by forming a to/from fraction.

Column B

$$\text{New mAs} = 22.4 \times \frac{2}{1}$$

$$\text{New mAs} = 44.8$$

Column D

$$\text{New mAs} = 70.6 \times \frac{2}{1}$$

$$\text{New mAs} = 141.2$$

	A	B	C	D
	100 mA .35 sec 6:1 grid 100 RSV Single phase	300 mA 25 msec 8:1 grid 400 RSV Three phase	500 mA .15 sec 16:1 grid 200 RSV Single phase	200 mA $\frac{1}{10}$ sec 12:1 grid 600 RSV Three phase
mAs	35 mAs	7.5 mAs	75 mAs	20 mAs
Grid	35 mAs	5.6 mAs	37.5 mAs	12 mAs
Screen	35 mAs	22.4 mAs	75 mAs	70.6 mAs
Gen	35 mAs	44.8 mAs	75 mAs	141.2 mAs

Column D, with the highest mAs, will produce the greatest density. Column A, with the least mAs, will produce the least density.

PERFORM ACTIVITY 16.C

PERFORM ACTIVITY 16.D

SUMMARY

When the radiographer is confronted with multiple changes in exposure conditions, each change is analyzed individually. The new mAs for the first change is calculated, and this mAs is used as the old mAs for the next calculation until all the changes are accounted for. The last answer is the new mAs to be used because of all the changes.

Several exposure conditions can be compared to see which will produce the most density and which will produce the least density.

CHAPTER 17

RADIOGRAPHIC TECHNIQUE CHARTS

CHAPTER OUTLINE

OBJECTIVES

At the end of this chapter you will be able to:

- State what should be included on a good radiographic technique chart.
- Describe the characteristics of a variable kVp technique chart.
- Describe the characteristics of a fixed kVp technique chart.
- Explain the advantages of a fixed kVp chart over a variable kVp chart.
- Given a working radiographic technique chart, produce a chart for another x-ray facility.
- Describe the two main reasons why the technique as listed on the chart might be changed.
- List some pathologies that may require the technique as listed on the chart to be decreased in order to produce a good-quality image.
- List some pathologies that may require the technique as listed on the chart to be increased in order to produce a good-quality image.

Most x-ray facilities have written technique charts of some type. Technique charts tell the radiographer what mA, time, and kVp to use for a body part of a particular size. The charts can range from a well-developed one that has a technique for every procedure and every view to hand-written pieces of paper stuck to the wall near the control panels that have techniques written on them for procedures that are not performed very often.

Some facilities require technologists to use the technique charts for every exposure, and some facilities have the charts there only for a reference. Technique charts should be used regularly so that radiographs are of consistent good quality and the number of repeat radiographs is reduced.

It is important for the radiographer to understand how technique charts are developed in order to be able to use one effectively. Technique charts don't work in every situation, so technologists must also be able to change the technique that is listed on the chart when necessary. The general condition of the patient's body and the pathology that a patient may have are sometimes an indication that the technique as listed on the chart should be changed.

There are two main types of technique charts, a variable kVp chart and a fixed kVp chart. This chapter will explain how both types of charts are developed and how they are used. There are several reasons why the fixed kVp chart is preferred over the variable kVp chart.

TECHNIQUE CHARTS

A good technique chart has techniques listed for each view of each exam that is performed in the x-ray facility. For instance, in the chest category there might be techniques listed for PA, lateral, oblique, decubitus, and lordotic chests.

A technique should be listed for any variations that might be used within the exam category. There might be techniques listed for when the exposure is made with and without a grid. If different source-image distances are used for any reason, the techniques for the different distances might also be listed. If intensifying screens of different relative speed values can be used, there should be suggested techniques for each speed. Instructions for automatic exposure control or phototimed exposures should also be listed.

Within a particular category such as the chest, there will be several techniques listed under each view for patients of different size. Some charts are divided into three different technique sections for each view, one technique for a small patient, one technique for a medium-sized patient, and another technique for a large patient. The exposures in this type of chart usually vary by a factor of 2 for each category. Table 17–1 shows an example of this type of chart.

On other charts the measurements of the patient's body are listed by groups, and a technique is given for each measurement group. About a 30% technique change is made for each measurement group because it takes about a 30% change to see a change in density. This type of chart requires the technologist to measure the patient's body with a device called a caliper (Fig. 17–1). It is important for consistency that each technologist using this type of chart measure the patient in the same manner. Tables 17–2 and 17–3 show examples of this type of chart.

There are two general types of technique charts used in radiography. One is a variable kVp chart and one is a fixed kVp chart.

VARIABLE kVp TECHNIQUE CHARTS

When using a variable kVp chart, the mAs is kept the same for a particular body part, and the kVp is varied for patients of different sizes to produce the right density on the

Table 17–1. A Technique Chart Using Small, Medium, and Large Patient Size Categories

Position	Size	kVp	mA	Time	mAs	SID
KUB	Small	70	600	.025	15	40″
	Medium	70	600	.05	30	40″
	Large	70	600	.1	60	40″

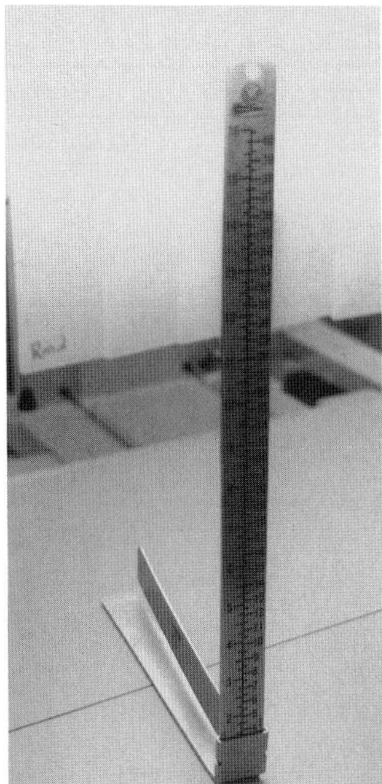

FIGURE 17–1. A caliper is used to measure the patient's body part to determine which technique to select from the technique chart.

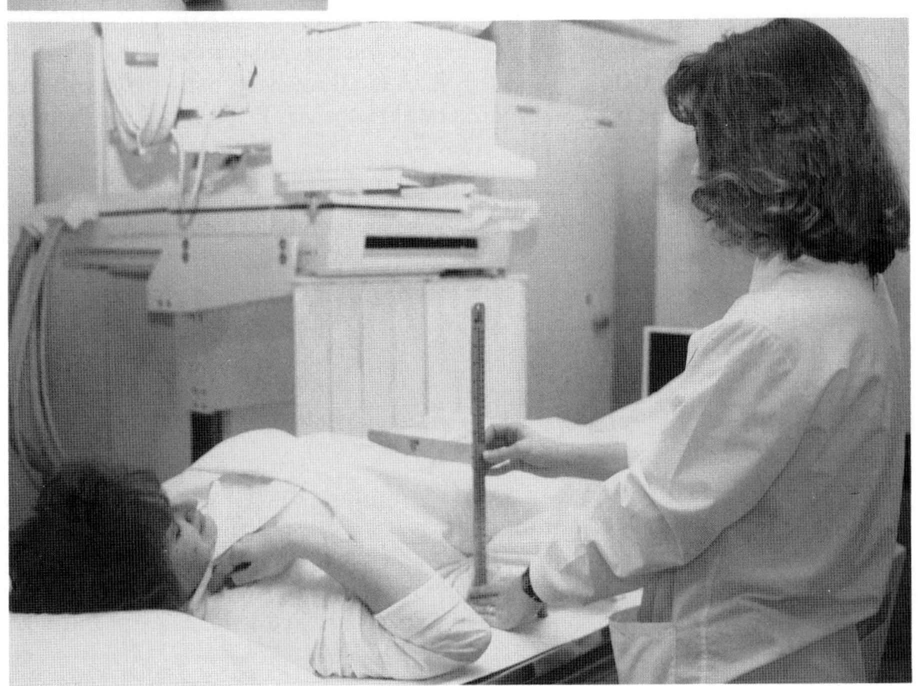

radiograph. For instance, 10 mAs might be used for all patients for a PA skull. For a small patient, a kVp of 60 might be used; for a medium-sized patient, a kVp of 70 might be used; and for a large patient, a kVp of 80 might be used. For the type of chart in which the patient's body part is measured, a difference of 1 cm in part measurement requires a change of 2 kVp. Table 17–2 shows an example of a variable kVp chart.

Table 17–2. A Variable kVp Technique Chart

Position	CM	kVp	mA	Time	mAs	SID	Comments
KUB	14	64	600	.04	24	40″	Measure at naval
	15	66	600	.04	24	40″	
	16	68	600	.04	24	40″	
	17	70	600	.04	24	40″	
	18	72	600	.04	24	40″	
	19	74	600	.04	24	40″	

In a variable kVp chart the mAs is kept the same for a body part and the kVp is varied according to the patient's size

FIXED kVp TECHNIQUE CHARTS

When using a fixed kVp chart, the kVp is kept the same for a particular body part, and the mAs is varied for patients of different sizes to produce the right density on the radiograph. For instance, 80 kVp might be used for all patients for a PA skull. For a small patient, 5 mAs might be used; for a medium-sized patient, 10 mAs might be used; and for a large patient, 15 mAs might be used. Table 17–3 shows an example of a fixed kVp chart.

In a fixed kVp chart the kVp is kept the same for a body part and the mAs is varied according to the patient's size

ADVANTAGES OF FIXED kVp CHARTS

There are several advantages of the fixed kVp chart over the variable kVp chart. Since mAs is the controlling factor for density, it makes sense to adjust only the mAs and not the kVp when the density needs to be changed for a larger or smaller patient. The fixed kVp chart allows the technologist to use the optimum kVp for the body part, since the optimum kVp should be chosen as the fixed kVp. The optimum kVp will

Table 17–3. A Fixed kVp Technique Chart

Position	CM	kVp	mA	Time	mAs	SID	Comments
KUB	14–16	70	600	.02	12	40″	Measure at naval
	17–19	70	600	.03	18	40″	
	20–22	70	600	.04	24	40″	
	23–25	70	600	.05	30	40″	
	26–28	70	600	.07	42	40″	
	29–31	70	600	.1	60	40″	

always be able to penetrate through the body part, it will produce sufficient radiographic contrast, and it will produce an acceptable level of scattered radiation. Optimum kVp was discussed in Chapter 8.

Fixed kVp charts are generally preferred over variable kVp charts.

Penetration of the Body Part

In order for a radiographic image to be produced, the kVp must be high enough to be able to penetrate through the body part. If the body part is not penetrated, the image will be very light (see Fig. 8–1).

When the kVp is varied to change the film density for a patient of a small size, the kVp is reduced. With a variable kVp chart, it is possible to reduce the kVp so far on a very small patient that the part would not be penetrated. The smallest body measurement group on a variable kVp chart usually calls for the minimum kVp that should be used for that body part. If a patient measures below the lowest measurement on the chart and the kVp is reduced further, that kVp will not be able to penetrate through the body part and the radiograph will be too light to show the image.

Since the optimum kVp is used for a fixed kVp chart, the kVp will always be able to penetrate through the body part.

Optimum kVp on a fixed kVp chart will always be able to penetrate through the body part.

Sufficient Radiographic Contrast

kVp is the controlling factor for radiographic contrast. If a low kVp is used, the image produced will show high contrast, which is a mostly black-and-white image. If a high kVp is used, the image produced will show low contrast, which is many gray tones.

When radiographs are produced of the same body part with a different kVp used for each exposure, as happens with a variable kVp chart, the contrast on each radiograph will be different. This results in images in which areas are penetrated too much when a high kVp is used and these same areas are not penetrated enough when a low kVp is used. Thus on one patient it would be possible to see some structures and on another patient these same structures would not be seen because the sizes of the patients varied and the kVp used on each patient was different.

Since the optimum kVp is used for a fixed kVp chart, the kVp will produce approximately the same radiographic contrast on every image of the same body part.

Optimum kVp on a fixed kVp chart produces a consistent radiographic contrast for a body part.

Acceptable Level of Scattered Radiation

The kVp is a major factor in determining the amount of scattered radiation produced on a radiograph. A high kVp generates more scattered radiation than a low kVp.

With a variable kVp chart, the kVp is varied for each radiograph within a body part category, and so the amount of scattered radiation will change for each radiograph.

A grid is used to control the amount of scattered radiation reaching the film. If a low kVp is used, it may not be necessary to use a grid; and if a high kVp is used, it will be necessary to use a grid. If a grid is necessary, a lower ratio grid should be used with a low kVp and a higher-ratio grid should be used with a high kVp. It could become confusing to decide whether a grid is necessary and what grid ratio should be used since the kVp is varied for each radiograph with a variable kVp chart.

Changing the grid or grid ratio for each exposure produces a varying amount of contrast for each radiograph. This changes the structures within the body that are penetrated and imaged on the radiograph. It is also necessary to change the exposure factors when a grid or different grid ratio is used.

Since the optimum kVp is used for a fixed kVp chart, the amount of scattered radiation produced is about the same for each radiograph in a body part category. Then it becomes a standard decision whether or not a grid is necessary, and if it is necessary, what grid ratio to use.

Optimum kVp on a fixed kVp chart produces about the same amount of scattered radiation for each radiograph, making the use of a grid a standard decision.

Other Advantages

Some other advantages of using a fixed kVp chart result from the fact that fixed kVp charts ordinarily use a higher kVp for the same body part than variable kVp charts. This higher kVp gives the patient a lower radiation dose, gives the radiographer more exposure latitude, and also achieves less chance of motion on the radiograph.

A higher kVp gives the patient a lower radiation dose because the photons in a high kVp beam have a higher energy than the photons in a low kVp beam. Photons with more energy, produced by a high kVp beam, tend to pass right through the patient's body without interacting with the atoms in the body. Photons with less energy, produced by a low kVp beam, are more easily absorbed by the atoms of the body. When photons are absorbed, the photons ionize the atoms of the body. Ionization, the removal of an electron from an atom, is what initiates radiation damage to the patient's body.

A higher kVp that is usually used with a fixed kVp chart gives the radiographer more exposure latitude than a lower kVp. Exposure latitude is room for error. This means that the exposure factors can be varied somewhat from what would be the ideal exposure, and the radiograph will still be diagnostic.

According to the 15% rule, the density on a radiograph will be doubled or halved if the kVp is changed by 15%. At 60 kVp it takes only a 9-kVp change (60 × 15% = 9) to double or halve the density. At 80 kVp, it takes a 14-kVp change (80 × 15% = 14) to double or halve the density. Therefore, if a radiographer uses a kVp that produces a density mistake of 9 kVp away from what would be the ideal kVp, the density mistake would have a greater effect on the radiograph with a low kVp beam than with a high kVp beam.

A higher kVp that is usually used with a fixed kVp chart will help control motion on the radiograph. According to the 15% rule, if a radiograph is produced with 70 kVp and 10 mAs, a radiograph with the same density can be produced with 80 kVp and 5 mAs. If the 500-mA station is used for both radiographs, the exposure time is only .01 second (500 mA × .01 = 5 mAs) with the technique of 80 kVp and 5 mAs. It will be .02 second (500 mA × .02 = 10 mAs) with the technique of 70 kVp and 10 mAs. The shorter time of .01 second achieves less chance of producing a radiograph with motion than the longer time of .02 second.

PRODUCING A TECHNIQUE CHART

What if your worst nightmare came true and you got a job in an x-ray facility and then found out that the facility did not have technique charts at all? How could you compensate for all the variations that exist among x-ray facilities, like different x-ray tubes, generators, intensifying screens, grid ratios, processor chemicals and temperatures, and many others? There is an easy way to produce a new technique chart from any working technique chart that compensates for all the variations with only one calculation.

At the new x-ray facility use a radiographic phantom and produce a radiograph with the suggested mAs and kVp from a working technique chart used in another x-ray facility. Then make a second exposure using one half of the suggested mAs. Then make a third exposure using two times the suggested mAs. Develop all three films and evaluate the radiographs to see which one produces the best density.

If the radiograph taken at double the suggested mAs is the best density, then all that needs to be done to produce a new technique chart is to double the mAs listed on the working technique chart for all exposures, assuming that all exposure conditions are the same. If the radiograph taken at half the suggested mAs is the best density, then the techniques on the working technique chart should all be cut in half for the new chart.

If the best density falls somewhere between the three phantom exposures, a correction factor needs to be calculated. Suppose the suggested mAs from the working technique chart is 6 mAs. One half of this mAs would be 3, and two times this mAs would be 12. After analyzing the three radiographs, let's say that the radiograph produced with 6 mAs is close to the correct density, but an mAs of 5 would be the best.

To calculate the correction factor, divide the corrected mAs of 5 by the suggested mAs of 6.

$$\frac{5}{6} = .83 \qquad \text{(the correction factor)}$$

To use this correction factor, multiply all the techniques from the working technique chart by .83 to get the techniques for the new chart. A conversion like this is not foolproof. The new technique chart will still need some fine tuning to perfect it.

ALTERING THE TECHNIQUE FROM THE CHART

A correctly formulated technique chart will only work about 85% of the time. A good technologist knows how to assess the patient and change the technique that is listed on the chart if necessary. The most common reasons for changing the technique listed on the chart are the patient's physical condition or possible pathology.

Patient's Physical Condition

The body part of a small patient will measure less, and the fixed kVp technique chart will call for a lower mAs. However, if a small patient has a high degree of muscular development, the radiograph may be light because it takes more mAs to produce an adequate density on a patient with a high degree of muscular development. If another patient is emaciated because of chronic disease, using the technique as listed on the chart may result in a radiograph that is too dark.

It takes some experience in judging the physique of a patient to learn when to make these adjustments. One easy way to make the changes is to go up or down to the next measurement category listed on the technique chart.

Pathology

Some pathology or disease conditions can alter the tissue density of patients' bones and can alter the tissue density of the contents in their chests and abdomens. Some of this pathology may require the technologist to increase the technique as listed on the chart to produce a good radiograph, and some pathology may require a technologist to decrease the technique as listed on the chart. Often the patient's pathology is indicated in the clinical history for the exam.

Decrease in Technique

Any disease the patient may have that results in bony destruction will require the technologist to reduce the technique as listed on the chart. Some of these diseases are osteoporosis, osteomyelitis, degenerative arthritis, sarcoma, multiple myeloma, bony metastasis, and osteomalacia.

Patients with emphysema retain stale air in their lungs. This increase in air in the lungs reduces the tissue density of the lungs and requires a reduction in technique.

Patients with a bowel obstruction may have a lot of trapped gas in their abdomens. This gas reduces the tissue density of the abdomen and requires a reduction in technique. The conditions requiring a decrease in technique are summarized in Table 17–4.

Increase in Technique

Any disease the patient may have that results in an addition of fluid to the body will require the technologist to increase the technique as listed on the chart. Any type of edema or swelling will require an increase in technique.

Many chest conditions result in extra fluid in the lungs, which requires an increase in technique. Some of these conditions are pulmonary edema, pleural effusion, pneumonia, congestive heart failure, and atelectasis.

Ascites is a condition that results in increased fluid in the abdomen and requires

Table 17–4. Conditions Requiring a Decrease in Technique

Osteoporosis	Bony metastasis
Osteomyelitis	Osteomalacia
Degenerative arthritis	Emphysema
Sarcoma	Bowel obstruction due to air
Multiple myeloma	

Table 17–5. Conditions Requiring an Increase in Technique

Edema	Congestive heart failure
Pulmonary edema	Atelectasis
Pleural effusion	Ascites
Pneumonia	Paget's disease

an increase in technique. A patient with ascites will have a distended abdomen that will feel spongy. A patient with a bowel obstruction who has trapped air will also have a distended abdomen but it will usually feel tight like a drum.

Paget's disease will require an increase in technique when bony parts are being radiographed because in this disease the bones become very dense. The conditions requiring an increase in technique are summarized in Table 17–5.

SUMMARY

The fixed kVp technique chart has some definite advantages over the variable kVp chart. The advantages are that the part will always be penetrated, a sufficient amount of radiographic contrast is produced, and an acceptable level of scattered radiation is produced. Fixed kVp charts require a higher kVp than variable kVp charts, which results in these advantages: the patient absorbs less radiation, a wider exposure latitude is achieved, and there is less chance of motion appearing in a radiograph.

To develop a technique chart, find a working technique chart and calculate a corrected mAs. Then multiply the corrected mAs by the suggested mAs as listed on the working technique chart.

About 15% of the time the technique as listed on the chart must be changed. This is because of an increase or decrease in the average physical development of the patient, or because the patient may have a type of pathology. Some of the pathologies require an increase in the technique as listed on the chart and some pathologies require a decrease in the technique.

PERFORM ACTIVITY 17.A

CHAPTER 18

AUTOMATIC EXPOSURE CONTROL

CHAPTER OUTLINE

OBJECTIVES

At the end of this chapter you should be able to:

- Define automatic exposure control.
- Explain how the photocell stops the exposure at the correct time for patients of different sizes.
- Determine how high to set the backup time.
- Explain why the optimum kVp should be used with automatic exposure control.
- Determine what photocell arrangement should be used for a body part.
- Explain what happens to radiographic density if the body part is not correctly positioned over the photocell.
- Describe how to change the density of an exposure made with automatic exposure control.
- Explain why the backup time must be set above the minimum reaction time.

Learning about the principles of radiographic exposure can be difficult. The end result of all this learning is the ability of the radiographer to choose the right accessories like grids and collimation, set the correct technique factors on the control panel, and evaluate the quality of the radiograph produced. Even with all this knowledge, sometimes the technique factors the radiographer sets on the control panel are not quite right because of the patient's size, tissue composition, or pathology. In this case the radiograph may not be the best, or it may even need to be repeated.

Wouldn't it be great if there were one button on the control panel that the radiographer could press that would compensate for variations in patients and produce a good radiograph each time? There is! It is called automatic exposure control or phototiming.

Automatic exposure control automatically stops the exposure at the right time so that a radiograph with good density is produced. The device used to do this is called a photocell.

If it sounds too good to be true, it is. When used correctly, automatic exposure control produces good radiographs. However, there are a lot of pitfalls that the radiographer must learn to avoid.

PHOTOCELLS

A photocell is the device used for automatic exposure control. A photocell is either an ionization chamber or a photomultiplier tube. Photocells are placed in or near the Bucky and cannot be seen. With automatic exposure control, the photocell instead of the x-ray timer determines the length of the x-ray exposure.

When exit radiation from the patient hits the photocell, a current is produced inside the photocell corresponding to how much exit radiation hit the photocell. A large current is produced with a large amount of exit radiation and a small current is produced with a small amount of exit radiation. The current produced inside the photocell charges the x-ray timer. When the x-ray timer receives a predetermined amount of charge from the photocell, the x-ray exposure is stopped.

The predetermined amount of charge is set so that the densities of the image will fall between .25 and 2.0 above base-plus-fog. This is the usual range of radiographic densities within the image.

If automatic exposure control is used on a large patient, it would take a long time for enough exit radiation to get through the patient and into the photocell to charge the x-ray timer to the predetermined amount of charge. The length of the x-ray exposure would then be long. For a smaller patient, it wouldn't take much time for enough radiation to get through the patient to charge the x-ray timer. In this case the length of the x-ray exposure would be short.

Photocells are usually arranged in a group of three (Fig. 18–1). A device on the control panel allows the radiographer to activate the photocells. The most common use is to activate both outside cells together, or just the center photocell by itself.

USING AUTOMATIC EXPOSURE CONTROL

When using automatic exposure control, several buttons or dials must be set on the control panel and these are very important for radiographic quality. These settings are the backup time, the kVp, the mA, the photocell arrangement, and the automatic exposure control density. Positioning the body part correctly is also very important.

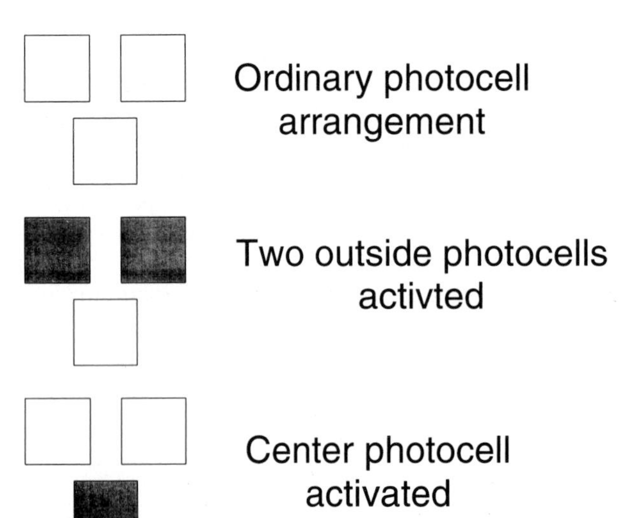

FIGURE 18–1. The two most common arrangements for activating the photocells are selecting the two outside photocells together or the center photocell by itself.

Backup Time

Automatic exposure control acts only on the exposure time. The length of the x-ray exposure is determined by how long it takes the exit radiation to charge the x-ray timer. When automatic exposure is used, the ordinary timer used for an exposure made without automatic exposure control is called a backup timer. The backup time must be set above the length of the expected exposure time.

The backup time must be set above the expected exposure time.

If the ordinary exposure time for a PA chest radiograph is .20 second, the backup time must be set above .20 second and the automatic exposure control will stop the exposure at .20 second. If the backup time is set at only .15 second, the exposure will be stopped at .15 second and the radiograph will turn out too light.

Some radiographers respond to this by setting the backup time very high so that it will always be above the expected exposure time. It is good radiation safety practice not to set the backup time too high since the backup time acts as a safety device. If the automatic exposure control does not work, the exposure will be stopped at the backup time setting. If the backup time is set very high, the patient would get a large exposure if the automatic exposure control fails to work properly. If the backup time is set low, the exposure to the patient is less if the automatic exposure control fails to work.

kVp

Automatic exposure control affects only the exposure time, and time controls density. kVp controls contrast and affects density. If the kVp is changed, the automatic exposure control will compensate with an adjustment in exposure time to adjust density. If the kVp is decreased, density decreases, so the automatic exposure control will increase the time to compensate for the decrease in kVp. If the kVp is increased, density increases, so the automatic exposure control will decrease the time to compensate for the increase in kVp. An increase or decrease in kVp when using automatic exposure control only changes the contrast on the radiograph, not density, so the kVp should not be varied when using automatic exposure control.

The optimum kVp for the body part being radiographed should always be selected. kVp determines the penetration of the body part, the contrast on the radiograph, and the amount of scattered radiation produced. The part may not be penetrated with a kVp that is too low, and too much scattered radiation will be produced with a kVp that is too high.

Optimum kVp should be used with automatic exposure control.

---

mA

Theoretically, any mA can be selected when using automatic exposure control and the radiograph will turn out all right. If a low mA is selected, the length of the exposure time will be increased by the photocell to produce adequate density. If a high mA is selected, the length of the exposure time will be decreased by the photocell to produce adequate density.

Ordinarily the best mA to choose is a high mA. This causes the actual exposure time to be as short as possible, which helps control motion on the radiograph. If a small focal spot is required, the mA must be low enough to be in the small focal spot range, and the exposure time will be long.

Use a high mA to keep the exposure time short.

Photocell Arrangement

The radiographer must decide which photocells to activate. Either the two outside photocells together or the center photocell alone is usually chosen. The two outside photocells should be used when the density of the body part over the two photocells is close to the same for each photocell. For example, the two outside photocells should be chosen for a PA chest, KUB, AP ribs, and pelvis radiographs.

The center photocell should be used for a body part whose center section is to be demonstrated on the radiograph. For example, the center photocell should be used for a lateral chest, AP or lateral spine, AP hip, and AP shoulder radiographs.

Activating the wrong photocell can cause the radiograph to turn out too light or too dark. If the center photocell is activated for a PA chest instead of the two outside photocells, the tissue density of the spine and mediastinum will lie over the activated photocell, and this tissue density will determine the actual length of the exposure rather than the tissue density in the two lungs. In this case the radiograph will be too dark (Fig. 18–2). If the center photocell is used for a KUB, the spine will determine the length of the exposure rather than the soft tissues of the abdomen and the radiograph will be too dark (Fig. 18–3).

PERFORM ACTIVITY 18.A

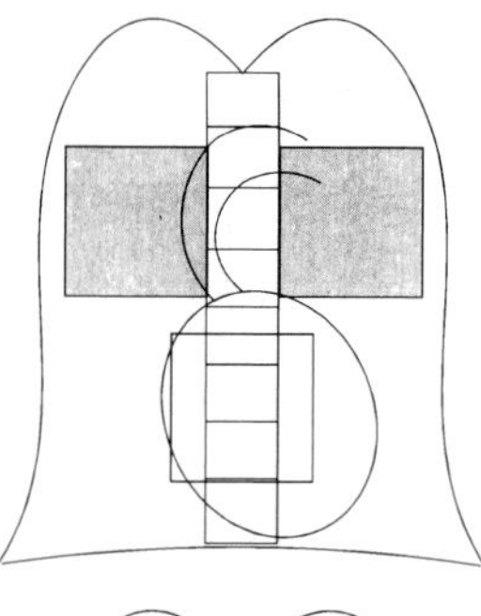

2 outside photocells activated

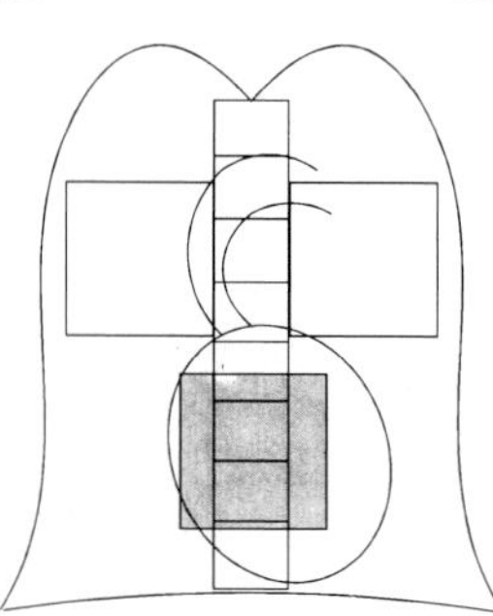

Center photocell activated

FIGURE 18–2. Selecting the two outside photocells for a PA chest causes the tissue density of the lungs to determine the length of the exposure. This is the correct arrangement. Selecting the center photocell for a PA chest causes the tissue density of the mediastinum and thoracic spine to determine the length of the exposure. In this case the radiograph will be too dark.

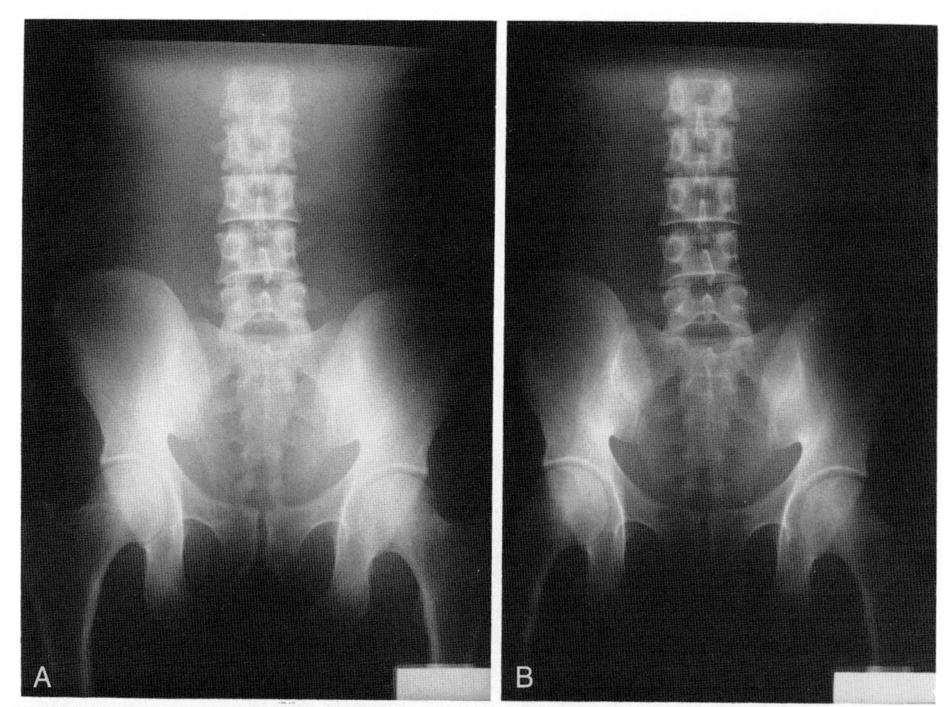

FIGURE 18–3. Selecting the two outside photocells for a KUB causes the soft tissues of the abdomen to determine the length of the exposure. This is the correct arrangement. (*A*) Radiograph was taken with the two outside photocells activated. Selecting the center photocell causes the spine to determine the length of the exposure. In this case the radiograph will be too dark. (*B*) Radiograph was taken with the center photocell activated and the radiograph is too dark to show the soft tissues of the abdomen.

Positioning the Body Part

Several factors need to be considered when positioning the body part over the photocell. A photocell determines the length of the exposure by averaging the tissue densities it detects, so the entire photocell must be covered by the body part. If the edge of a body part such as a shoulder or hip is positioned over the photocell, the photocell will detect some of the body part and some blank space. When the photocell averages the length of the exposure, the exposure will be too short and the radiograph will be light (Fig. 18–4).

The photocell must be completely covered by the body part.

PERFORM ACTIVITY 18.B

Proper positioning of the body part is very important when using automatic exposure control. The body part to be demonstrated on the radiograph must be placed directly over the photocell that is activated. If the body part is not over the photocell, the radiograph could be too light or too dark.

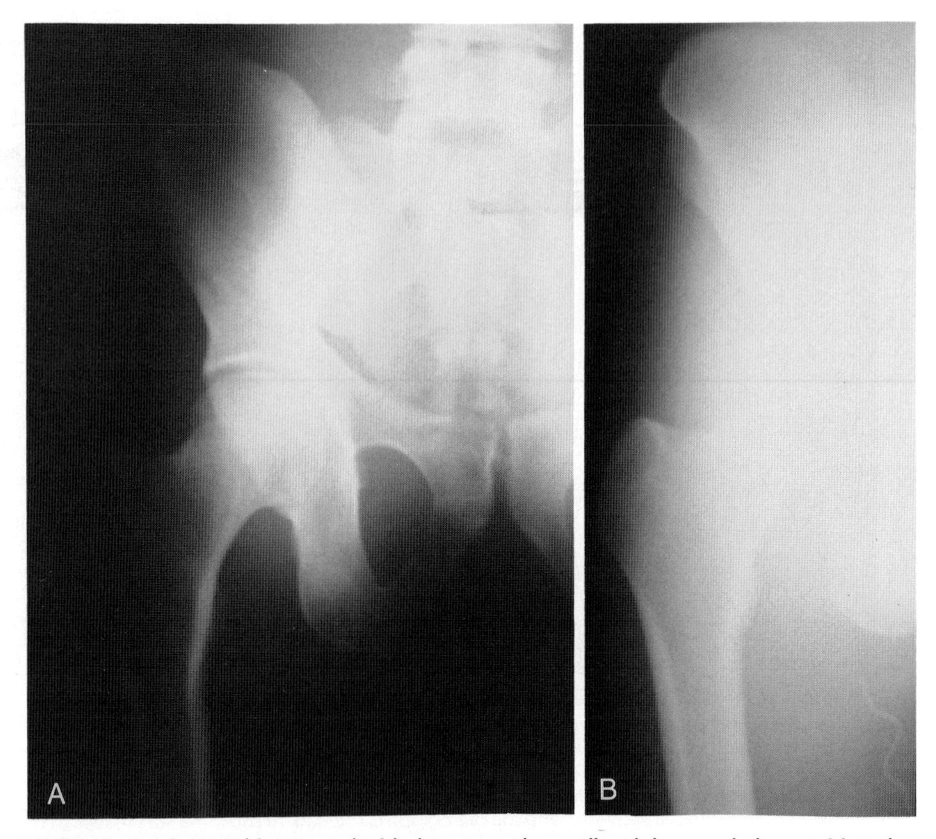

FIGURE 18–4. (*A*) An AP hip exposed with the center photocell and the acetabulum positioned over the center photocell. The density is correct. (*B*) An AP hip exposed with the center photocell and the greater trochanter positioned over the center photocell. Placing the edge of the body part over the photocell causes the radiograph to be too light.

For example, for an AP and lateral lumbar spine, the center photocell should be selected. If the spine is not positioned directly over this photocell, the radiograph will be too light (Fig. 18–5).

The body part to be demonstrated must be positioned over the photocell.

PERFORM ACTIVITY 18.C

Using the correct centering point for an exam is important with automatic exposure control. If the centering point for a PA chest is placed too low, the tissue that determines the length of the exposure will be the abdomen instead of the chest, and the radiograph will be too dark. If the centering point is placed too high, the tissue that determines the length of the exposure will be the thin upper part of the chest and the radiograph will be too light.

When using automatic exposure control for body parts that have had barium added to them, it is necessary to position the barium over the photocell that is activated. For example, the center photocell should be used for lateral and oblique stomach films during an upper gastrointestinal series. If the abdomen instead of the barium is over the photocell, the radiograph will be too light (Fig. 18–6).

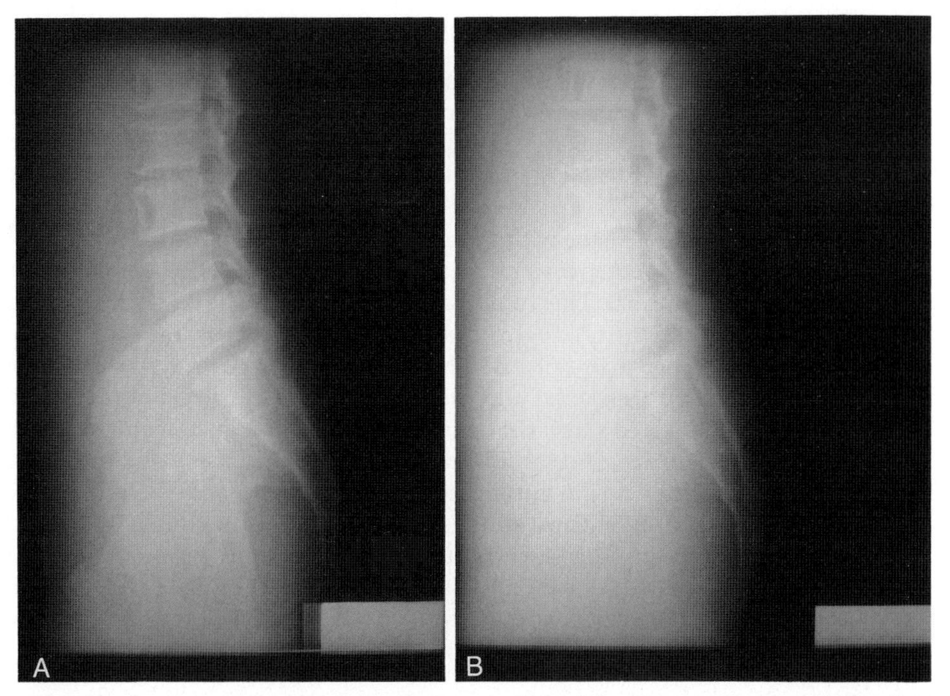

FIGURE 18–5. (*A*) A lateral lumbar spine that was positioned directly over the center photocell. (*B*) When radiograph was exposed, the spine was not over the center photocell and the radiograph is too light.

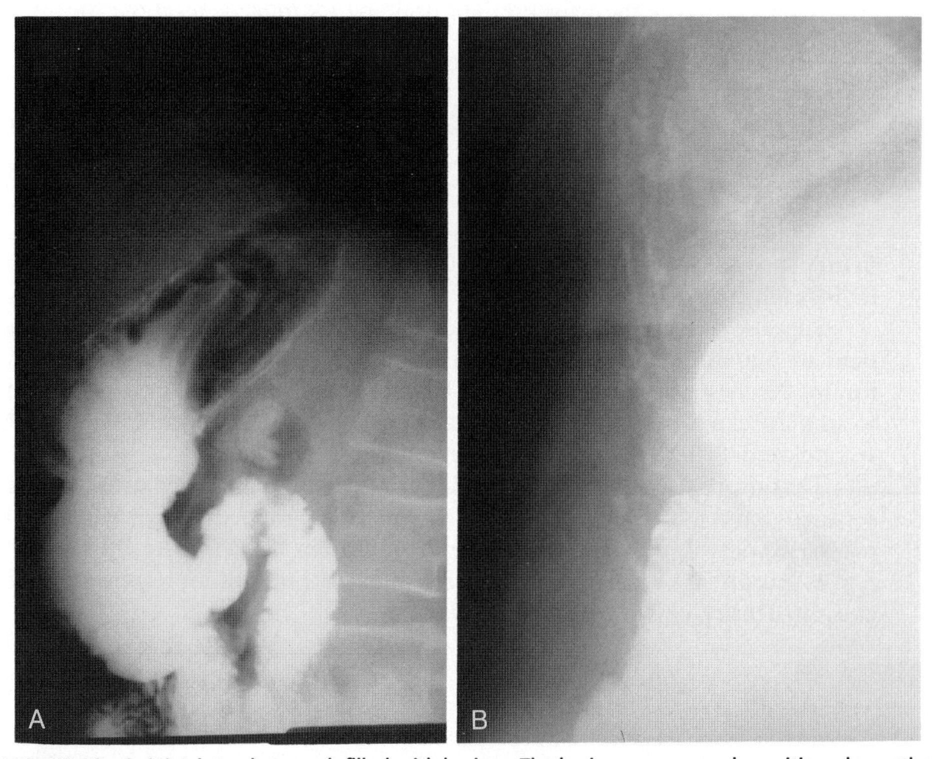

FIGURE 18–6. (*A*) A lateral stomach filled with barium. The barium was properly positioned over the center photocell. (*B*) Radiograph was taken with the barium not positioned over the center photocell, and the radiograph is too light.

Automatic Exposure Control Density

The density of the radiograph with automatic exposure control is determined by the predetermined charge setting on the timer. Under ordinary circumstances this normal setting works well. However, if the radiographer is presented with a patient who is extremely small or extremely large, the predetermined charge may need to be adjusted.

The adjustment is made with the automatic exposure control density settings. Setting the density one step lower than normal causes the exposure time to be about 30% shorter than normal. This could be used in the case of a very small or emaciated patient. Setting the density one step higher than normal causes the exposure time to be about 30% higher than normal. This could be used for a very large patient.

The only way to make an automatic exposure control radiograph darker or lighter than normal is to adjust the density settings. The adjustments normally used for an x-ray exposure have no effect when using automatic exposure control. Adjusting the mA up or down with automatic exposure control only forces the exposure time to be adjusted up or down by the photocells. Adjusting the timer up or down doesn't change the length of the exposure because the timer is only a backup timer. Adjusting the kVp up or down only changes the contrast on the radiograph not the density, since the automatic exposure control will adjust the exposure time to bring the density back to normal if the kVp is changed.

MINIMUM REACTION TIME

Another factor to consider when using automatic exposure control is the minimum reaction time. The minimum reaction time is the shortest time it takes for the photocells to decide to stop the exposure. The backup time must be set above the minimum reaction time.

The minimum reaction time is the shortest time it takes for the photocells to decide to stop the exposure.

If the minimum reaction time is .01 second, every exposure made with automatic exposure control will be at least .01 second long. Sometimes this can produce a radiograph that is too dark.

Suppose the very best exposure factors for a PA chest radiograph on a small patient are 600 mA, .005 second, and 110 kVp. If automatic exposure control is used for this PA chest, it would take at least .01 second for the automatic exposure control to stop the exposure. The exposure factors for the PA chest would be 600 mA, .01 second, and 110 kVp, and the image would be too dark.

The only way to avoid this is to reduce the mA on small patients. 600 mA at .005 second is 3 mAs. If the mA is reduced to 100 for the exposure made with automatic exposure control, the exposure factors would then be 100 mA, .03 second (also 3 mAs), and 110 kVp. The time of .03 is above the minimum reaction time of .01 and the density would be acceptable.

SUMMARY

Automatic exposure control automatically stops the exposure after a predetermined charge is reached on the exposure timer. This produces a radiograph with adequate density.

The ordinary exposure time is a backup time and it must be set above the expected exposure time. If the small focal spot is necessary, a low mA should be chosen. Otherwise a high mA should be used to keep the time short. The optimum kVp should be used to produce good contrast. Either the two outside photocells or the center photocell should be activated depending on the body part being radiographed. The normal density setting should be used except with an extremely large or small patient.

The entire body part must cover the photocell. Also, the area of interest in the body part must be positioned over the photocell that is activated.

With a very small patient, a lower mA should be used. This forces a compensating increase in exposure time, which puts the exposure time above the minimum reaction time of the automatic exposure control.

PERFORM ACTIVITY 18.D

APPENDIX A

BASIC MATH REVIEW

FRACTIONS

A fraction is a part of a whole unit. A fraction is written with one number over the other such as $\frac{1}{4}$, $\frac{2}{3}$, or $\frac{5}{8}$. The number above the line is called the numerator and the number below the line is called the denominator. If a whole unit is divided into four parts, the number 4 would be placed in the denominator. If the fraction is only dealing with three of the four parts, the number 3 would be placed in the numerator. This would form the fraction $\frac{3}{4}$.

Multiplying a Whole Number by a Fraction

To multiply a whole number by a fraction, first multiply the whole number by the numerator, then divide this answer by the denominator.

To multiply 300 by the fraction $\frac{2}{3}$:

$$300 \times \frac{2}{3} = \frac{600}{3} = 200$$

On a calculator:
Enter 300, multiply sign, 2, divide sign, 3, equal sign.

Dividing a Whole Number by a Fraction

To divide a whole number by a fraction, first invert the fraction so that the denominator is on top of the fraction and the numerator is on the bottom. Then multiply as shown above.

To divide 300 by the fraction $\frac{2}{3}$:
Invert the fraction: $\frac{2}{3}$ becomes $\frac{3}{2}$
Then multiply

$$300 \times \frac{3}{2} = \frac{900}{2} = 450$$

On a calculator:
Enter 300, multiply sign, 3, divide sign, 2, equal sign.

Finding the Least Common Denominator

In order to add or subtract several fractions with different denominators, the least common denominator must first be found. This is the lowest number that all the denominators will divide into evenly. You can find it experimentally or multiply all the denominators together. This, however, may yield a very large number that might not be the "least."

$$\frac{1}{2}\ \frac{2}{3}\ \frac{5}{6}\ \frac{3}{4} = \text{(The least common denominator is 12)}$$

$$\frac{5}{8}\ \frac{7}{12}\ \frac{3}{16}\ \frac{7}{24} = \text{(The least common denominator is 48)}$$

All the above fractions must be converted to a new fraction with the least common denominator in the denominator of all the new fractions. To do this, divide the denominator of each old fraction into the least common denominator, multiply the numerator of the old fraction by this number, and place the answer in the numerator of the new fraction.

$$\frac{1}{2}\ \frac{2}{3}\ \frac{5}{6}\ \frac{3}{4} = \frac{6}{12}\ \frac{8}{12}\ \frac{10}{12}\ \frac{9}{12}$$

$$\frac{5}{8}\ \frac{7}{12}\ \frac{3}{16}\ \frac{7}{24} = \frac{30}{48}\ \frac{28}{48}\ \frac{9}{48}\ \frac{14}{48}$$

Reducing Fractions

Reducing a fraction places the lowest number possible in both the numerator and denominator. First find the largest number that will divide equally into both the numerator and denominator. This is done by trial and error. Perform the division and form the new fraction.

$\frac{25}{45}$ reduces to $\frac{5}{9}$ (Each number was divided by 5)

$\frac{36}{48}$ reduces to $\frac{3}{4}$ (Each number was divided by 12)

Adding Fractions

After finding the least common denominator, adding the fractions is easy. Just add up all the numerators, place this answer in the numerator and the least common denominator in the denominator.

$\frac{6}{12}+\frac{8}{12}+\frac{10}{12}+\frac{9}{12}=\frac{33}{12}$ (This can be changed to $2\frac{3}{4}$)

$\frac{30}{48}+\frac{28}{48}+\frac{9}{48}+\frac{14}{48}=\frac{81}{48}$ (This can be changed to $1\frac{11}{16}$)

Subtracting Fractions

After finding the least common denominator, subtract the numerators, place this answer in the numerator, and the least common denominator in the denominator.

$\frac{2}{5}-\frac{1}{15}=\frac{6}{15}-\frac{1}{15}=\frac{5}{15}$ (Reduces to $\frac{1}{3}$)

Multiplying Fractions

To multiply one fraction by the other, multiply the numerators by each other, and place this answer in the numerator. Then do the same for the denominator.

$\frac{12}{17}\times\frac{5}{6}=\frac{12\times 5}{17\times 6}=\frac{60}{102}$ (Reduces to $\frac{10}{17}$)

Dividing Fractions

To divide one fraction by the other, the fraction that is doing the dividing (the divisor) must be inverted first. Then the two fractions are multiplied by each other as above.

$\frac{3}{4}\div\frac{2}{3}=\frac{3}{4}\times\frac{3}{2}=\frac{3\times 3}{4\times 2}=\frac{9}{8}$ (Reduces to $1\frac{1}{8}$)

DECIMALS

A decimal, like a fraction, is a way of expressing a part of a whole number. A number that has a period or decimal point in it is a decimal number. For example, .05, 1.08, and .45 are all decimals. The first number to the right of the decimal point holds the ten's place, the second number to the right holds the hundred's place, the third number to the right holds the thousand's place, and so on. The number or numbers to the left of the decimal point are whole numbers.

$$.5 = \frac{5}{10} \qquad .05 = \frac{5}{100} \qquad .005 = \frac{5}{1000}$$

Adding and Subtracting Decimals

When adding or subtracting decimals, it is essential to arrange the numbers so that the decimal points are lined up vertically before adding or subtracting the column of numbers.

$$\begin{array}{r} 1.57 \\ .30 \\ .02 \\ +\underline{21.39} \\ 23.28 \end{array} \qquad \begin{array}{r} 239.45 \\ \underline{-8.56} \\ 230.89 \end{array}$$

Multiplying Decimals

To multiply a decimal, arrange the numbers in columns. Perform the multiplications from right to left and line up each answer. Then add the column of answers. Count the total number of digits to the right of the decimal point in the numbers you are multiplying. Count this same number of places in the answer from the right to the left. Put the decimal point there in the answer.

Problem 1

$$\begin{array}{r} .835 \\ \times\ \underline{.902} \\ 1670 \\ \underline{75150\ \ } \\ 753170 \end{array} = .75317$$

(six decimal points)

Problem 2

$$\begin{array}{r} 7.53 \\ \times\ \underline{.87} \\ 5271 \\ \underline{6024\ \ } \\ 65511 \end{array} = 6.5511$$

(four decimal points)

On a calculator, for Problem 1, enter decimal point, 8, 3, 5, multiply sign, decimal point 9, 0, 2, equal sign; .75317 should be displayed. For Problem 2, enter 7, decimal point, 5, 3, multiply sign, decimal point, 8, 7, equal sign; 6.5511 should be displayed.

Dividing Decimals

When dividing decimals, swing the decimal point in the number you are dividing by from left to right to the end of the number. Then swing the decimal point in the number you are dividing into an equal number of places. You may need to fill this number in with zeros. Place the decimal point in the answer directly above where it is in the number you are dividing into. Then perform long division.

Problem 1

$$
\begin{array}{r}
8.75 \\
.20\overline{)1.75} = 20\overline{)175.00} \\
\underline{160} \\
150 \\
\underline{140} \\
100 \\
\underline{100} \\
0
\end{array}
$$

Problem 2

$$
\begin{array}{r}
6000 \\
.05\overline{)300} = 5\overline{)30000} \\
\underline{30} \\
0
\end{array}
$$

On a calculator, for Problem 1, enter 1.75, divide sign, .20, equal sign; 8.75 should be displayed. For Problem 2, enter 300, divide sign, .05, equal sign; 6000 should be displayed.

Converting Decimals to Fractions

To convert a decimal to a fraction, place the number in the decimal over 10, 100, 1000, etc., depending on how many places there are in the decimal. The fraction can then be reduced.

$$.15 = \frac{15}{100} \qquad 1.685 = \frac{1685}{1000} \qquad .02 = \frac{2}{100} \qquad .5 = \frac{5}{10}$$

To convert a fraction to a decimal, divide the denominator into the numerator.

$$\frac{1}{2} = .5 \qquad \frac{80}{250} = .32 \qquad \frac{2}{3} = .667 \qquad \frac{185}{368} = .503$$

PERCENTAGE

A percent is also a way of expressing a part of a whole number. Percent means per hundred or how many parts out of a hundred. Percents are always written with a percent sign (%) to the right of the number: 100%, 85%, 3%, 1500%. To perform calculations, the percent must first be converted to a decimal or a fraction. Then the calculations are performed just as if the percent were an ordinary decimal or fraction.

Converting Percentages to Decimals

To convert a percentage to a decimal, place a decimal point to the right of the numbers in the percent, move it to the left two places, and fill in zeros if necessary.

100% = 1.00   85% = .85   3% = .03   1500% = 15.00

To convert a decimal to a percentage, move the decimal point two places to the right, fill in zeros if necessary, and add a percent sign.

.53 = 53%   .1 = 10%   .002 = .2%   2.67 = 267%

Converting Percentages to Fractions

To convert a percentage to a fraction, first convert it to a decimal, then place the decimal without the decimal point over the corresponding 10, 100, or 1000 place it is holding.

$$53\% = .53 = \frac{53}{100} \qquad 10\% = .1 = \frac{1}{10}$$

To convert a fraction to a percentage, convert the fraction to a decimal, then move the decimal point two places to the right, and add a percent sign.

$$\frac{5}{8} = .625 = 62.5\% \qquad \frac{15}{32} = .47 = 47\%$$

Percentage Increase or Decrease

To increase or decrease a number by a certain percentage, first convert the percentage to a decimal. Then multiply the number by this decimal. This answer must be added to the original number to increase it or subtracted from the original number to decrease it.

Increase 300 by 30%

$$30\% = .30 \qquad 300 \times .30 = 90 \qquad 300 + 90 = 390$$

Increase 80 by 15%

$$15\% = .25 \qquad 80 \times .15 = 12 \qquad 80 + 12 = 92$$

Decrease 25 by 6%

$$6\% = .06 \qquad 25 \times .06 = 1.5 \qquad 25 - 1.5 = 23.5$$

Decrease 70 by 25%

$$25\% = .25 \qquad 70 \times .25 = 17.5 \qquad 70 - 17.5 = 52.5$$

ALGEBRA

Math operations can be performed with numbers or letters using algebra. A letter in algebra signifies an unknown quantity called a variable. The value of the unknown quantity can be discovered by solving an equation. In an equation all parts on one side of the equal sign are equal to all parts on the other side of the equal sign. When performing math functions on an equation, this equal relationship must be maintained by performing the same function on both sides of the equation or equal sign.

Subtract 5 from both sides or

$$\begin{aligned} x + 5 &= 42 \\ x + 5 - 5 &= 42 - 5 \\ x &= 37 \end{aligned} \qquad \begin{aligned} x + 5 &= 42 \\ x &= 42 - 5 \\ x &= 37 \end{aligned}$$

Divide both sides by 5 or

$$\begin{aligned} 5x &= 40 \\ \frac{5x}{5} &= \frac{40}{5} \\ x &= 8 \end{aligned} \qquad \begin{aligned} 5x &= 40 \\ x &= \frac{40}{5} \\ x &= 8 \end{aligned}$$

Order of Operations

In some algebraic expressions, several math functions need to be performed. It is important to perform them in the right order or the answer will be wrong. Always multiply and divide first, then add and subtract.

$x = 5(2) + 25$ (Multiply 5×2 first)
$x = 10 + 25$ (then add)
$x = 35$

Functions written inside parentheses are always performed before the functions outside the parentheses.

$x = 5(40 - 6 + 12)$ (Perform functions inside parentheses)
$x = 5(46)$
$x = 230$

RATIOS AND PROPORTIONS

A ratio is a fixed relationship between two quantities. It is written like a fraction, and actually is a fraction. All fractions are ratios. A ratio indicates how many times larger or smaller one number is than the other. In the ratio $\frac{1}{2}$, the denominator is always twice as big as the numerator.

$$\frac{1}{2} = \frac{2}{4} = \frac{5}{10} = \frac{20}{40} = \frac{50}{100}$$

A proportion is a statement showing that two ratios are equal.

$$\frac{a}{b} = \frac{c}{d}$$ (a is to b as c is to d)

A proportion is an equation, and an unknown value in the proportion can be found by solving like algebra. The easiest way to find the unknown is to cross-multiply first, then solve the equation. When cross-multiplying, an equation is formed. Cross-multiply by multiplying the factor in the top left of the proportion by the factor in the bottom right of the proportion, and place this answer on the left side of the equation. Then multiply the factor in the top right of the proportion by the factor in the bottom left of the proportion, and place this answer on the right side of the equation. Then solve the equation.

Cross-multiply:

$\frac{a}{b} = \frac{c}{d}$ becomes $ad = cb$

$\frac{2}{5} = \frac{4}{d}$ becomes $2d = 5(4) = 2d = 20$ $d = 10$

$\frac{x}{12} = \frac{3}{8}$ becomes $8x = 12(3) = 8x = 36$ $x = 4.5$

Two numbers can be directly proportional or inversely proportional. If they are directly proportional, they both change in the same direction. If one is increased, the other is increased by the same amount. If they are inversely proportional, they change in opposite directions. If one is increased, the other is decreased by the same amount.

Direct proportion

1 increase this number by 3 times = 3
2 this number also increases by 3 times = 6

Inverse proportion

4 increase this number by 3 times = 12
6 decrease this number by 3 times = 2

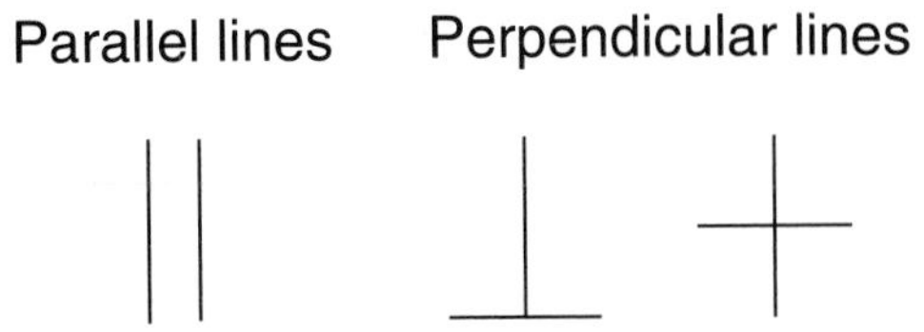

Parallel lines Perpendicular lines

FIGURE A–1. Parallel and perpendicular lines.

EXPONENTS

An exponent is written above another number called the base. The exponent indicates how many times the base is multiplied by itself. If the exponent 2 is used, this is called squaring the number.

(exponent)
10^2 (base) (multiply $10 \times 10 = 100$)

(exponent)
10^3 (base) (multiply $10 \times 10 \times 10 = 1000$)

GEOMETRY

Geometry is the science of lines and planes. It deals with angles and figures that are formed by lines. If two lines are parallel to each other, they are equidistant from each other at every point and therefore will never meet or cross each other. If two lines are perpendicular to each other, they meet or cross each other and form a 90 degree angle (Fig. A–1).

If two straight lines meet at a point, they form an angle. The number of degrees in the angle is measured at the point where the two lines meet (Fig. A–2). The maximum number of degrees in an angle is 360, which is the same number of degrees in a circle. A straight line measures 180 degrees.

Triangles

A triangle is a three-sided figure. The total number of degrees in a triangle is always equal to 180. A right triangle has one angle that is a right angle or 90 degrees (Fig. A–3). The sum of the degrees in the other two angles must equal 90 degrees.

Two triangles are similar if all three pairs of corresponding angles are equal. Similar means that the two triangles are the same shape but not necessarily the same

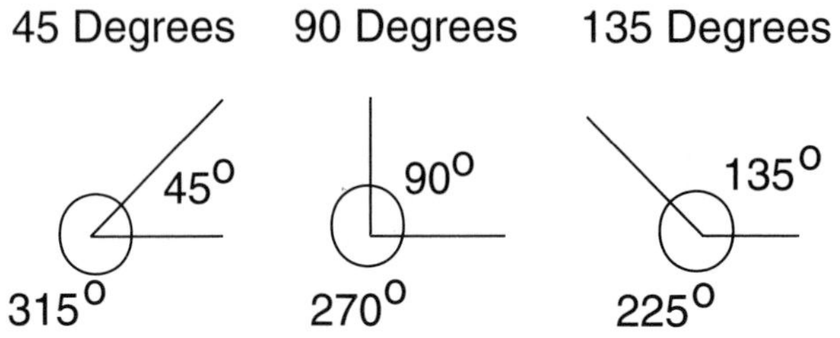

45 Degrees 90 Degrees 135 Degrees

45° 90° 135°

315° 270° 225°

FIGURE A–2. Angles.

A triangle

A right triangle

FIGURE A–3. Triangles.

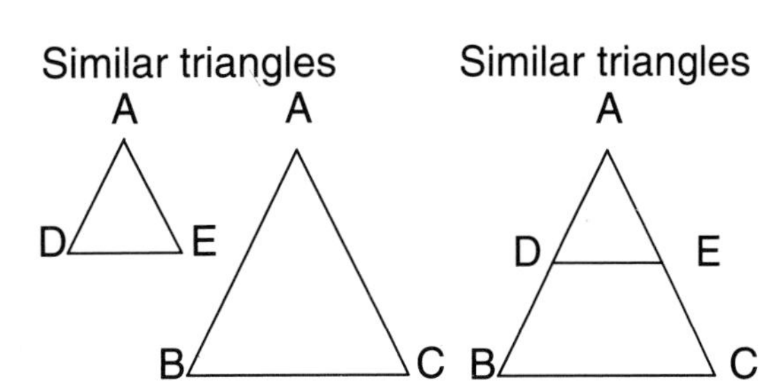

FIGURE A–4. Similar triangles.

size. One triangle may look larger than the other but they are still similar. If a line (line *DE*) is drawn that passes through a triangle (triangle *ABC*), and the line is parallel to the base of the triangle, two triangles are formed that are similar to each other (Fig. A–4).

Triangle *ADE* is similar to triangle *ABC*. Line *BC* is longer than line *DE*. In radiography, line *DE* represents the object being radiographed and line *BC* represents the image of the object. The image of the object is always larger than the actual object.

APPENDIX B

ANSWERS TO ACTIVITIES

ACTIVITY 1.D

1. c	5. c	8. d
2. b	6. b	9. a
3. a	7. d	10. b
4. a		

ACTIVITY 2.B

Puzzle Solution

```
           E H C M
       R COLLIMATOR
   WINDOW  E G T L
  F    T   C H H Y
  I FILAMENTS  O B
  L O  T   R   D D
  A C LEAD O C E E
  M U  S   N O   N
  E S   EMISSION U
  N I        L   M
  TUNGSTEN      M
    G   N   TARGET
        V B   H T
    G  NEGATIVE A
  V L   L K   N L
  A A PROTECT I   A
FOCUS   P D CURRENT
  U SAUCER    M   O
  U               D
  M            PYREX
```

ACTIVITY 2.C

10 electrons lose energy
4 the filament boils off electrons
____ a vacuum is created in the metal housing
____ electrons are aimed at the patient
12 the focal spot is formed
5 electrons form a space charge

2 the filament gets hot
___ the focusing cup becomes positive
3 the filament glows
13 x-rays are emitted isotropically
1 current runs through the filament circuit
___ the large focal spot changes into the small focal spot
___ the tungsten filament wire melts
7 electrons are attracted by the anode
11 light, heat, and x-rays are produced
___ the anode repels the electrons
___ 98% of the electron energy is converted to x-ray energy
___ the electrons in the space charge fly out of the tube
___ the other filament gets heated
9 electrons slam into the anode at the target
8 electrons move over to the anode
6 electrons are repelled from the focusing cup
14 x-rays are absorbed by the glass and metal housings

ACTIVITY 2.D

```
+ + + + D I V E R G E T I H W
L + + I N V I S I B L E + + +
I P + H E T E R O G E N O U S
G E O B I O L O G I C + E F R
H N D L T H G I A R T S L + O
T E O E Y + + + + N R U C + H
S T + I B E + + O + O L I I P
C R + + T R N T + R M A T S S
A A + Y + A O E E + A C R O O
T T S + R H Z S R + G O A T H
T I + S P A C I B G N F P R P
E N X + E E M L N A E + M O +
R G + E N T A I + O T T L P +
+ + + C + C T + R + I + I I +
D A E L K + + E + P C + F C +
```

ACTIVITY 2.E

1. b	6. c	11. d	16. b	21. b
2. c	7. c	12. c	17. c	22. d
3. a	8. a	13. b	18. a	23. c
4. b	9. b	14. c	19. c	24. a
5. d	10. d	15. a	20. a	25. d

ACTIVITY 3.A

1. SID; source-image distance
2. FFD; focus-film distance
3. OID; object-image distance
4. OFD; object-film distance
5. SOD; source-object distance
6. FOD; focus-object distance
7. 44
8. 5
9. 65
10. 64
11. 44
12. 14
13. 4
14. 68
15. 55

ACTIVITY 3.E

1. 6.35	6. 1.09	11. 96	16. 167%
2. 4.29	7. 1.16	12. 3.6 × 6	17. 25%
3. 2.86	8. 1.25	13. 2	18. 171%
4. 4.57	9. 1.17	14. 7.2	19. 100%
5. 6.89	10. 1.75	15. 10	20. 5.3%

ACTIVITY 3.H

1. b	6. d	11. 50	16. 63
2. c	7. c	12. 68	17. 33%
3. d	8. b	13. 2	18. 2
4. a	9. d	14. 7.84	19. 1.125
5. a	10. d	15. 7.84	20. 5.2

ACTIVITY 4.F

1. d	6. b	11. a
2. c	7. c	12. a
3. a	8. d	13. c
4. d	9. b	14. b
5. c	10. a	15. d

ACTIVITY 4.G

Crossword Puzzle Solution

```
     OID
     B  SOD F I
     J   I  O N
     E FFD  R C
   D C  I  HEART  M
  CENTRAL   S E   A
   C    M   H A   G
 E R        O SEVEN
DIVERGENT THREE   I
 G A        T   M F
 H S      F E S O I
 T ELONGATION H R C
      I   F IMAGE A
S A   N   TEN P   T
PARALLEL  Y G E  SID
A E      S        O
T A SUPERIMPOSITION
I        Z
A    PERPENDICULAR
L
```

ACTIVITY 4.H

Definitions and Sentence Completion

1. four
2. angle
3. short
4. three
5. SID
6. elongated
7. fifty
8. close
9. increases
10. edge
11. long, OID
12. superimposed, separated
13. spatial
14. larger
15. ideal, parallel, perpendicular
16. shape
17. SOD
18. fifteen
19. less
20. film

ACTIVITY 4.H

Puzzle Solution

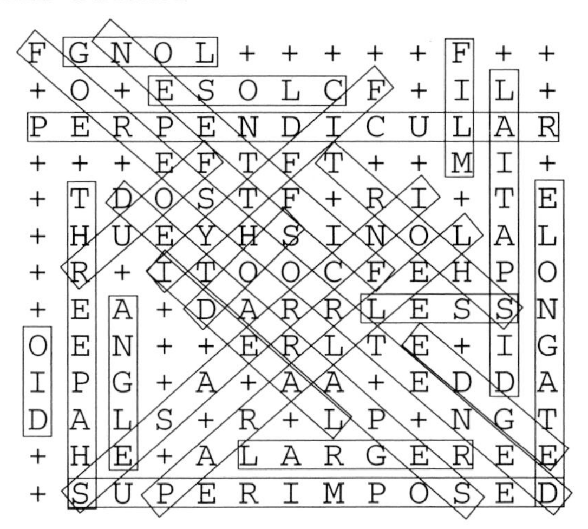

ACTIVITY 4.I

1. a
2. a
3. b
4. d
5. c
6. a
7. b
8. b
9. d
10. c
11. a
12. b
13. d
14. a
15. a
16. c
17. d
18. b
19. a
20. b

ACTIVITY 5.D

1. .010
2. .250
3. .008
4. .400
5. 1.250
6. .620
7. .015
8. .005
9. 10.000
10. .180
11. $\frac{320}{1000}$; $\frac{8}{25}$
12. $\frac{5}{1000}$; $\frac{1}{200}$
13. $\frac{1000}{1000}$; 1
14. $\frac{12}{1000}$; $\frac{3}{250}$
15. $\frac{15000}{1000}$; 15
16. $\frac{80}{1000}$; $\frac{2}{25}$
17. $\frac{25}{1000}$; $\frac{1}{40}$
18. $\frac{480}{1000}$; $\frac{12}{25}$
19. $\frac{6}{1000}$; $\frac{3}{500}$
20. $\frac{90}{1000}$; $\frac{9}{100}$
21. 450
22. 800
23. 1000
24. 28
25. 4
26. 16
27. 200
28. 180
29. 380
30. 1500
31. 20
32. 300
33. 15
34. 8
35. 1200
36. 10
37. 200
38. 80
39. 40
40. 500

ACTIVITY 5.E

1. 35
2. 25
3. 3
4. 20
5. 75
6. 2.8
7. 17.5
8. 20
9. 150
10. 12.5
11. 10
12. 80
13. 50
14. 120
15. 40
16. 150
17. 45
18. 100
19. 10
20. 100
21. 15
22. 64
23. 96
24. 1.5
25. 2.5
26. 200
27. 5
28. 35
29. 20
30. 2.4

ACTIVITY 5.G

1. 2.5
2. 75
3. 12.5
4. 50
5. 75
6. 250
7. 100
8. 17.5
9. 100
10. 2.5
11. 5
12. 2.5
13. 10
14. 30
15. 60
16. 15
17. 25
18. 5
19. 20
20. 30

ACTIVITY 5.H

1. 10
2. 75
3. 12.5
4. 3.33
5. 30
6. 15
7. 10
8. 20
9. 10
10. 3
11. 50
12. 50
13. 200
14. 300
15. 600
16. 400
17. 600
18. 400
19. 200
20. 1200
21. .03
22. .5
23. .05
24. .025
25. .075
26. .04
27. .10
28. .008
29. .06
30. .10

ACTIVITY 5.I

	mA	Time		mA	Time
1.	1200	.01	16.	1000	$\frac{1}{20}$
2.	800	.005	17.	600	$\frac{1}{40}$
3.	1000	.02	18.	1000	$\frac{1}{120}$
4.	800	.02	19.	300	$\frac{1}{40}$
5.	1200	.005	20.	1200	$\frac{1}{60}$
6.	1200	.025	21.	1000	5
7.	1000	.01	22.	1200	10
8.	1000	.015	23.	1000	10
9.	1000	.005	24.	1000	4
10.	1200	.015	25.	1000	32
11.	1200	$\frac{1}{120}$	26.	1200	12.5
12.	800	$\frac{1}{120}$	27.	1200	2.5
13.	1200	$\frac{1}{30}$	28.	1000	25
14.	1200	$\frac{1}{40}$	29.	1000	8
15.	600	$\frac{1}{120}$	30.	1000	16

ACTIVITY 5.J

	mA	Time		mA	Time
1.	200	.07	16.	200	$\frac{1}{10}$
2.	200	.02	17.	200	$\frac{1}{5}$
3.	200	.10	18.	200	$\frac{1}{4}$
4.	100	.15	19.	200	$\frac{1}{120}$
5.	200	.03	20.	200	$\frac{1}{30}$
6.	200	.015	21.	200	25
7.	200	.05	22.	200	12.5
8.	25	3.0	23.	200	50
9.	100	.25	24.	200	20
10.	200	.025	25.	200	10
11.	50	$\frac{1}{4}$	26.	100	150
12.	200	$\frac{1}{20}$	27.	200	25
13.	100	$\frac{1}{40}$	28.	200	2
14.	200	$\frac{1}{40}$	29.	200	40
15.	200	$\frac{1}{60}$	30.	200	80

ACTIVITY 5.K

	mA	Time		mA	Time
1.	50	.3	11.	25	$\frac{4}{5}$
2.	25	2	12.	50	$\frac{3}{5}$
3.	25	.4	13.	25	$\frac{3}{5}$
4.	25	.2	14.	100	$\frac{4}{5}$
5.	100	.4	15.	25	$\frac{1}{2}$
6.	25	.5	16.	25	3
7.	25	1	17.	25	1
8.	50	.4	18.	25	2
9.	25	.7	19.	25	$\frac{2}{5}$
10.	25	.30	20.	50	$\frac{4}{5}$

ACTIVITY 5.L

1. 7.5
2. 3.5
3. 6.0
4. 1.25
5. 18
6. 20
7. 3.0
8. .75
9. 9.96
10. 3.33
11. 50
12. 200
13. 200
14. 25
15. 600
16. 100
17. 300
18. 400
19. 100
20. 500
21. 7 msec; .007
22. 15 msec; .015
23. 8.3 msec; $\frac{1}{120}$; .0083
24. 5 msec; .005
25. 30 msec; .030
26. 20 msec; .02
27. 35 msec; .035
28. 16.6 msec; $\frac{1}{60}$; .0166
29. 25 msec; $\frac{1}{40}$; .025
30. 20 msec; .020

ACTIVITY 5.M

1. a
2. c
3. d
4. b
5. c
6. b
7. d
8. a
9. b
10. a
11. d
12. b
13. a
14. d
15. a
16. a
17. c
18. c
19. a
20. d
21. 7.5 mAs
22. .03 sec; $\frac{3}{100}$; 30 msec
23. 1000 mA
24. .2 sec; $\frac{2}{10}$; 200 msec
25. 10 mAs
26. .02 sec; $\frac{2}{100}$; 20 msec
27. 600 mA
28. 10 mAs; 10 mAs
29. 200 mA
30. .10 sec; $\frac{10}{100}$; 100 msec

ACTIVITY 6.B

1. 27.8 mR
2. 81.4 mR
3. 19.3 mR
4. .67 mR
5. 14.9 mR
6. 6.5 mR
7. 44.4 mR
8. 98 mR
9. 116 mR
10. 360 mR
11. 400 mR
12. 43 mR
13. 276 mR
14. 7.8 mR
15. 242 mR

ACTIVITY 6.C

1. 2.5 mR
2. 37.5 mR
3. 11.3 mR
4. 3.75 mR
5. 1.25 mR
6. 80 mR
7. 100 mR
8. 200 mR
9. 32 mR
10. 1440 mR
11. 7.5 mR
12. 12.5 mR
13. 1.5 mR
14. 3 mR
15. .75 mR
16. 160 mR
17. 240 mR
18. 88 mR
19. 72 mR
20. 600 mR

ACTIVITY 6.E

1. 9.3 mAs
2. 7.9 mAs
3. 5.7 mAs
4. 1.4 mAs
5. 22.5 mAs
6. 13 mAs
7. 38.4 mAs
8. 408 mAs
9. 21.3 mAs
10. 288 mAs
11. 7.5 mAs
12. 5.7 mAs
13. 11 mAs
14. 3.9 mAs
15. 67.5 mAs
16. 126 mAs
17. 240 mAs
18. 79 mAs
19. 86.4 mAs
20. 338 mAs

ACTIVITY 6.G

1. .015 sec
2. $\frac{1}{5}$ sec
3. 11.3 msec
4. .07 sec
5. $\frac{1}{20}$ sec
6. 13 msec
7. .22 sec
8. 234 msec
9. $\frac{1}{10}$ sec
10. .07 sec

ACTIVITY 6.H

1. 12.5
2. 40
3. 2
4. 25
5. 6.25
6. 64
7. 280
8. 3
9. 16
10. 128
11. .025
12. $\frac{1}{10}$
13. 5 msec
14. .10
15. $\frac{1}{8}$
16. 60 msec
17. $\frac{1}{20}$
18. .28
19. 1.0
20. 144 msec

ACTIVITY 6.I

1. 40.8 mAs
2. 4.4 mAs
3. 13.5 mAs
4. 288 mAs
5. 11.3 mAs
6. 8.3 mAs
7. 67.5 mAs
8. 6.7 mAs
9. 31.6 mAs
10. 45.4 mAs

ACTIVITY 6.J

1. a	11. 4.6 mR
2. d	12. 4.1 mR
3. b	13. 13.5 mR
4. c	14. 238 mR
5. d	15. 14.9 mR
6. a	16. 26 mAs
7. d	17. 14.4 mAs
8. b	18. 235 mAs
9. d	19. 45.3 mAs
10. d	20. 144 mAs

ACTIVITY 7.D

1. c	6. a	11. b	16. a	21. a
2. a	7. b	12. a	17. c	22. a
3. a	8. c	13. b	18. c	23. c
4. b	9. a	14. a	19. a	
5. d	10. a	15. b	20. a	

kVp	Photon Energy	Radiographic Contrast	Contrast Scale	Penetrating Ability
High	**High**/Low	High/**Low**	Short/**Long**	**High**/Low
High/**Low**	High/**Low**	**High**/Low	Short	High/**Low**

ACTIVITY 8.B

1. 80	6. 46	11. 6	16. 15
2. 77	7. 98	12. 20	17. 200
3. 64	8. 59	13. 7.5	18. 36
4. 69	9. 61	14. 14	19. 20
5. 85	10. 76	15. 60	20. 120

ACTIVITY 8.C

1. 30 mAs; 68 kVp	11. 5 mAs; 103 kVp
2. 40 mAs; 77 kVp	12. 7.5 mAs; 80 kVp
3. 64 mAs; 72 kVp	13. 4.5 mAs; 78 kVp
4. 240 mAs; 70 kVp	14. 25 mAs; 85 kVp
5. 48 mAs; 94 kVp	15. 50 mAs; 69 kVp
6. 2.5 mAs; 69 kVp	16. 19 mAs; 63 kVp
7. 25 mAs; 84 kVp	17. 13 mAs; 98 kVp
8. 6 mAs; 101 kVp	18. 7 mAs; 88 kVp
9. 12.5 mAs; 90 kVp	19. 21 mAs; 76 kVp
10. 4 mAs; 76 kVp	20. 20 mAs; 90 kVp

ACTIVITY 8.E

1. 60 kVp	6. 80 kVp	11. 5 mAs	16. 12.5 mAs
2. 80 kVp	7. 90 kVp	12. 30 mAs	17. 180 mAs
3. 85 kVp	8. 68 kVp	13. 3.5 mAs	18. 16 mAs
4. 70 kVp	9. 62 kVp	14. 80 mAs	19. 28 mAs
5. 75 kVp	10. 66 kVp	15. 220 mAs	20. 12 mAs

ACTIVITY 8.F

1. b	11. a	21. 70 kVp
2. a	12. b	22. 80 kVp
3. e	13. a	23. 57 kVp
4. e	14. d	24. 70 kVp
5. c	15. b	25. 85 kVp
6. b	16. a	26. 7.5 kVp
7. d	17. b	27. 12 mAs
8. c	18. a	28. 10 mAs
9. a	19. d	29. 34 mAs
10. d	20. b	30. 6.25 mAs

ACTIVITY 8.G

1. b	21. c	41. 50 mAs
2. a	22. a	42. .15 sec
3. a	23. b	43. 50 mA
4. b	24. b	44. 40 mAs
5. c	25. c	45. .10 sec
6. a	26. a	46. 82.7 mR
7. c	27. b	47. 12.5 mR
8. b	28. b	48. 56 mR
9. a	29. b	49. 18 mR
10. a	30. d	50. 3.75 mR
11. c	31. d	51. 40.5 mAs
12. a	32. a	52. 53.3 mAs
13. c	33. d	53. 2.2 mAs
14. d	34. a	54. 21.3 mAs
15. d	35. b	55. 400 mAs
16. c	36. d	56. 8.5 mAs
17. b	37. d	57. 110 mAs
18. a	38. a	58. 85 kVp
19. b	39. b	59. 85 kVp
20. a	40. b	60. 70 kVp

ACTIVITY 8.H

Definitions and Sentence Completions

1. eight
2. direct
3. ten
4. iodine
5. four
6. high
7. bone
8. thirty
9. reciprocity
10. five
11. forty
12. mAs
13. attenuation
14. kVp
15. low
16. motion
17. decrease
18. primary
19. quantity
20. half

ACTIVITY 8.H

Puzzle Solution

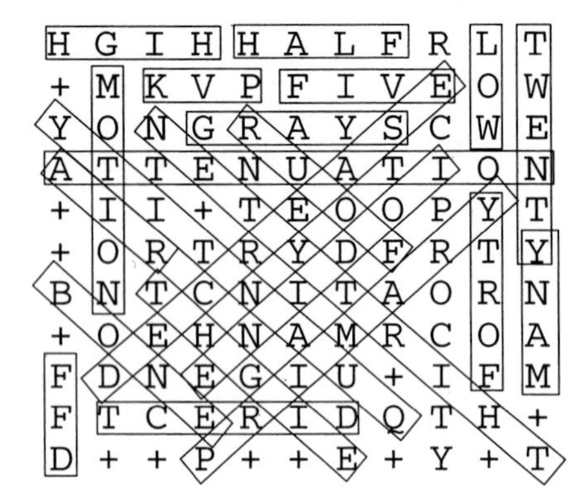

ACTIVITY 8.I

Crossword Puzzle Solution

```
 S  SIMILAR
 H      O  BEAM  E
 AFFECT W  A     L L
 D   O  E  R     E O
 E PENETRATING SEVEN
 S   T     U   U E G
  SHORT    M   B N
K    O         J  I
I  MILLIAMPERAGE ONE
L  I     A     C  T
O  LESS  S SCATTERED
V  L  A   B       N
OPTIMUM MORE   K  S
L  S  E   E  D V  I
TIME      A COMPACT
A  CONTRAST  W    Y
G  O I    H ENERGY
E  N N    I     R
 SID E  DENSITY A
          G     Y
```

ACTIVITY 9.H

1. 30 mAs
2. 2.5 mAs
3. 4 mAs
4. 13.3 mAs
5. 7.5 mAs
6. 25 mAs
7. 4.8 mAs
8. 24 mAs
9. 30 mAs
10. 62.5 mAs
11. 26.7 mAs
12. 70 mAs
13. 1.6 mAs
14. 10 mAs
15. 72 mAs

ACTIVITY 9.J

1. c
2. a
3. c
4. d
5. a
6. d
7. a
8. b
9. d
10. b
11. c
12. a
13. c
14. d
15. a
16. c
17. b
18. b
19. c
20. a
21. d
22. a
23. b
24. c
25. d
26. 33.3 mAs
27. 2.3 mAs
28. 2.4 mAs
29. 80 mAs
30. 7.5 mAs

ACTIVITY 10.A

1. 18.75 mAs	6. 8.93 mAs	11. 21 mAs
2. 6.44 mAs	7. 2.8 mAs	12. 16 mAs
3. 9.6 mAs	8. 13.6 mAs	13. 5.6 mAs
4. 71.4 mAs	9. 2.2 mAs	
5. 8.96 mAs	10. 3.57 mAs	

ACTIVITY 10.F

1. b	6. c	11. a	16. a	21. a
2. b	7. b	12. b	17. d	22. d
3. d	8. b	13. a	18. d	23. b
4. a	9. b	14. c	19. c	24. a
5. b	10. a	15. a	20. b	25. b

ACTIVITY 10.G

1. d	11. a	21. c	31. c
2. b	12. c	22. d	32. d
3. c	13. c	23. a	33. d
4. b	14. a	24. d	34. c
5. a	15. c	25. a	35. c
6. a	16. d	26. b	
7. a	17. b	27. b	
8. c	18. c	28. a	
9. d	19. a	29. b	
10. a	20. d	30. b	

ACTIVITY 10.H

Crossword Puzzle Solution

```
  FOCAL  AIRGAP
     C       D
MIRROR LOW   D  T
     O E   P EIGHT
     SCATTERED  I
 BLURS D   I    N
      H    M D
S     INCREASE  F
H C   G  A R CUTOFF
U O  SHORT Y R  C
T L  C   I   E BUCKY
T L  A   O   A  S
E I  T    C  S WEDGE
R M  T  TWELVE  D
SMALLER   N
  T  R CONTRAST
  O       E   ELEVEN
THREE     R   N    I
       FIVE        N
          DENSITY  E
```

ACTIVITY 11.D

1. .106
2. .053 − +
3. .035 − +
4. .095 − +
5. .090 − +
6. .353 + −
7. .064 − +
8. .211 + −
9. .055 − +
10. .282 + −
11. .053 − +
12. .120 + −
13. .067 − +
14. .141 + −
15. .212 + −

ACTIVITY 11.F

1. SID
   OID
   focal spot
   screen speed
   film speed
   contact of film and screen
   motion
2. SID
   OID
   focal spot
3. + −
4. − +
5. 0 0
6. + −
7. 0 0
8. + −
9. − +
10. + −
11. − +
12. − +
13. a
14. d
15. b
16. b
17. c
18. b
19. b
20. a
21. .009
22. .041
23. .071
24. .088
25. .060

ACTIVITY 12.B

1. base, emulsion
2. polyester
3. no
4. .007 inches
5. .0005 inches
6. .0075 inches
7. .008 inches
8. the base
9. 85%
10. dimensional stability
11. silver bromide
12. amphoteric
13. supercoating
14. colloid
15. supercoating, emulsion, adhesive, base, adhesive, emulsion, supercoating
16. supercoating, emulsion, adhesive, base

ACTIVITY 12.D

1. developer
2. latent
3. sodium sulfite
4. 45–90 seconds
5. 93–98 degrees
6. glutaraldehyde
7. fixer
8. phenidone
9. fixing, clearing
10. fixer
11. fog
12. hydroquinone
13. potassium bromide
14. developer
15. wash
16. activator, acid
17. ammonium thiosulfate, hypo
18. dryer
19. restrainer
20. potassium alum

ACTIVITY 12.G

1. c
2. e
3. h
4. f
5. j
6. b
7. d
8. i
9. a
10. g
11. b
12. c
13. d
14. c
15. a
16. d
17. b
18. d
19. a
20. b
21. b
22. c
23. c
24. a
25. d

ACTIVITY 13.C

1.	.25	11.	5 mAs
2.	.17	12.	2 mAs
3.	2	13.	66 mAs
4.	1	14.	24 mAs
5.	.5	15.	.5 mAs
6.	.2	16.	5.8 mAs
7.	.125	17.	3 mAs
8.	.33	18.	1.5 mAs
9.	.14	19.	2.5 mAs
10.	.4	20.	2.8 mAs

ACTIVITY 13.E

1.	c	11.	a	21.	a
2.	b	12.	c	22.	b
3.	a	13.	c	23.	b
4.	b	14.	b	24.	c
5.	d	15.	c	25.	b
6.	b	16.	b	26.	.25
7.	a	17.	a	27.	2.4
8.	b	18.	a	28.	.17
9.	d	19.	b	29.	20
10.	b	20.	c	30.	3

ACTIVITY 13.F

1. SID
   OID
   focal spot
   screen speed
   film speed
   film/screen contact
   motion
2. a. decreases
   b. decreases
   c. decreases
   d. no change
   e. decreases
   f. decreases
   g. increases
   h. no change
3. b
4. c
5. d
6. b
7. c
8. c
9. c
10. b
11. c
12. b
13. d
14. c
15. a
16. d
17. c
18. b
19. a
20. a
21. b
22. b
23. c
24. d
25. d
26. c
27. a
28. b
29. a
30. b
31. d
32. b
33. a
34. c
35. .04
36. 8.5
37. a
38. d
39. c
40. b

ACTIVITY 13.G

Crossword Puzzle Solution

```
 SUPERCOATING      F
 L      M    BLACK I
 O PERIAPICAL A    X
 P      H     T C  E
RESOLUTION DEVELOPER
   I N  T  E  N N N
 SID SPEED C  T T T
 M   H  R CRT   A R
BASE A  I  E    M A
  L  R  C WASH  I N
  L  P     S    N C
    INCREASES   A E
 H   E  M  S WHITE
LAYERS  U       I
 R   S  L      TOE
 D P    SINGLE  N
MEDIUM  I   A
 N X   FOG  REDUCING
 E E    N   G
 R L     THRESHOLD
```

ACTIVITY 13.H

Definitions and Sentence Completion

1. phenidone
2. gadolinium
3. glutaraldehyde
4. matrix
5. fluorescence
6. six
7. wire mesh
8. restrainer
9. accelerator
10. contrast
11. yellow-green
12. sensitometer
13. steep
14. adhesive
15. crossover
16. two
17. fixer
18. increases
19. polyester
20. large
21. phosphor
22. developer
23. SID
24. rare earth
25. OID

ACTIVITY 13.H

Puzzle Solution

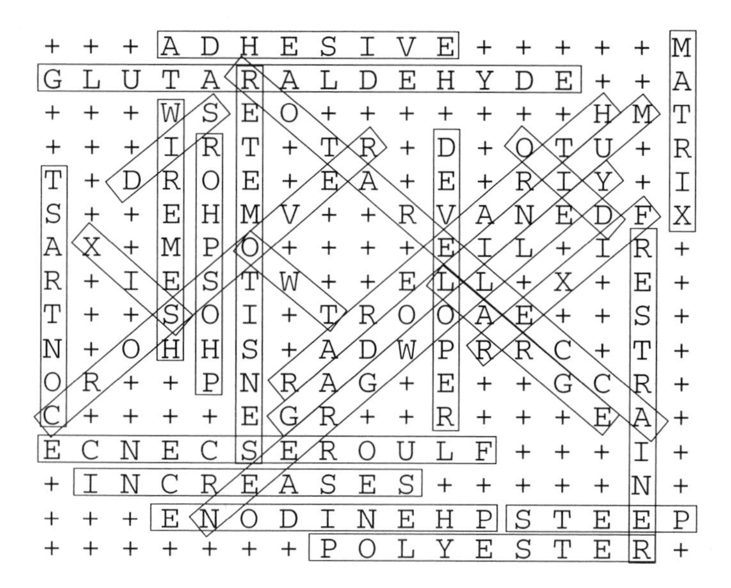

ACTIVITY 14.A

Density

Factors Changed	Effect on Density
200 mA	−
$\frac{1}{15}$ sec	−
30 mAs	−
70 kVp	+
68″ SID	−
4″ OID	+
1.5-mm focal spot	0
6:1 grid ratio	+
10 × 12 coll. field size	+
2.5 mm filtration	−
100-speed screen	−
96° developer temperature	+

ACTIVITY 14.B

Density

Factors Changed	Effect on Density
600 mA	+
25 msec	+
3 mAs	−
80 kVp	+
56″ SID	−
10″ OID	−
2.0-mm focal spot	0
12:1 grid ratio	−
8 × 10 coll. field size	−
2.0-mm filtration	+
50-speed screen	−
88° developer temperature	−

ACTIVITY 14.C

Density

Factors Changed	Effect on Density
100 mA	−
.04 sec	+
12 mAs	+
85 kVp	+
56″ SID	−
2″ OID	+
.6-mm focal spot	0
12:1 grid ratio	+
14 × 17 coll. field size	+
3.5-mm filtration	−
100-speed screen	−
89° developer temperature	−

ACTIVITY 14.D

Contrast

Factors Changed	Effect on Contrast
200 mA	0
$\frac{1}{40}$ sec	0
4 mAs	0
70 kVp	+
62″ SID	0
6″ OID	+
1.2-mm focal spot	0
12:1 grid ratio	+
8 × 10 coll. field size	+
3.5-mm filtration	−
200-speed screen	0
96° developer temperature	−

ACTIVITY 14.E

Contrast

Factors Changed	Effect on Contrast
400 mA	0
$\frac{3}{5}$ sec	0
140 mAs	0
70 kVp	+
40″ SID	0
6″ OID	+
1.2-mm focal spot	0
6:1 grid ratio	+
8 × 10 coll. field size	+
2.5-mm filtration	+
100-speed screen	0
88° developer temperature	−

ACTIVITY 14.F

Contrast

Factors Changed	Effect on Contrast
400 mA	0
.4 sec	0
15 mAs	0
75 kVp	−
60″ SID	0
9″ OID	+
.3-mm focal spot	0
6:1 grid ratio	−
14 × 17 coll. field size	−
3.0-mm filtration	−
300-speed screen	0
100° developer temperature	−

ACTIVITY 14.G

Recorded Detail

Factors Changed	Effect on Recorded Detail
500 mA	0
45 msec	0
40 mAs	0
74 kVp	0
40″ SID	−
1″ OID	+
.6-mm focal spot	+
12:1 grid ratio	0
8 × 10 coll. field size	0
3.5-mm filtration	0
400-speed screen	−
95° developer temperature	0

ACTIVITY 14.H

Recorded Detail

Factors Changed	Effect on Recorded Detail
200 mA	0
$\frac{1}{60}$ sec	0
4 mAs	0
60 kVp	0
72″ SID	+
6″ OID	−
1.2-mm focal spot	−
12:1 grid ratio	0
10 × 12 coll. field size	0
3.0-mm filtration	0
100-speed screen	−
92° developer temperature	0

ACTIVITY 14.I

Recorded Detail

Factors Changed	Effect on Recorded Detail
100 mA	0
.035 sec	0
7 mAs	0
72 kVp	0
40″ SID	−
3″ OID	+
.6 mm focal spot 8 : 1 grid ratio	+ 0
10 × 12 coll. field size	0
2.0-mm filtration	0
200-speed screen	+
92° developer temperature	0

ACTIVITY 14.J

Distortion

Factors Changed	Effect on Distortion
200 mA	0
.02 sec	0
5.8 mAs	0
68 kVp	0
68″ SID	−
4″ OID	−
1.0-mm focal spot	0
16 : 1 grid ratio	0
14 × 17 coll. field size	0
2.5-mm filtration	0
200-speed screen	0
92° developer temperature	0

ACTIVITY 14.K

Distortion

Factors Changed	Effect on Distortion
500 mA	0
.15 sec	0
16 mAs	0
70 kVp	0
32″ SID	+
6″ OID	+
.3-mm focal spot	0
6:1 grid ratio	0
10 × 12 coll. field size	0
2.0-mm filtration	0
800-speed screen	0
96° developer temperature	0

ACTIVITY 14.L

Relationship of All Factors

Factors	Density	Contrast	Recorded Detail	Distortion
200 mA	–	0	0	0
.07 sec	+	0	0	0
10 mAs	–	0	0	0
80 kVp	+	–	0	0
40″ SID	+	0	–	+
7″ OID	–	+	–	+
.3-mm focal spot	0	0	+	0
12:1 grid ratio	–	+	0	0
8 × 10 field size	–	+	0	0
2.5-mm filtration	+	+	0	0
100-speed screen	–	0	+	0
88° dev. temp.	–	–	0	0

ACTIVITY 14.M

Relationship of all Factors

Factors	Density	Contrast	Recorded Detail	Distortion
500 mA	−	0	0	0
$\frac{1}{40}$ sec	−	0	0	0
40 mAs	+	0	0	0
75 kVp	−	+	0	0
60″ SID	−	0	+	−
4″ OID	+	−	+	−
1.2-mm focal spot	0	0	−	0
5:1 grid ratio	+	−	0	0
14 × 17 field size	+	−	0	0
3.0-mm filtration	−	−	0	0
200-speed screen	−	0	+	0
98° dev. temp.	+	−	0	0

ACTIVITY 14.N

Relationship of All Factors

Factors	Density	Contrast	Recorded Detail	Distortion
100 mA	+	0	0	0
25 msec	+	0	0	0
1 mAs	+	0	0	0
60 kVp	−	+	0	0
40″ SID	+	0	−	+
9″ OID	−	+	−	+
.6 mm focal spot	0	0	+	0
12:1 grid ratio	−	+	0	0
10 × 12 field size	+	−	0	0
2.0-mm filtration	+	+	0	0
500-speed screen	+	0	−	0
98° dev. temp.	+	−	0	0

ACTIVITY 14.0

Relationship of All Factors

Factors	Density	Contrast	Recorded Detail	Distortion
200 mA	−	0	0	0
.04 sec	+	0	0	0
2 mAs	−	0	0	0
60 kVp	−	+	0	0
56″ SID	−	0	+	−
3″ OID	+	−	+	−
2.0 mm focal spot	0	0	−	0
12:1 grid ratio	−	+	0	0
8 × 10 field size	−	+	0	0
1.2-mm filtration	+	+	0	0
100-speed screen	+	0	−	0
87° dev. temp.	−	−	0	0

ACTIVITY 15.A

1. 10
2. 120
3. 12
4. 150
5. 400
6. 400
7. .06
8. .016
9. .05
10. 24
11. any mA and time that equals 24
12. 25
13. any mA and time that equals 25
14. 19.4
15. 19.1
16. 8.1
17. 78
18. 65
19. 24
20. 3
21. 40
22. 5.6
23. 5.3
24. 48
25. 8.9
26. 8.4
27. 17.6
28. .2
29. .33
30. .125
31. 2.5
32. 26.4
33. 129
34. 3
35. 9

ACTIVITY 15.B

1. 10
2. 20
3. 10
4. 200
5. 800
6. 600
7. .02
8. .04
9. .05
10. any three sets of mA and time that equal 10 mAs
11. 25 mA, 3 sec
12. 500 mA, .05 sec
13. 200 mA, .15 sec
14. 39
15. 6.8
16. 7.2
17. 80
18. 15
19. 10 mAs, 80 kVp
20. 500 mA, .25 sec, 80 kVp
21. 30
22. 4.5
23. 1.7
24. 50
25. 18.8
26. 3.6
27. 9.4
28. .17
29. .5
30. 5.7
31. 15
32. 500 mA, .01 sec
33. 10
34. 10
35. 3.5

ACTIVITY 15.C

1. 100 mA, .025 sec, 70 kVp
2. 25 mA, 2 sec, 70 kVp
3. 500 mA, .01 sec
4. 400 mA, .2 sec, 70 kVp
5. 400 mA, .04 sec, 80 kVp
6. 400 mA, .02 sec, 75 kVp
7. 500 mA, .15 sec, 80 kVp
8. 200 mA, .05 sec, 60 kVp
9. 500 mA, .01 sec, 90 kVp
10. 100 mA, .01 sec, 70 kVp

ACTIVITY 16.A

1. .6 sec
2. 200 mA
3. .02 sec
4. 400 mA
5. 16 mAs
6. 1/20 sec
7. 47 mAs
8. 162 mAs
9. .15 sec
10. 700 mA
11. 500 mA
12. 1/3 sec
13. 250 msec
14. 374 mAs
15. 7.75 mAs

ACTIVITY 16.B

1. 500 mA, .2 sec, 70 kVp
2. 500 mA, .01 sec, 90 kVp
3. 200 mA, .7 sec, 70 kVp
4. 200 mA, .01 sec, 70 kVp
5. 200 mA, .10 sec, 70 kVp

ACTIVITY 16.C

1. Greatest density is column D.

	A		B		C		D	
	100	mA	200	mA	200	mA	300	mA
	$\frac{3}{4}$	sec	2	sec	$\frac{1}{2}$	sec	1	sec
	80	kVp	70	kVp	80	kVp	70	kVp
	40″	SID	72″	SID	42″	SID	36″	SID
To	75	mAs	400	mAs	100	mAs	300	mAs
80	75	mAs	200	mAs	100	mAs	150	mAs
40″	75	mAs	62	mAs	91	mAs	185	mAs

2. Greatest density is column D.

	A		B		C		D	
	200	mA	500	mA	500	mA	400	mA
	.4	sec	.12	sec	.25	sec	.3	sec
	72″	SID	60″	SID	72″	SID	64″	SID
	6:1	grid	8:1	grid	16:1	grid	12:1	grid
To	80	mAs	60	mAs	125	mAs	120	mAs
72″	80	mAs	86	mAs	125	mAs	152	mAs
6:1	80	mAs	65	mAs	63	mAs	91	mAs

3. Least density is column D.

	A		B		C		D	
	300	mA	400	mA	1000	mA	800	mA
	40	msec	30	msec	10	msec	20	msec
	70	kVp	80	kVp	80	kVp	60	kVp
	50	RSV	100	RSV	200	RSV	100	RSV
	Three	phase	Single	phase	Three	phase	Single	phase
To	12	mAs	12	mAs	10	mAs	16	mAs
80	6	mAs	12	mAs	10	mAs	4	mAs
100	3	mAs	12	mAs	20	mAs	4	mAs
3 pH	3	mAs	6	mAs	20	mAs	2	mAs

4. Greatest density is column D.

	A		B		C		D	
	200	mA	100	mA	500	mA	600	mA
	$\frac{3}{10}$	sec	$\frac{1}{2}$	sec	$\frac{3}{10}$	sec	$\frac{2}{10}$	sec
	80	kVp	90	kVp	80	kVp	105	kVp
	8:1	grid	6:1	grid	16:1	grid	8:1	grid
	40″	SID	50″	SID	36″	SID	72″	SID
To	60	mAs	50	mAs	150	mAs	120	mAs
80	60	mAs	100	mAs	150	mAs	480	mAs
8:1	60	mAs	133	mAs	100	mAs	480	mAs
40″	60	mAs	85	mAs	123	mAs	148	mAs

5. Greatest density is column B.

	A		B		C		D	
	400	mA	300	mA	600	mA	500	mA
	.05	sec	.07	sec	.02	sec	.03	sec
	70	kVp	90	kVp	80	kVp	70	kVp
	5:1	grid	12:1	grid	8:1	grid	16:1	grid
	14 × 17	coll.	10 × 12	coll.	14 × 17	coll.	10 × 12	coll.
To	20	mAs	21	mAs	12	mAs	15	mAs
70	20	mAs	84	mAs	24	mAs	15	mAs
5:1	20	mAs	34	mAs	12	mAs	5	mAs
14	20	mAs	27	mAs	12	mAs	4	mAs

6. Greatest density is column C.

	A		B		C		D	
	200	mA	100	mA	300	mA	100	mA
	$\frac{1}{2}$	sec	$\frac{2}{10}$	sec	$\frac{2}{15}$	sec	$\frac{3}{5}$	sec
	70	kVp	80	kVp	90	kVp	70	kVp
	40″	SID	72″	SID	54″	SID	62″	SID
	100	RSV	50	RSV	200	RSV	400	RSV
To	100	mAs	20	mAs	40	mAs	60	mAs
70	100	mAs	40	mAs	160	mAs	60	mAs
40″	100	mAs	12	mAs	88	mAs	25	mAs
100	100	mAs	6	mAs	176	mAs	100	mAs

ACTIVITY 16.D

1. Greatest density is column A.

	A		B		C		D	
	500	mA	500	mA	100	mA	200	mAs
	.2	sec	.1	sec	1	sec	1	sec
	90	kVp	80	kVp	80	kVp	90	kVp
	12:1	grid	16:1	grid	16:1	grid	8:1	grid
	40″	SID	48″	SID	36″	SID	72″	SID
To	100	mAs	50	mAs	100	mAs	200	mAs
90	100	mAs	25	mAs	50	mAs	200	mAs
16	120	mAs	25	mAs	50	mAs	300	mAs
40″	120	mAs	17	mAs	62	mAs	93	mAs

2. Greatest density is column B.

	A		B		C		D	
	100	mA	200	mA	400	mA	500	mA
	$\frac{1}{2}$	sec	$\frac{1}{4}$	sec	$\frac{1}{8}$	sec	$\frac{1}{10}$	sec
	48″	SID	36″	SID	40″	SID	62″	SID
	80	kVp	80	kVp	70	kVp	80	kVp
	12:1	grid	12:1	grid	16:1	grid	8:1	grid
	100	RSV	100	RSV	50	RSV	200	RSV
To	50	mAs	50	mAs	50	mAs	50	mAs
48″	50	mAs	89	mAs	72	mAs	30	mAs
80	50	mAs	89	mAs	36	mAs	30	mAs
12	50	mAs	89	mAs	30	mAs	38	mAs
100	50	mAs	89	mAs	15	mAs	76	mAs

3. Least density is column D.

	A		B		C		D	
	400	mA	300	mA	200	mA	500	mA
	40	msec	60	msec	30	msec	10	msec
	70	kVp	80	kVp	90	kVp	80	kVp
	36″	SID	54″	SID	48″	SID	68″	SID
	100	RSV	500	RSV	100	RSV	400	RSV
To	16	mAs	18	mAs	6	mAs	5	mAs
80	8	mAs	18	mAs	12	mAs	5	mAs
36″	8	mAs	8	mAs	7	mAs	1	mAs
100	8	mAs	40	mAs	7	mAs	4	mAs

4. Least density is column D.

	A		B		C		D	
	200	mA	300	mA	50	mA	200	mA
	$\frac{1}{2}$	sec	$\frac{1}{6}$	sec	1	sec	$\frac{1}{8}$	sec
	70	kVp	80	kVp	70	kVp	80	kVp
	40″	SID	50″	SID	40″	SID	60″	SID
	Single	phase	Three	phase	Single	phase	Three	phase
To	100	mAs	50	mAs	50	mAs	25	mAs
70	100	mAs	100	mAs	50	mAs	50	mAs
40″	100	mAs	64	mAs	50	mAs	22	mAs
sin	100	mAs	128	mAs	50	mAs	44	mAs

5. Greatest density is column A.

	A		B		C		D	
	1000	mA	100	mA	800	mA	400	mA
	.1	sec	.5	sec	.1	sec	.25	sec
	90	kVp	104	kVp	80	kVp	80	kVp
	12:1	grid	16:1	grid	8:1	grid	8:1	grid
	14 × 17	coll.	8 × 10	coll.	10 × 12	coll.	14 × 17	coll.
To	100	mAs	50	mAs	80	mAs	100	mAs
90	100	mAs	100	mAs	40	mAs	50	mAs
8:1	80	mAs	66	mAs	40	mAs	50	mAs
14	80	mAs	47	mAs	32	mAs	50	mAs

6. Greatest density is column C.

	A		B		C		D	
	500	mA	600	mA	400	mA	500	mA
	.05	sec	.03	sec	.015	sec	.01	sec
	70	kVp	80	kVp	90	kVp	80	kVp
	40″	SID	50″	SID	48″	SID	72″	SID
	100	RSV	200	RSV	600	RSV	400	RSV
To	25	mAs	18	mAs	6	mAs	5	mAs
80	13	mAs	18	mAs	12	mAs	5	mAs
40″	13	mAs	11	mAs	8	mAs	1.5	mAs
100	13	mAs	22	mAs	47	mAs	6	mAs

ACTIVITY 17.A

1. b
2. c
3. a
4. b
5. c
6. a
7. b
8. a
9. b
10. a
11. a
12. c
13. b
14. I
15. D
16. I
17. I
18. D
19. D
20. D

ACTIVITY 18.D

1. d
2. a
3. a
4. b
5. d
6. b
7. c
8. c
9. b
10. a
11. c
12. c
13. d
14. c
15. a
16. b
17. a
18. b
19. a
20. a

ACTIVITIES

NAME ________________________

DATE ________________________

ACTIVITY 1.A

Fill in the blanks on this chart.

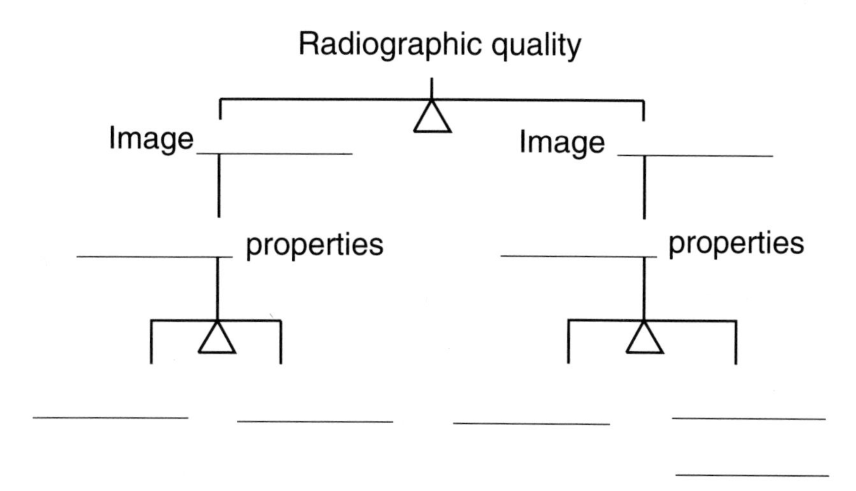

NAME ______________________

DATE ______________________

ACTIVITY 1.B

FACTORS AFFECTING THE FOUR RADIOGRAPHIC QUALITIES

Fill in the blanks on this chart.

Density

mAs (milliampere-seconds)
kVp (kilovolts)

____

Film

____

____

Beam restriction
Processing
Filtration

____

OID (used in air gap)
Patient

Distortion

OID (object image distance)

____

Object alignment
Film alignment

____

Contrast

kVp

____

Grid
Processing

____

OID (used in air gap)

____

Film

Recorded Detail

SID
OID

____

Screen

____

Contact

____

NAME ______________________________

DATE ______________________________

ACTIVITY 1.B

FACTORS AFFECTING THE FOUR RADIOGRAPHIC QUALITIES

Fill in the blanks on this chart.

Density

mAs (milliampere-seconds)
kVp (kilovolts)

____

Film

____

____

Beam restriction
Processing
Filtration

____

OID (used in air gap)
Patient

Distortion

OID (object image distance)

____

Object alignment
Film alignment

____

Contrast

kVp

____

Grid
Processing

____

OID (used in air gap)

____

Film

Recorded Detail

SID
OID

____

Screen

____

Contact

____

NAME ____________________

DATE ____________________

ACTIVITY 1.C

In Box A, draw a house. Then take a marker or crayon and color over it so that you can no longer see the house. Draw another house in Box B, making the lines on the outside very dark and the lines on the windows and doors very light. Draw a third house in Box C with very wiggly lines. Draw a fourth house in Box D with one half larger than the other. Now, thinking about the four radiographic qualities of density, contrast, recorded detail, and distortion, label each box according to which quality it represents.

NAME ______________________

DATE ______________________

ACTIVITY 1.D

CHAPTER REVIEW

MULTIPLE CHOICE

_____ 1. The four radiographic qualities that work together to produce a good quality radiograph are:
    1. visibility
    2. density
    3. recorded detail
    4. geometric
    5. distortion
    6. photographic
    7. contrast
    8. sharpness
  a. 1, 3, 4, 6
  b. 3, 5, 6, 7
  c. 2, 3, 5, 7
  d. 1, 4, 6, 8

_____ 2. The radiographic qualities that affect the sharpness of the image are:
  a. density and contrast
  b. recorded detail and distortion
  c. density and distortion
  d. the geometric and photographic properties

_____ 3. The radiographic qualities that affect the visibility of the image are:
  a. contrast and density
  b. distortion and contrast
  c. recorded detail and distortion
  d. density and recorded detail

_____ 4. The overall blackness of a radiograph is called:
  a. density
  b. contrast
  c. recorded detail
  d. distortion

_____ 5. The sharpness of the lines of the image is called:
  a. density
  b. contrast
  c. recorded detail
  d. distortion

_____ 6. The difference between adjacent densities on the radiograph is called:
  a. density
  b. contrast
  c. recorded detail
  d. distortion

____ 7. The misrepresentation of the true size or shape of the image as compared with the object is called:
a. density
b. contrast
c. recorded detail
d. distortion

____ 8. According to the chart in Table 1–2, SID controls or influences:
1. density
2. contrast
3. recorded detail
4. distortion

a. 1, 2
b. 1, 2, 4
c. 3, 4
d. 1, 3, 4,

____ 9. According to the chart in Table 1–2, kVp controls or influences:
1. density
2. contrast
3. recorded detail
4. distortion

a. 1, 2
b. 3
c. 2
d. 3, 4

____ 10. Which table shown in this chapter do you think will be most important throughout this book?
a. Table 1–1
b. Table 1–2
c. Table 1–3

NAME ____________________

DATE ____________________

ACTIVITY 2.A

Draw a diagram of the following:

1. A filament as viewed from the side
2. A focusing cup as viewed from the side
3. A dual focus cathode as viewed from the front
4. A rotating anode as viewed from both the side and front
5. A glass envelope with the window
6. The entire assembled x-ray tubes as viewed from the side
7. Label these parts on drawing 6:

the cathode	the focal track
the anode	the glass envelope
the focusing cup	the window
the filament	

ACTIVITY 2.B

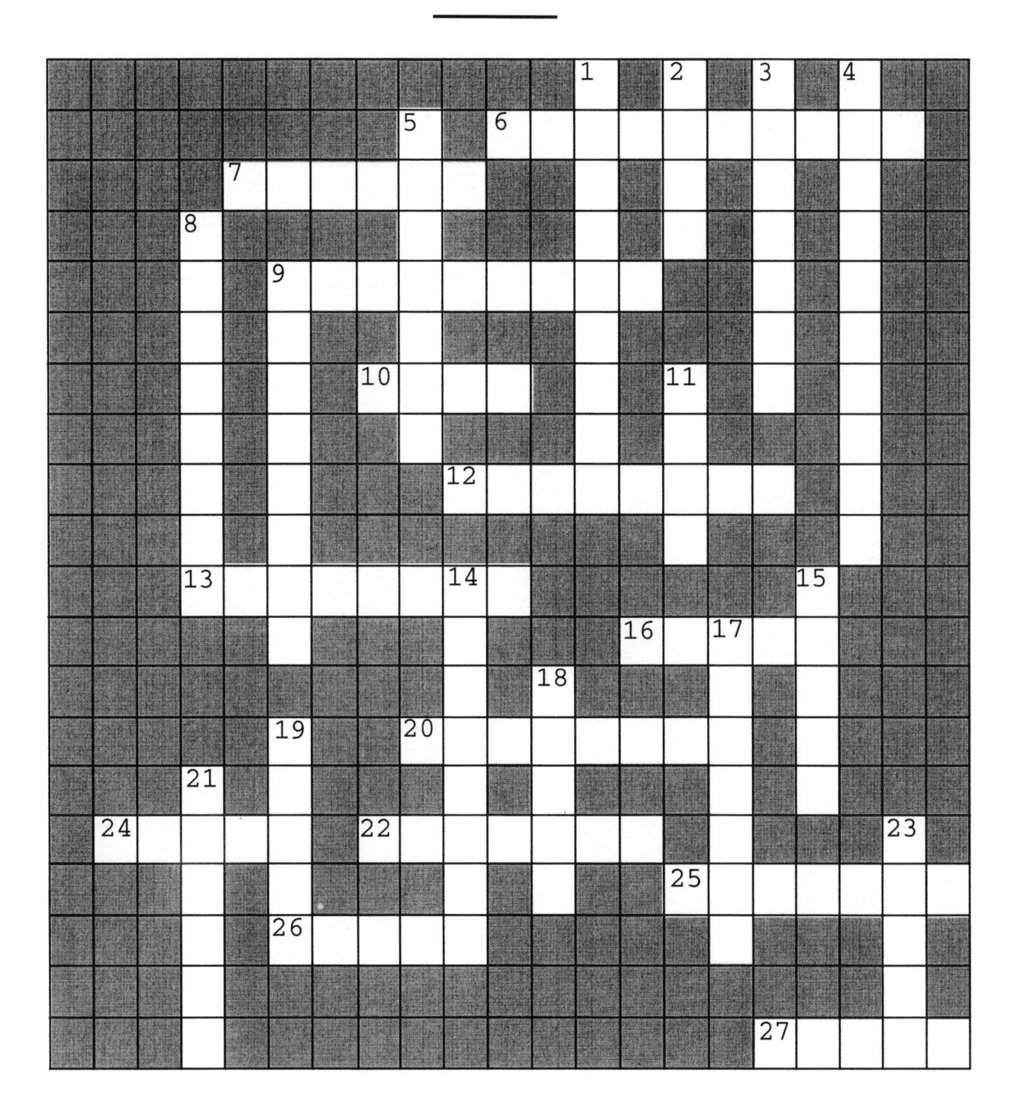

Across Clues

6. This device sits below the x-ray tube.
7. The thin spot in the glass envelope.
9. A dual-focus x-ray tube has two of these.
10. This absorbing material is added to the glass for the housing.
12. The process of thermionic ______________.
13. This is what the filament is made of.
16. The electrons are aimed at this.
20. The cathode has this charge.
22. One job of the metal housing is to ______________ the glass housing.
24. A dual ______________ x-ray tube.
25. This runs through the filament circuit to heat it.
26. This is the shape of the anode.
27. A special type of heat-resistant glass used in the glass envelope.

Down clues continued on following page.

Down Clues

1. These are boiled off at the filament.
2. Electrons must travel at ____________ speed.
3. The negative electrode of the x-ray tube.
4. The focusing cup is made of this.
5. How the anode moves.
8. Thermionic emission takes place at the ____________.
9. A negatively charged ____________ cup.
11. This is the shape of the filament.
14. The glass housing is also called a glass ____________.
15. The exterior housing of the x-ray tube is made of this.
17. This is added to the target material.
18. The glass envelope gets ____________ during manufacturing.
19. The envelope is made of this.
21. This exists inside the glass housing.
23. X-rays are produced on this side of the x-ray tube.

NAME ______________________

DATE ______________________

ACTIVITY 2.C

Decide which of the events listed in this activity really do take place in the production of x-rays. Place only these events in chronological order by numbering them on the line.

_____ electrons lose energy
_____ the filament boils off electrons
_____ a vacuum is created in the metal house
_____ electrons are aimed at the patient
_____ the focal spot is formed
_____ electrons form a space charge
_____ the filament gets hot
_____ the focusing cup becomes positive
_____ the filament glows
_____ x-rays are emitted isotropically
_____ current runs through the filament circuit
_____ the large focal spot changes into the small focal spot
_____ the tungsten filament wire melts
_____ electrons are attracted by the anode
_____ light, heat, and x-rays are produced
_____ the anode repels the electrons
_____ 98% of the electron energy is converted to x-ray energy
_____ the electrons in the space charge fly out of the tube
_____ the other filament gets heated
_____ electrons slam into the anode at the target
_____ electrons move over to the anode
_____ electrons are repelled from the focusing cup
_____ x-rays are absorbed by the glass and metal housings

ACTIVITY 2.D

V O Q Q D I V E R G E T I H W

L V N I N V I S I B L E W E U

I P X H E T E R O G E N O U S

G E O B I O L O G I C L E F R

H N D L T H G I A R T S L H O

T E O E Y V P P H N R U C C H

S T Y I B E G D O S O L I I P

C R L S T R N T K R M A T S S

A A R Y X A O E E N A C R O O

T T S J R H Z S R E G O A T H

T I H S P A C I B G N F P R P

E N X O E E M L N A E Y M O P

R G J E N T A I Z O T T L P L

V X W C Z C T K R K I T I I V

D A E L K R A E T P C Z F C V

See questions on following page.

NAME ______________________

DATE ______________________

ACTIVITY 2.D

WORD SEARCH—PROPERTIES OF X-RAYS

Decide which word best matches the definition or completes the sentence. Write the word on the line, and then find it in the word search puzzle and circle it.

______________ 1. Intensifying screens are in this.

______________ 2. X-rays are produced at a ______________ spot.

______________ 3. Can you see x-rays? They are ______________.

______________ 4. One word meaning many energies.

______________ 5. Another word meaning many energies.

______________ 6. P______________ radiation is directed at the patient.

______________ 7. Another name for x-ray energy.

______________ 8. X-rays hit phosphors and produce ______________.

______________ 9. Low energy x-rays are more easily a______________ by the patient's body.

______________ 10. Areas of the film that receive a lot of x-rays will be developed as what color.

______________ 11. Areas of the film that receive no x-rays will be developed as what color.

______________ 12. X-rays are highly p______________.

______________ 13. Photons are a pa______________ of energy.

______________ 14. This material is in the walls of x-ray rooms to absorb radiation.

______________ 15. X-rays are emitted in all directions. This is called i______________ emission.

______________ 16. X-rays d______________ from the focal spot.

______________ 17. X-rays cause ______________ damage.

______________ 18. X-rays are a form of e______________ radiation.

______________ 19. X-rays affect photographic ______________.

______________ 20. The process of removing electrons from atoms.

______________ 21. This type of radiation gets through the patient and puts density on the film.

______________ 22. X-rays travel in ______________ lines.

______________ 23. P______________ light up when hit with x-rays.

______________ 24. X-rays cause f______________ of some materials.

______________ 25. X-rays that bounce off the patient's body are called s______________.

NAME ______________________

DATE ______________________

ACTIVITY 2.E

CHAPTER REVIEW

MULTIPLE CHOICE

_____ 1. The positive electrode of the x-ray tube is the ____________ and the negative electrode is the ____________.
a. cathode, anode
b. anode, cathode

_____ 2. The two parts of the cathode are the:
a. focusing cup and anode
b. glass envelope and metal housing
c. filament and focusing cup
d. focal spot and filament

_____ 3. The term for the radiation that leaves the x-ray tube and is directed at the patient's body is:
a. primary radiation
b. scattered radiation
c. exit radiation
d. secondary radiation

_____ 4. Which one of these is *not* a property of x-rays?
a. they are invisible
b. they are all the same energy
c. they are highly penetrating
d. they are heterogeneous

_____ 5. Which one of these statements is *not* true concerning the production of x-rays?
a. the filament gets heated by current
b. electrons are freed from the filament
c. electrons move at high speed to the anode
d. most electrons penetrate the anode

_____ 6. Of these parts of the x-ray tube, which have tungsten in them:
1. the filament
2. the focusing cup
3. the glass housing
4. the anode
a. 1
b. 2, 3
c. 1, 4
d. 1, 2, 4

_____ 7. The ability of phosphors to light up when hit by x-rays is called:
a. ionization
b. thermionic emission
c. fluorescence
d. isotropic emission

_____ 8. X-rays damage biologic matter by the process of:
   a. ionization
   b. thermionic emission
   c. fluorescence
   d. incandescence

_____ 9. Photons that bounce off the patient's body parts and fly out in a new direction are called:
   a. primary radiation
   b. scattered radiation
   c. exit radiation
   d. fluorescence

_____ 10. Which part of the x-ray tube rotates?
   a. cathode
   b. filament
   c. focusing cup
   d. anode

_____ 11. Radiographers are able to see x-rays when they:
   a. are produced
   b. leave the tube
   c. enter the patient's body
   d. none of the above

_____ 12. Which one of these terms means the size of the area from which the x-rays originate?
   a. the anode
   b. the target
   c. the focal spot
   d. the window

_____ 13. A dual-focus x-ray tube has two:
   a. anodes
   b. filaments
   c. focusing cups
   d. cathodes

_____ 14. The group of electrons sitting beyond the filament after thermionic emission is called:
   a. scattered radiation
   b. a thermion group
   c. a space charge
   d. the filament current

_____ 15. The job of the focusing cup is to:
   a. repel electrons
   b. release the electrons
   c. stop the electrons
   d. heat the filament

_____ 16. The job of the filament is to:
   a. repel electrons
   b. release electrons
   c. stop electrons
   d. heat the filament

_____ 17. The job of the anode is to:
   a. repel electrons

b. release the electrons
c. stop the electrons
d. heat the filament

_____ 18. The glass envelope has lead in it to:
a. absorb leakage radiation
b. keep the glass from cracking
c. absorb heat
d. create the space charge

_____ 19. X-rays leave the tube at a spot called the:
a. focal spot
b. focal track
c. window
d. target

_____ 20. If the small filament is heated, which size focal spot would be produced?
a. small
b. large
c. neither of these

_____ 21. When the electrons lose energy at the anode, which of these energy types is produced in the greatest amount?
a. light
b. heat
c. x-ray
d. nuclear

_____ 22. When the x-rays travel toward the patient's body, the beam takes this shape?
a. a rectangle
b. a helix
c. a triangle
d. a cone

_____ 23. X-rays travel at the speed of light, which is approximately:
a. 75,000 meters per second
b. 125,000 miles per minute
c. 186,000 miles per second
d. 212,982 meters per nanosecond

_____ 24. Scattered radiation does what to radiographic contrast?
a. it reduces it
b. it increases it
c. it has no effect on it

_____ 25. Which of these increases recorded detail?
a. a large space charge
b. a strongly positive anode
c. fluorescence
d. a small focal spot

NAME ____________________

DATE ____________________

ACTIVITY 3.A

List the abbreviations and write out the distance names for the distances listed.

Abbreviation	**Distance**
From the x-ray tube to the film.	
1. ______	______
2. ______	______
From the object to the film.	
3. ______	______
4. ______	______
From the x-ray tube to the object.	
5. ______	______
6. ______	______

Calculate the following:

______ 7. If the OID is 8 inches and the SID is 52 inches, what is the SOD?

______ 8. If the SID is 72 inches and the SOD is 67 inches, what is the OID?

______ 9. If the SOD is 53 inches and the OID is 12 inches, what is the SID?

______ 10. If the SID is 68 inches and the OID is 4 inches, what is the SOD?

______ 11. If the SOD is 36 inches and the OID is 8 inches, what is the SID?

______ 12. If the SOD is 58 inches and the SID is 72 inches, what is the OID?

______ 13. If the SID is 72 inches and the SOD is 68 inches, what is the OID?

______ 14. If the SOD is 56 inches and the OID is 12 inches, what is the SID?

______ 15. If the OID is 15 inches and the SOD is 40 inches, what is the SID?

NAME ______________________

DATE ______________________

ACTIVITY 3.B

The x-ray beam and a light beam have some similar characteristics. This activity will help you see size distortion or magnification caused by light. Although x-rays penetrate through matter and light rays don't, x-rays and light rays both cause size distortion in the same manner.

MATERIALS

A radiographic room
A small solid rectangular object
An assistant if necessary to hold the object

PROCEDURE

1. Measure the length and width of the rectangular object and record it.
   length ____________ width ____________
2. Suspend the rectangular object 4 inches from the x-ray table top. You may have an assistant hold it or prop it up on something that is smaller than the object is. Position the x-ray tube so that it is over the object at a distance of 25 inches from the table top. Do not angle the x-ray tube. Shine the light from the collimator onto the object. You should be able to see the shadow of all four edges of the object on the table in the collimator light.
3. Measure the length and width of the shadow cast by the object and record it.
   length ____________ width ____________
4. Subtract the length and width of the actual object from the length and width of the shadow produced in procedure 3 and record it.
   length difference ____________ width difference ____________
5. Move the object to 8 inches from the table and measure the length and width of the shadow it casts.
   length ____________ width ____________
6. Subtract the length and width of the actual object from the length and width of the shadow produced in procedure 5 and record it.
   length difference ____________ width difference ____________
7. Which shadow was larger, the one from procedure 3 or 5? ____________
8. Explain what you think the reason is for the answer you gave in question number 7.

   ____

   ____

   ____
9. Move the rectangular object up and down, changing its distance from the table top, and observe what happens to the sharpness of the edges of the shadow. Is

there a relationship between the distance of the object from the table top and the sharpness of the shadow? Explain.

____

____

____

10. Repeat procedure 2 and 3, but change the distance of the x-ray tube from the table top to 50 inches.

    length ____________ width ____________

11. Subtract the length and width of the actual object from the length and width of the shadow of procedure 10 and record it.

    length difference ____________ width difference ____________

12. Calculate the difference between the measurements from procedure 3 and procedure 10 and record it.

    length difference ____________ width difference ____________

13. What do you conclude from the differences measured in procedure 12?

    ____

    ____

    ____

    ____

14. Did the image of the object ever get smaller than the actual object in any of the procedures? ____________

15. What do you expect to learn about size distortion produced by x-rays from these procedures?

    ____

    ____

    ____

ACTIVITY 3.C

LAB ASSIGNMENT—SIZE DISTORTION AND OBJECT-IMAGE DISTANCE

MATERIALS

A step wedge; a flat heavy metallic object; a radiographic phantom of a small body part that is exposed table top; or a flat, skeletal bone
Three loaded cassettes big enough to fit an image of the step wedge, metallic object, phantom, or bone. You can also use a large cassette and divide it into three sections.
A radiographic room
A processor
A ruler
Several rectangular or square radiographic sponges

PROCEDURE

You can use the same exposure factors for all three exposures. You may need to ask your instructor what technique to use for the exposures. For the step wedge and metallic object, the technique you would use for a foot will probably work. For the dry bone, the technique you would use for a hand will probably work. For the phantom, use the technique you would ordinarily use for that body part.

For all exposures, place the cassette on top of the x-ray table. Place the step wedge, metallic object, phantom, or bone directly on the cassette in the center of the cassette or section of the cassette you are using. Keep the object parallel to the cassette. Use a 40-inch source-image distance, and position the center of the x-ray beam directly over the center of the object. Do not angle the x-ray tube. Adjust the collimation so that all four edges of the object will be included on the film.

Exposure 1. Make the first exposure with the object flat on the cassette. Label this image exposure 1.

Exposure 2. Make the second exposure using the same conditions used for exposure 1. The only thing you need to change is to place a 3-inch radiographic sponge between the cassette and the object. The object must remain parallel to the cassette. Label this image exposure 2.

Exposure 3. Make the third exposure using the same conditions used for exposure 1. The only thing you need to change is to place one 6-inch or two 3-inch sponges between the cassette and the object. The object must remain parallel to the cassette. Label this image exposure 3.

Answer the lab analysis questions. Save the radiographs, data, and lab analysis for use with Activities 3.F and 3.G.

NAME ______________________

DATE ______________________

ACTIVITY 3.C

LAB ANALYSIS—SIZE DISTORTION AND OBJECT-IMAGE DISTANCE

1. Measure the actual length and width of the step wedge, metallic object, phantom, or bone you used and record it. If you are using an object that is irregular in shape, pick two spots along its length and width and make your measurements there. Measure in exactly these same spots for the subsequent procedures.

   length ____________ width ____________

2. Measure the length and width of the image on the radiographs from exposure 1, 2, and 3 and record it.

   Exposure 1 length ____________ width ____________

   Exposure 2 length ____________ width ____________

   Exposure 3 length ____________ width ____________

3. Calculate the difference between the length and width from procedure number 1 (actual measurements) and procedure number 2 (image measurements) and record it.

   Exposure 1 length ____________ width ____________

   Exposure 2 length ____________ width ____________

   Exposure 3 length ____________ width ____________

4. As the object-image distance increased, what happened to the image size?

   ____

   ____

5. Which image size varies the least from the actual object size?

   ____

6. Which image size varies the most from the actual object size?

   ____

7. What do you conclude about the relationship between object-image distance and size distortion from this lab assignment?

   ____

   ____

   ____

ACTIVITY 3.D

LAB ASSIGNMENT—SIZE DISTORTION AND SOURCE-IMAGE DISTANCE

MATERIALS

A step wedge; a flat, heavy metallic object; a radiographic phantom of a small body part that is exposed table top; or a flat, skeletal bone.
Three loaded cassettes big enough to fit an image of the step wedge, metallic object, phantom, or bone. You may also use a large cassette and divide it into three sections.
A radiographic room
A processor
A ruler
Several rectangular or square radiographic sponges

PROCEDURE

For all exposures, place the cassette on the x-ray table top and put a 2- to 3-inch radiographic sponge on top of the cassette. The sponge creates a small object-image distance, which is necessary to produce the lab results. Place the step wedge, metallic object, phantom, or bone directly on top of the sponge in the center of the cassette or section of the cassette you are using. Keep the object parallel to the cassette. Use a 40-inch source-image distance and position the center of the x-ray beam directly over the center of the object. Do not angle the x-ray tube. Adjust the collimation so that all four edges of the object will be included on the film.

Exposure 1. Make the first exposure using a 40-inch source-image distance. You may need to ask your instructor what technique to use for the exposures. For the step wedge and metallic object, the technique you would use for a foot will probably work. For the bone, the technique you would use for a hand will probably work. For the phantom, use the technique you would ordinarily use for that body part. Label this image exposure 1.

Exposure 2. Make the second exposure using the same conditions used for exposure 1. For this exposure, use a 56-inch source-image distance. You also need to double the mAs that was used for exposure 1. Ask for help with the technique if you need it. Label this image exposure 2.

Exposure 3. Make the third exposure using the same conditions used for exposure 1. For this exposure use a 28-inch source-image distance. You also need to cut the mAs from exposure 1 in half. Ask for help with the technique if you need it. Label this image exposure 3.

Answer the lab analysis questions. Save the radiographs, data, and lab analysis for use with Activity 3.F and 3.G.

NAME ______________________

DATE ______________________

ACTIVITY 3.D

LAB ANALYSIS—SIZE DISTORTION AND SOURCE-IMAGE DISTANCE

1. Measure the actual length and width of the step wedge, metallic object, phantom or bone you used and record it. If you are using an object that is irregular in shape, pick two spots along its length and width and make your measurements there. Measure in exactly these same spots for the subsequent procedures.

   length ____________ width ____________

2. Measure the length and width of the image on the radiographs from exposures 1, 2, and 3 and record the measurements.

   Exposure 1 length ____________ width ____________
   Exposure 2 length ____________ width ____________
   Exposure 3 length ____________ width ____________

3. Calculate the difference between the length and width from procedure number 1 (actual measurements) and procedure number 2 (image measurements) and record the differences.

   Exposure 1 length ____________ width ____________
   Exposure 2 length ____________ width ____________
   Exposure 3 length ____________ width ____________

4. As the source-image distance is increased and decreased, what happened to the image size?

   ____

   ____

5. Which image size varies the least from the actual object size?

   ____

6. Which image size varies the most from the actual object size?

   ____

7. What do you conclude about the relationship between source-image distance and size distortion from this lab assignment?

   ____

   ____

   ____

NAME ______________________

DATE ______________________

ACTIVITY 3.E

CALCULATION OF SIZE DISTORTION

IMAGE SIZE OR OBJECT SIZE

_____ 1. If the SID is 72 inches, the SOD 68 inches, and the object length 6 inches, what is the image length?

_____ 2. If the SID is 56 inches, the SOD 48 inches, and the image width 5 inches, what is the object width?

_____ 3. If the SID is 44 inches, the OID 2 inches, and the image length 3 inches, what is the object length?

_____ 4. If the SID is 48 inches, the OID 6 inches, and the object width 4 inches, what is the image width?

_____ 5. If the SOD is 54 inches, the OID 8 inches, and the object length 6 inches, what is the image length?

MAGNIFICATION FACTOR

Calculate the magnification factor for the following:

_____ 6. The SID is 72 inches and the SOD is 66 inches.

_____ 7. The SID is 44 inches and the OID is 6 inches.

_____ 8. The image is 10 inches long and the object is 8 inches long.

_____ 9. The SID is 56 inches and the SOD is 48 inches.

_____ 10. The image is 7 inches wide and the object is 4 inches wide.

_____ 11. If the area of an object is 24 inches and the image has a magnification factor of 2, what is the area of the image?

_____ 12. If the object measures 3 cm by 5 cm, what will the image measure if the magnification factor is 1.2?

_____ 13. If the image is 8 inches long and 4 inches wide, and the object is 4 inches long, what is the width of the object?

_____ 14. If the length of the object is 6 inches, the SID is 72 inches, and the SOD is 60 inches, what is the length of the image?

_____ 15. If the magnification factor is 2 and the area of the image is 40 inches, what is the area of the object?

PERCENT OF MAGNIFICATION

Calculate the percentage of magnification for the following:

_____ 16. The image is 8 inches long and the object is 3 inches long.

_____ 17. The image is 10 inches wide and the object is 8 inches wide.

_____ 18. The image is 19 inches long and the object is 7 inches long.

_____ 19. The image is 12 inches wide and the object is 6 inches wide.

_____ 20. The image is 10 inches long and the object is 9.5 inches long.

NAME ____________________

DATE ____________________

ACTIVITY 3.F

For this activity, you will need to use the radiographs, data, and lab analyses from Activities 3.C and 3.D.

RADIOGRAPHS FROM ACTIVITY 3.C

Use the radiographs from exposure 1.

____ 1. Calculate the image length as if you didn't know what it is and see if it is the same as what you measured.

____ 2. Calculate the magnification factor.

____ 3. Calculate the percent of magnification.

Use the radiographs from exposure 2.

____ 4. Calculate the image width as if you didn't know what it is and see if it is the same as what you measured.

____ 5. Calculate the magnification factor.

____ 6. Calculate the percent of magnification.

Use the radiographs from exposure 3.

____ 7. Calculate the image length as if you didn't know what it is and see if it is the same as what you measured.

____ 8. Calculate the magnification factor.

____ 9. Calculate the percent of magnification.

RADIOGRAPHS FROM ACTIVITY 3.D

Use the radiographs from exposure 1.

____ 10. Calculate the image width as if you didn't know what it is and see if it is the same as what you measured.

____ 11. Calculate the magnification factor.

____ 12. Calculate the percentage of magnification.

Use the radiographs from exposure 2.

____ 13. Calculate the image length as if you didn't know what it is and see if it is the same as what you measured.

____ 14. Calculate the magnification factor.

____ 15. Calculate the percent of magnification.

Use the radiographs from exposure 3.

____ 16. Calculate the image width as if you didn't know what it is and see if it is the same as what you measured.

____ 17. Calculate the magnification factor.

____ 18. Calculate the percent of magnification.

NAME ______________________________

DATE ______________________________

ACTIVITY 3.G

SID, OID, AND THE FOUR RADIOGRAPHIC QUALITIES

This activity uses the radiographs from Activities 3.C and 3.D.

Look at the radiographs from Activity 3.C

1. Do you see any differences in density between the radiographs? If you do, what do you think accounts for this? Explain.

   ____

   ____

2. Do you see any differences in contrast between the radiographs? If you do, what do you think accounts for this? Explain.

   ____

   ____

3. Do you see any differences in recorded detail between the radiographs? If you do, what do you think accounts for this? Explain.

   ____

   ____

Look at the radiographs from Activity 3.D.

4. Do you see any differences in density between the radiographs? If you do, what do you think accounts for this? Explain.

   ____

   ____

5. Do you see any differences in contrast between the radiographs? If you do, what do you think accounts for this? Explain.

   ____

   ____

6. Do you see any differences in recorded detail between the radiographs? If you do, what do you think accounts for this? Explain.

   ____

   ____

NAME ________________

DATE ________________

ACTIVITY 3.H

CHAPTER REVIEW

MULTIPLE CHOICE

_____ 1. Which one of these is *not* a term for the distance from the x-ray tube to the film?
a. source-image distance
b. tube film distance
c. focus-film distance

_____ 2. To calculate the SOD:
a. subtract the SID from the FOD
b. add the SID and OID
c. subtract the OID from the SID
d. divide the image size by the object size

_____ 3. To calculate the magnification factor:
a. divide the SID by the OID
b. subtract the OID from the SID
c. divide the object size by the image size
d. divide the SID by the SOD

_____ 4. Size distortion occurs when the:
a. image is larger than the object
b. object is larger than the image
c. image and object sizes are exactly the same

_____ 5. Which one of these is the major factor for controlling size distortion?
a. OID
b. SID

_____ 6. Which one of these maneuvers would cause the least magnification of the spine on a radiograph?
a. placing the patient on the x-ray table face down
b. placing the patient on the x-ray table on his or her right side
c. placing the patient on the x-ray table on his or her left side
d. placing the patient on the x-ray table face up

_____ 7. Which one of these would produce the least magnification?
a. using a long SID and long OID
b. using a short SID and short OID
c. using a long SID and short OID
d. using a short SID and long OID

_____ 8. Which one of these are the most common source-image distances used in clinical situations?
a. 56 inches, 36 inches
b. 72 inches, 40 inches
c. 66 inches, 44 inches
d. 84 inches, 42 inches

_____ 9. If the OID is large in a clinical situation, which one of these maneuvers would decrease the magnification?
a. reduce the SID
b. reduce the SOD
c. increase the OID
d. increase the SID

_____ 10. Which of these source-image distances would be best to see the truest size of the heart on a chest radiograph?
a. 36 inches
b. 44 inches
c. 56 inches
d. 72 inches

Calculate the following:

_____ 11. If the SID is 56 inches, and the OID is 6 inches, what is the SOD?

_____ 12. If the OID is 4 inches, and the SOD is 64 inches, what is the SID?

_____ 13. If the SID is 72 inches, and the SOD is 70 inches, what is the OID?

_____ 14. If the object length is 7 inches, the SID 56 inches, and the OID 6 inches, what is the image length?

_____ 15. If the image is 9 inches wide, the SID 62 inches, and the OID 8 inches, what is the object width?

_____ 16. If the image is 10 inches long, the object 9 inches long, and the SID 70 inches, what is the SOD?

_____ 17. If the image is 6 inches wide and the object is 4.5 inches wide, what is the percent of magnification?

_____ 18. If the image has an area of 20 inches and the object has an area of 5 inches, what is the magnification factor?

_____ 19. If the OID is 8 inches and the SID is 72 inches, what is the magnification factor?

_____ 20. If the magnification factor is 1.3 and the object is 4 inches long, what is the image length?

NAME ______________________________

DATE ______________________________

ACTIVITY 4.A

The x-ray beam and a light beam have some similar characteristics. This activity will help you see shape distortion caused by light. Although x-rays penetrate through matter and light rays don't, x-rays and light rays both cause shape distortion in the same manner.

MATERIALS

A radiographic room
A small heavy metal object with holes in it (examples are a small wrench, a key, a tool)
An assistant if necessary to hold the object
A ruler

PROCEDURE

1. Measure the length and width of the metal object and record it. If you are using an object that is irregular in shape, pick two spots along its length and width and make your measurements there. Measure in exactly these same spots for the subsequent procedures.

   length ____________ width ____________

2. Suspend the object 2 inches from the x-ray tabletop so that the longest part of the object corresponds with the long part of the x-ray table. You may have an assistant hold it or prop it up on something that is smaller than the object. Position the x-ray tube so that it is directly over the object at a distance of 40 inches from the tabletop. Do not angle the x-ray beam. Shine the light from the collimator on the object. You should be able to see the shadow of all four edges of the object on the table in the collimator light.
3. Measure the length and width of the shadow cast by the object and record it.

   length ____________ width ____________

4. Tilt or angle the object in the collimator light so that the middle of the object stays at a 2-inch distance from the table top, but one part of the object is lower and one part is higher. Angle the object about 10 degrees. Measure the length and width of the shadow cast by the object and record it.

   length ____________ width ____________

5. Repeat procedure 4, but angle the object 45 degrees. Measure the length and width of the shadow cast by the object and record it.

   length ____________ width ____________

6. Did you record any difference in the measurements from procedures 3, 4, and 5? If so, what were the differences?

   ____

   ____

   ____

7. Did you see any difference in the appearance of the shadow of the object at the

different object angles? Did you see any difference in the appearance of the holes in the object when using the different angles?

____

____

____

8. Now repeat procedure 2, but this time angle the central ray 10 degrees from left to right along the length of the object, keeping the object parallel to the film. Measure the length and width of the shadow cast by the object and record it.

   length ____________ width ____________

9. Repeat procedure 8, but angle the central ray 45 degrees this time. Measure the length and width of the shadow cast by the object and record it.

   length ____________ width ____________

10. Did you record any difference in the measurements from procedures 8 and 9? If so, what were the differences?

____

____

____

11. Did you see any difference in the appearance of the shadow of the object at the different angles of the central ray? Did you see any difference in the appearance of the holes in the object when using the different central ray angles?

____

____

____

12. What do you expect to learn about shape distortion caused by x-rays from this activity?

____

____

____

ACTIVITY 4.B

LAB ASSIGNMENT—FORESHORTENING

MATERIALS

A small heavy metal object with holes in it (examples are a small wrench, a key, a tool)
Three loaded cassettes big enough to fit an image of the object you are using. You may also use a large cassette and divide it into three sections.
A radiographic room
A processor
Several angled radiographic sponges
A ruler

PROCEDURE

You can use the same exposure factors for all three exposures. You may need help from your instructor with the technique. The technique you would use for a foot will probably work.

For all exposures, place the cassette on the x-ray tabletop. Place the metal object in the center of the cassette or section of the cassette you are using. Keep the object parallel to the cassette. Use a 40-inch source-image distance, and position the center of the x-ray beam directly over the center of the metal object. Do not angle the x-ray tube. Adjust the collimation so that all four edges of the object will be included on the film.

Exposure 1. Make the first exposure with the object directly on top of the cassette. Keep the object parallel to the film. Label this image exposure 1.

Exposure 2. Make the second exposure using the same conditions used for exposure 1. The only thing you need to change is to prop the object up on a radiographic sponge so that it is at about a 15 degree angle to the film. Label this image exposure 2.

Exposure 3. Make the third exposure using the same conditions used for exposure 1. The only thing you need to change is to prop the object up on radiographic sponge so that it is at about a 30 degree angle to the film. Label this image exposure 3.

Answer the questions on the lab analysis.

NAME ____________________

DATE ____________________

ACTIVITY 4.B

LAB ANALYSIS—FORESHORTENING

1. Measure the length and width of the object you used and record it. If you are using an object that is irregular in shape, pick two spots along its length and width and make your measurements there. Measure in exactly these same spots for the subsequent procedures.

   length ____________ width ____________

2. Measure the length and width of the image on the radiographs from each exposure and record the measurements.

   Exposure 1 length ____________ width ____________

   Exposure 2 length ____________ width ____________

   Exposure 3 length ____________ width ____________

3. Did you measure any differences in the measurements from exposures 1, 2, and 3? Explain.

   ____

   ____

   ____

4. If you measured any differences from procedure 2, explain why you think these occurred?

   ____

   ____

   ____

5. Do you see any differences in the shape of the holes of your metal object on the images from exposures 1, 2, and 3? If you do, why do you think these occurred?

   ____

   ____

   ____

6. What do you conclude concerning foreshortening from this activity?

   ____

   ____

   ____

ACTIVITY 4.C

LAB ASSIGNMENT—ELONGATION

MATERIALS

A small heavy metal object with holes in it (examples are a small wrench, a key, a tool)
Three loaded cassettes big enough to fit an image of the object you are using. You may also use a large cassette and divide it into three sections.
A radiographic room
A processor
Several rectangular or square radiographic sponges
A ruler

PROCEDURE

You can use the same exposure factors for all three exposures. You may need help from your instructor with the technique. The technique you would use for a foot will probably work.

For all exposures, place the cassette on the x-ray table top and put a 2- to 3-inch radiographic sponge on top of the cassette. The sponge creates a small object-image distance, which is necessary to produce the lab results. Place the metal object directly on top of the sponge in the center of the cassette or section of the cassette you are using. Keep the object parallel to the cassette. Position the longest part of the object to correspond with the long part of the x-ray table. Use a 40-inch source-image distance, and position the center of the x-ray beam directly over the center of the metal object. Adjust the collimation so that all four edges of the object will be included on the film.

Exposure 1. Make the first exposure with the conditions listed for all exposures. Do not angle the central ray. Label this image exposure 1.

Exposure 2. Make the second exposure using the same conditions used for exposure 1. The only thing you need to change is to angle the central ray so that it is a 20 degree angle along the longest portion of the object. Label this image exposure 2.

Exposure 3. Make the third exposure using the same conditions used for exposure 1. The only thing you need to change is to angle the central ray so that it is at a 40 degree angle along the longest portion of the object. Label this image 3. Answer the questions on the lab analysis.

NAME ____________________

DATE ____________________

ACTIVITY 4.C

LAB ANALYSIS ELONGATION

1. Measure the length and width of the object you used and record it. If you are using an object that is irregular in shape, pick two spots along its length and width and make your measurements there. Measure in exactly these spots for the subsequent procedures.

   length ____________ width ____________

2. Measure the length and width of the image on the radiographs from each exposure and record the measurements.

   Exposure 1 length ____________ width ____________

   Exposure 2 length ____________ width ____________

   Exposure 3 length ____________ width ____________

3. Did you measure any differences in the measurements from exposure 1, 2, and 3? Explain.

   ____

   ____

   ____

4. If you measured any differences from procedure 2, explain why you think these occurred.

   ____

   ____

   ____

5. Do you see any differences in the shape of the holes of your metal object on the images from exposures 1, 2, and 3? If you do, why do you think these occurred?

   ____

   ____

   ____

6. What do you conclude concerning elongation from this activity?

   ____

   ____

   ____

ACTIVITY 4.D

LAB ASSIGNMENT—BEAM CENTERING

MATERIALS

Two small heavy metal objects that can stand on edge. They should be approximately the same length and width. (Examples are a small wrench, a key, a tool.)
Three loaded cassettes big enough to fit an image of the object you are using. You may also use a large cassette and divide it into three sections.
A radiographic room
A processor
A ruler

PROCEDURE

For all exposures; place the cassette directly on top of the x-ray table. Use a 40-inch source-image distance. Place the two objects directly on the cassette. The longest part of each object should correspond with the shortest part of the x-ray table. Stand the objects on edge and place them exactly 1 inch apart. Place the objects in the center of the cassette or section of the cassette you are using. Adjust the collimation so that all four edges of the two objects will be included on the film. You will use the same technique for each exposure. The technique you would use for a foot will probably work.

Exposure 1. Make the first exposure with the central ray perpendicular to the film and objects. Keep the central ray over the center of the two objects and center it in the middle of the 1-inch space between the objects. Label this image exposure 1.

Exposure 2. Use the same conditions as for exposure 1. The only thing you need to change is to move the central ray to the right along the longest part of the x-ray table. Move it about 6 inches. Be sure to include the two objects in the x-ray beam. They will be toward the edge of the beam. Some of the beam may extend beyond the edges of the cassette. Label this image exposure 2.

Exposure 3. Use the same conditions as for exposure 1. The only thing you need to change is to move the central ray to the left along the longest part of the x-ray table. Move it about 6 inches. Be sure to include the two objects in the x-ray beam. They will be toward the edge of the beam. Some of the beam may extend beyond the edges of the cassette. Label this image exposure 3.

Answer the questions on the lab analysis.

NAME ___________________________

DATE ___________________________

ACTIVITY 4.D

LAB ANALYSIS—BEAM CENTERING

1. Measure on the image the distance between the inside edges of the images of the two objects from exposures 1, 2, and 3. Record these measurements.

	Exposure 1	**Exposure 2**	**Exposure 3**
distance measured	____________	____________	____________

2. Did you record any differences in these measurements?

____

____

____

3. If you recorded differences in the measurements, what do you think caused the differences?

____

____

____

4. What do you conclude concerning beam centering from this activity?

____

____

____

ACTIVITY 4.E

LAB ASSIGNMENT—SPATIAL DISTORTION

MATERIALS

2 small heavy metal objects with holes in them. They should be approximately the same length and width. (Examples are a small wrench, a key, a tool.)
3 loaded cassettes big enough to fit an image of both of the objects you are using. You may also use a large cassette and divide it into 3 sections.
A radiographic room
A processor
A square or rectangle radiographic sponge
A ruler
Tape

PROCEDURE

Tape 1 of the metal objects (object 1) onto the center of a square or rectangular radiographic sponge. Tape the other metal object (object 2) onto the other side of the sponge, directly across from the first object. The distance between the two objects is determined by the thickness of the sponge. Object 1 should be turned 90 degrees from object 2 so that the two objects would form an "X" on the image if they were superimposed.

For all exposures, place the cassette directly on top of the x-ray table. Place the radiographic sponge with the two objects taped on it directly on the cassette so that object 1 has more object-image distance than object 2. Position the sponge so that the long portion of object 1 corresponds with the short part of the x-ray table. Place the center of the objects in the center of the cassette or section of the cassette you are using. Use a 40-inch source-image distance. Adjust the collimation so that all four edges of the objects will be included on the film. You will use the same technique for each exposure. The technique you would use for a foot will probably work.

Exposure 1. Make the first exposure with the central ray perpendicular to the film and objects. Label this image exposure 1.

Exposure 2. Use the same conditions as for exposure 1. The only thing you need to change is to angle the central ray so that it is at a 20 degree angle from left to right along the long portion of the x-ray table. Label this image exposure 2.

Exposure 3. Use the same conditions as for exposure 1. The only thing you need to change is to angle the central ray so that it is from right to left along the long portion of the x-ray table. Label this image exposure 3.

Answer the questions on the lab analysis.

NAME ______________________

DATE ______________________

ACTIVITY 4.E

LAB ANALYSIS—SPATIAL DISTORTION

1. Measure on the image from exposures 1, 2, and 3 from the center of object 1 to the left edge of object 2. Then measure from the center of object 1 to the right edge of object 2. Record these measurements.

	Exposure 1	**Exposure 2**	**Exposure 3**
center to left edge	________	________	________
center to right edge	________	________	________

2. Did you record any differences in these measurements?

   ____

   ____

   ____

3. If you recorded differences in the measurements, what do you think caused the differences?

   ____

   ____

   ____

4. What do you conclude concerning spatial distortion from this activity?

   ____

   ____

   ____

NAME ____________________

DATE ____________________

ACTIVITY 4.F

CHAPTER REVIEW

MULTIPLE CHOICE

_____ 1. Which one of these is *not* a type of shape distortion?
- a. foreshortening
- b. elongation
- c. spatial distortion
- d. cone distortion

_____ 2. The central ray is located in the center of the:
- a. film
- b. x-ray tube
- c. x-ray beam
- d. Bucky tray

_____ 3. With the x-ray beam pointed straight at the patient, the central ray is:
- a. perpendicular to the patient
- b. parallel to the patient
- c. at a 2 degree angle to the patient
- d. at a 5 degree angle to the patient

_____ 4. When all the body parts in a structure are on top of each other in the image, this is called:
- a. foreshortening
- b. elongation
- c. spatial distortion
- d. superimposition

_____ 5. Which one of these maneuvers will produce the least amount of shape distortion?
- a. place the central ray perpendicular to the object and parallel to the film
- b. place the object perpendicular to the film and parallel to the central ray
- c. place the central ray perpendicular to the object and film
- d. place the film perpendicular to the object and central ray

_____ 6. Foreshortening occurs when:
- a. the film is at an angle and the central ray is perpendicular to the film
- b. the object is at an angle and the central ray is perpendicular to the film
- c. the central ray is at an angle and the object is parallel to the film
- d. several body parts are each elongated differently

_____ 7. Elongation occurs when:
- a. the film is at an angle and the central ray is perpendicular to the film
- b. the object is at an angle and the central ray is perpendicular to the film
- c. the central ray is at an angle and the object is parallel to the film
- d. several body parts are each elongated differently

_____ 8. Spatial distortion occurs when:
- a. the film is at an angle and the central ray is perpendicular to the film
- b. the object is at an angle and the central ray is perpendicular to the film

c. the central ray is at an angle and the object is parallel to the film
d. several body parts are each elongated differently

_____ 9. To avoid shape distortion, it is important to keep the central ray:
a. parallel to the object
b. directly over the object
c. directly over the edge of the film
d. parallel to the film

_____ 10. Which one of these types of distortion might be best at hiding a small fracture?
a. foreshortening
b. elongation
c. spatial distortion

Use the following diagram to answer questions 11–15.

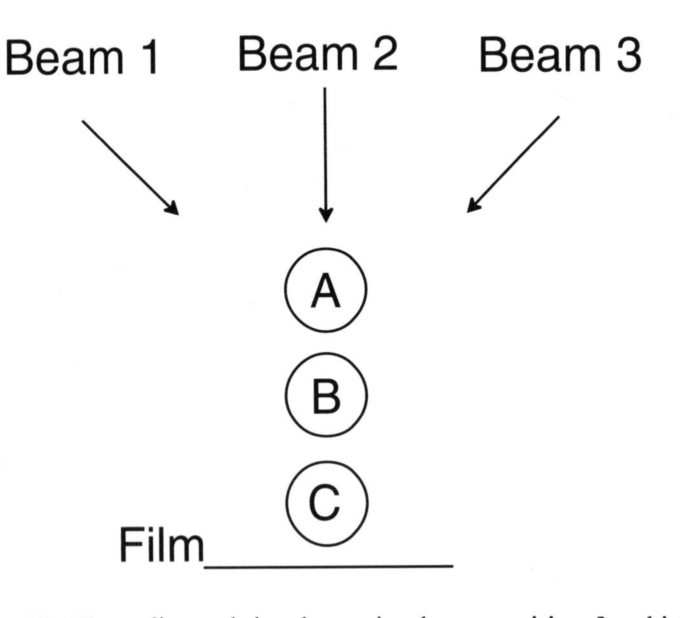

_____ 11. If a radiograph is taken using beam position 1, which part would be more spatially distorted?
a. part A
b. part B
c. part C
d. they would all be equally distorted

_____ 12. If a radiograph is taken using beam position 3, which part would appear on the left side of the image?
a. part A
b. part B
c. part C

_____ 13. If a radiograph is taken using beam position 1, which part would appear on the left side of the image?
a. part A
b. part B
c. part C

_____ 14. Which beam position would produce superimposition of parts A, B, and C on the image?
a. position 1

b. position 2
c. position 3
d. none of the positions

_____ 15. If a radiograph is taken using beam 1, which part would appear foreshortened on the image?
a. part A
b. part B
c. part C
d. none of the parts

ACTIVITY 4.G

REVIEW OF SIZE AND SHAPE DISTORTION

See clues on following page.

ACROSS CLUES

1. What is the major factor that causes size distortion?
2. SID minus OID.
6. The distance from the focal spot to the film.
9. A 72-inch SID is used during chest radiography to avoid magnification of the ______.
11. This ray is where the angle of the beam is measured.
13. If the image size is 12.84 and the object size is 12, what is the percent of magnification?
14. The elongation at the edges of an image results from these rays.
15. If the image length is 4, the SID 40, and the OID 10, what is the object length?
19. A type of shape distortion due to an angle of the beam.
21. The "I" in SID.
24. If the object width is 5 and the magnification factor is 2, the image width is ______.
25. In elongation the central ray is angled but the object and film are ______.
26. If this distance is increased, magnification is decreased.
28. Body parts on top of each other on the image.
29. To avoid shape distortion, the central ray should be ______ to the object and film.

DOWN CLUES

1. This is placed parallel to the film to avoid shape distortion.
3. A large ______ increases magnification.
4. Distortion in which the object is angled but the central ray and film are perpendicular.
5. With a large OID, magnification will ______.
7. To avoid shape distortion, this should be parallel to the object.
8. With a large SID, magnification will ______.
10. Another term for size distortion.
12. If the SID is 72″, the SOD 63″, and the object length is 7″, what is the image length?
16. A decrease in SID will cause ______ magnification.
17. If the object width is 6 and the image width is 9, what is the percent of magnification?
18. Using the ideal relationship between the central ray, object, and film avoids this distortion.
20. If the object length is 4.5 cm and the magnification factor is 2, what is the image length?
22. The type of distortion used when radiographing the clavicle.
23. With a magnification factor of 2, this in the image grows by a factor of 4.
27. This type of distortion is controlled by SID and OID.

ACTIVITY 4.H

F	G	N	O	L	E	G	J	A	Z	F	K	C
V	O	Q	E	S	O	L	C	F	P	I	L	D
P	E	R	P	E	N	D	I	C	U	L	A	R
Y	I	H	E	F	T	F	T	M	B	M	I	N
N	T	D	O	S	T	F	P	R	I	W	T	E
T	H	U	E	Y	H	S	I	N	O	L	A	L
Q	R	O	I	T	O	O	C	F	E	H	P	O
C	E	A	C	D	A	R	R	L	E	S	S	N
O	E	N	C	K	E	R	L	T	E	P	I	G
I	P	G	L	A	Y	A	A	S	E	D	D	A
D	A	L	S	L	R	H	L	P	O	N	G	T
Q	H	E	R	A	L	A	R	G	E	R	E	E
S	S	U	P	E	R	I	M	P	O	S	E	D

See questions on following page.

NAME ______________________

DATE ______________________

ACTIVITY 4.H

WORD SEARCH—DISTORTION

Decide which word best matches the definition or completes the sentence. Write the word on the line, and then find it in the word search puzzle and circle it.

__________ 1. OID affects this many of the four radiographic qualities.

__________ 2. Foreshortening occurs when the central ray is perpendicular to the film and the object is at an __________.

__________ 3. For the least magnification use a s__________ object-image distance.

__________ 4. If the object length is 3 and the image length is 9, what is the magnification factor?

__________ 5. OID plus SOD.

__________ 6. If the object and film are parallel but the central ray is angled, the image will be e__________

__________ 7. If the image width is 12 and the object width is 8, what is the percent of magnification?

__________ 8. To avoid magnification, place the object c__________ to the film.

__________ 9. If the OID increases, magnification __________.

__________ 10. In every image there is some elongation at the e__________ of the image.

__________ 11. To avoid size distortion, use a __________ SID, and a short __________. (Find two words.)

__________ 12. Two parts in the same object having different object-image distances would be s__________ with the central ray perpendicular. With an angle of the central ray off perpendicular they will appear s__________ on the image. (Find two words.)

__________ 13. Number 12 describes what kind of distortion?

__________ 14. In number 12, the part having the most object-image distance would appear l__________ on the image.

__________ 15. The i__________ relationship is to have the object and film p__________ to each other and have the central ray p__________ to the object and film. (Find three words.)

__________ 16. The relationship described in number 15 will avoid what type of distortion?

__________ 17. The magnification factor is calculated by dividing SID by __________.

_________________ 18. If the object size is 13.5, the SID 40, and the OID 4, what is the image size?

_________________ 19. A short OID will produce l____________ magnification than a long OID.

_________________ 20. To avoid foreshortening, the object should be parallel to the ____________.

NAME ______________________________

DATE ______________________________

ACTIVITY 4.1

DISTORTION REVIEW

MULTIPLE CHOICE

_____ 1. Magnification is the same as:
  a. size distortion
  b. shape distortion
  c. spatial distortion
  d. elongation

_____ 2. Using a short OID will avoid:
  a. size distortion
  b. shape distortion
  c. spatial distortion
  d. elongation

_____ 3. Placing the object parallel to the film will avoid:
  a. size distortion
  b. shape distortion
  c. spatial distortion
  d. elongation

_____ 4. Which one of these will avoid elongation?
  a. use a short OID
  b. use a long OID
  c. place the object parallel to the film
  d. place the central ray perpendicular to the object

_____ 5. Which one of these will avoid foreshortening?
  a. use a short OID
  b. use a long OID
  c. place the object parallel to the film
  d. place the central ray perpendicular to the object

_____ 6. Which one of these will avoid magnification?
  a. use a short OID
  b. use a long OID
  c. place the object parallel to the film
  d. place the central ray perpendicular to the object

_____ 7. Spatial distortion occurs for objects in which the body parts lie at a different:
  a. SID
  b. OID
  c. SOD
  d. angle

_____ 8. If the SID is 72 inches, the OID 12 inches, and the object width 10 inches, what is the image width?
  a. 8 inches
  b. 12 inches

c. 22.9 inches
d. 120 inches

_____ 9. If the area of the object is 10 inches, what is the area of the image with a magnification factor of 2?
a. 2 inches
b. 10 inches
c. 20 inches
d. 40 inches

_____ 10. When the object is at a large distance from the film, the image can be improved by:
a. decreasing the SOD
b. increasing the OID
c. increasing the SID
d. decreasing the SID

_____ 11. Which one of these is the best factor to control magnification?
a. OID
b. SID

_____ 12. The most commonly used source-image distances are:
a. 72 and 50 inches
b. 72 and 40 inches
c. 60 and 40 inches
d. 60 and 30 inches

_____ 13. If the object length is 12 and the image length is 24, the magnification factor is:
a. .5
b. 1
c. 1.5
d. 2

_____ 14. Which one of these is *not* a type of shape distortion?
a. magnification
b. foreshortening
c. elongation
d. spatial distortion

_____ 15. To avoid shape distortion, place the object _____________ to the film and the central ray _____________ to the object and film:
a. parallel, perpendicular
b. perpendicular, parallel

_____ 16. When body parts that lie at different OIDs appear on top of each other in the image, this is called:
a. foreshortening
b. elongation
c. superimposition
d. spatial distortion

_____ 17. Which one of these maneuvers would be most likely to show the size of the fracture space correctly?
a. place the fractured bone at an angle to the film
b. angle the central ray along the length of the fractured bone
c. place the fractured bone at an increased OID
d. place the fractured bone parallel and close to the film

_____ 18. With an angle of the central ray, which body part would be elongated the most?
a. one at a short OID
b. one at a long OID

_____ 19. If the object measures 12 inches and the image measures 15 inches, what is the percent of magnification?
a. 25%
b. 50%
c. 66%
d. 100%

_____ 20. To project the clavicle above the chest when the patient is lying on his or her back, the central ray should be angled:
a. toward the patient's feet
b. toward the patient's head

NAME ______________________

DATE ______________________

ACTIVITY 5.A

MATERIALS

A good-quality radiograph
A densitometer

Obtain any good-quality radiograph. You might have to get your instructor's advice on this. There are many types of densitometers, so you will need to get your instructor to show you how to use the one you have available. Then make the measurements on your own.

PROCEDURE

1. Measure the blackest area on the radiograph and record the measurement.

   ____________ Blackest area

2. Measure the whitest area on the radiograph and record the measurement.

   ____________ Whitest area

3. Measure four different areas within the image that appear to you to be different shades of gray. The first should be a light gray, the second should be a little darker shade of gray than the first, the third a little darker gray than the second, and the fourth a little darker gray than the third. Record these measurements.

   ____________ Gray area 1
   ____________ Gray area 2
   ____________ Gray area 3
   ____________ Gray area 4

4. What do you conclude about the different density values from your measurements?

   ____
   ____
   ____

5. Do you recall from Chapter 1 in the text what radiographic quality describes the various differences in density on a radiograph?

   ____

6. What do you think would happen to all of the density measurements if the entire radiograph were made darker or more dense? Explain.

   ____
   ____
   ____

ACTIVITY 5.B

LAB ASSIGNMENT—MILLIAMPERAGE (mA)

MATERIALS

A radiographic phantom of a small body part that can be exposed table top, a step wedge, or a skeletal bone
Three loaded cassettes big enough to fit an image of the phantom, step wedge, or bone you are using. You may also use a large cassette and divide it into three sections.
A radiographic room
A processor
A densitometer

PROCEDURE

You are going to take three different radiographs of your phantom, step wedge, or bone. You will need to ask your instructor for the first technique, which should produce a radiograph with an adequate amount of density. For a bone you can usually use about the same technique you would use for a hand exam. For a step wedge, the technique you would use for a foot will usually work. With the phantom, it will depend on the size and type of phantom.

For all exposures, place the cassette on top of the x-ray table. Place the step wedge, bone, or phantom directly on the cassette in the center of the cassette or section of the cassette you are using. Keep the object parallel to the cassette. Use a 40-inch SID, and position the center of the x-ray beam directly over the center of the object. Do not angle the x-ray tube. Adjust the collimation so that all four edges of the object will be included on the film.

Exposure 1. Make the first exposure using the technique specified by your instructor. Label this image exposure 1. Record the exposure factors used.

Exposure 1 factors mA ____________ time ____________

kVp ____________

Exposure 2. Make the second exposure using the same conditions used for exposure 1. The only thing you need to change is to cut the mA in half. For instance, if you used 200 mA on the first exposure, use 100 mA on this exposure. Label this image exposure 2. Record the exposure factors used.

Exposure 2 factors mA ____________ time ____________

kVp ____________

Exposure 3. Make the third exposure using the same conditions used for exposure 1. The only thing you need to change is to double the mA used for exposure 1. For instance, if you used 200 mA on the first exposure, use 400 mA on this exposure. Label this image exposure 3. Record the exposure factors used.

Exposure 3 factors mA ____________ time ____________

kVp ____________

Answer the lab analysis questions.

NAME ______________________

DATE ______________________

ACTIVITY 5.B

LAB ANALYSIS—MILLIAMPERE (mA)

1. What object (phantom, step wedge, or bone) did you use for your experiments?

 ____

2. What mA did you use for each exposure?

 Exposure 1 ____________

 Exposure 2 ____________

 Exposure 3 ____________

3. Select a medium gray spot within the first image to measure with a densitometer. Measure this same spot on all 3 images and record the numeric reading.

 Exposure 1 ____________

 Exposure 2 ____________

 Exposure 3 ____________

4. Do you see any relationship between the numeric readings from the densitometer and the mA used? Explain.

 ____

 ____

 ____

5. How did the density on the images appear to change as you changed the mA?

 ____

 ____

 ____

6. Did you see a direct relationship between mA and density on your three radiographs? Explain your answer.

 ____

 ____

 ____

ACTIVITY 5.C

LAB ASSIGNMENT—EXPOSURE TIME (sec)

MATERIALS

A radiographic phantom of a small body part that can be exposed table top, a step wedge, or a skeletal bone

Three loaded cassettes big enough to fit an image of the phantom, step wedge, or bone you are using. You may also use a large cassette and divide it into three sections

A radiographic room

A processor

A densitometer

PROCEDURE

You are going to take three different radiographs of your phantom, step wedge, or bone. You will need to ask your instructor for the first technique, which should produce a radiograph with an adequate amount of density. For a bone you can usually use about the same technique you would use for a hand exam. For a step wedge, the technique you would use for a foot will usually work. With the phantom, it will depend on the size and type of phantom.

For all exposures, place the cassette on top of the x-ray table. Place the step wedge, bone, or phantom directly on the cassette in the center of the cassette or section of the cassette you are using. Keep the object parallel to the cassette. Use a 40-inch SID, and position the center of the x-ray beam directly over the center of the object. Do not angle the x-ray tube. Adjust the collimation so that all four edges of the object will be included on the film.

Exposure 1. Make the first exposure using the technique specified by your instructor. Label this image exposure 1. Record the exposure factors used.

Exposure 1 factors mA ____________ time ____________

kVp ____________

Exposure 2. Make the second exposure using the same conditions used for exposure 1. The only thing you need to change is to cut the exposure time in half. For instance, if you used .01 second on the first exposure, use .005 second on this exposure. Label this image exposure 2. Record the exposure factors used.

Exposure 2 factors mA ____________ time ____________

kVp ____________

Exposure 3. Make the third exposure using the same conditions used for exposure 1. The only thing you need to change is to double the exposure time used for exposure 1. For instance, if you used .01 second on the first exposure, use .02 second on this exposure. Label this image exposure 3. Record the exposure factors used.

Exposure 3 factors mA ____________ time ____________

kVp ____________

Answer the lab analysis questions.

NAME ______________________

DATE ______________________

ACTIVITY 5.C

LAB ANALYSIS—EXPOSURE TIME (sec)

1. What object (phantom, step wedge, or bone) did you use for your experiments?

   ____

2. What exposure time did you use for each exposure?

   Exposure 1 __________

   Exposure 2 __________

   Exposure 3 __________

3. Select a medium-gray spot within the first image to measure with a densitometer. Measure this same spot on all three images and record the numeric reading.

   Exposure 1 __________

   Exposure 2 __________

   Exposure 3 __________

4. Do you see any relationship between the numeric readings from the densitometer and the time used? Explain.

   ____

   ____

   ____

5. How did the density on the images appear to change as you changed the time?

   ____

   ____

   ____

6. Did you see a direct relationship between the exposure time and density on your three radiographs? Explain your answer.

   ____

   ____

   ____

NAME ____________________

DATE ____________________

ACTIVITY 5.D

MILLISECONDS

Change the number of milliseconds to a decimal.

1. ____________ 10
2. ____________ 250
3. ____________ 8
4. ____________ 400
5. ____________ 1250
6. ____________ 620
7. ____________ 15
8. ____________ 5
9. ____________ 10,000
10. ____________ 180

Change the number of milliseconds to a fraction.

11. ____________ 320
12. ____________ 5
13. ____________ 1000
14. ____________ 12
15. ____________ 15,000
16. ____________ 80
17. ____________ 25
18. ____________ 480
19. ____________ 6
20. ____________ 90

Change the fraction or decimal numbers into milliseconds.

21. ____________ .450
22. ____________ .8
23. ____________ 1
24. ____________ .028
25. ____________ .004
26. ____________ .016
27. ____________ .20
28. ____________ .18
29. ____________ .380
30. ____________ 1.500

31. ____________ 20/1000
32. ____________ 300/1000
33. ____________ 15/1000
34. ____________ 8/1000
35. ____________ 1200/1000
36. ____________ 1/100
37. ____________ 1/5
38. ____________ 4/50
39. ____________ 1/25
40. ____________ 1/2

NAME ______________________

DATE ______________________

ACTIVITY 5.E

CALCULATION OF mAs

Calculate the mAs with these mA stations and *decimal* timers.

1.	100	mA	.35	sec	=	________	mAs
2.	500	mA	.05	sec	=	________	mAs
3.	600	mA	.005	sec	=	________	mAs
4.	1000	mA	.02	sec	=	________	mAs
5.	300	mA	.25	sec	=	________	mAs
6.	400	mA	.007	sec	=	________	mAs
7.	50	mA	.35	sec	=	________	mAs
8.	200	mA	.10	sec	=	________	mAs
9.	300	mA	.50	sec	=	________	mAs
10.	500	mA	.025	sec	=	________	mAs

Calculate the mAs with these mA stations and *fraction* timers.

11.	200	mA	1/20	sec	=	________	mAs
12.	400	mA	2/10	sec	=	________	mAs
13.	100	mA	1/2	sec	=	________	mAs
14.	1200	mA	1/10	sec	=	________	mAs
15.	600	mA	1/15	sec	=	________	mAs
16.	500	mA	3/10	sec	=	________	mAs
17.	300	mA	3/20	sec	=	________	mAs
18.	50	mA	2	sec	=	________	mAs
19.	100	mA	1/10	sec	=	________	mAs
20.	25	mA	4	sec	=	________	mAs

Calculate the mAs with these mA stations and *millisecond* timers.

21.	600	mA	25	msec	=	________	mAs
22.	100	mA	640	msec	=	________	mAs
23.	1200	mA	80	msec	=	________	mAs
24.	300	mA	5	msec	=	________	mAs
25.	25	mA	100	msec	=	________	mAs
26.	400	mA	500	msec	=	________	mAs
27.	500	mA	10	msec	=	________	mAs
28.	100	mA	350	msec	=	________	mAs
29.	400	mA	50	msec	=	________	mAs
30.	300	mA	8	msec	=	________	mAs

ACTIVITY 5.F

LAB ASSIGNMENT—MILLIAMPERE-SECONDS (mAs)

MATERIALS

A radiographic phantom of a small body part that can be exposed tabletop, a step wedge, or a skeletal bone
Three loaded cassettes big enough to fit an image of the phantom, step wedge, or bone you are using. You may also use a large cassette and divide it into three sections.
A radiographic room
A processor
A densitometer

PROCEDURE

You are going to take three different radiographs of your phantom, step wedge, or bone. You will need to ask your instructor for the first technique, which should produce a radiograph with an adequate amount of density. For a bone you can usually use about the same technique you would use for a hand exam. For a step wedge, the technique you would use for a foot will usually work. With the phantom, it will depend on the size and type of phantom.

For all exposures, place the cassette on top of the x-ray table. Place the step wedge, bone, or phantom directly on the cassette in the center of the cassette or section of the cassette you are using. Keep the object parallel to the cassette. Use a 40-inch SID, and position the center of the x-ray beam directly over the center of the object. Do not angle the x-ray tube. Adjust the collimation so that all four edges of the object will be included on the film.

Exposure 1. Make the first exposure using the technique specified by your instructor. Label this image exposure 1. Record the exposure factors.

Exposure 1 factors mA ____________ time ____________
kVp ____________

Exposure 2. Make the second exposure using the same conditions used for exposure 1. The only thing you need to change is to cut the mAs in half. For instance, if you used 10 mAs on the first exposure, use 5 mAs on this exposure. Label this image exposure 2. Record the exposure factors used.

Exposure 2 factors mA ____________ time ____________
kVp ____________

Exposure 3. Make the third exposure using the same conditions used for exposure 1. The only thing you need to change is to double the mAs used for exposure 1. For instance, if you used 10 mAs on the first exposure, use 20 mAs on this exposure. Label this image exposure 3. Record the exposure factors used.

Exposure 3 factors mA ____________ time ____________
kVp ____________

Answer the lab analysis questions.

NAME ____________________

DATE ____________________

ACTIVITY 5.F

LAB ANALYSIS—MILLIAMPERE-SECONDS (mAs)

1. What object (phantom, step wedge, or bone) did you use for your experiments?

   ____

2. What mAs did you use for each exposure?

   Exposure 1 ____________

   Exposure 2 ____________

   Exposure 3 ____________

3. Select a medium gray spot within the first image to measure with a densitometer. Measure this same spot on all 3 images and record the numeric reading.

   Exposure 1 ____________

   Exposure 2 ____________

   Exposure 3 ____________

4. Do you see any relationship between the numeric readings from the densitometer and the mAs used? Explain.

   ____

   ____

   ____

5. How did the density on the images change as you changed the mAs?

   ____

   ____

   ____

6. Did you see a direct relationship between mAs and density on your three radiographs? Explain your answer.

   ____

   ____

   ____

NAME ____________________

DATE ____________________

ACTIVITY 5.G

mAs CALCULATION WITH THE SAME mA OR TIME

Calculate the mAs with the mA listed, which is the same for all problems.

1.	500	mA	.005	sec	=	____________	mAs
2.	500	mA	.15	sec	=	____________	mAs
3.	500	mA	.025	sec	=	____________	mAs
4.	500	mA	1/10	sec	=	____________	mAs
5.	500	mA	3/20	sec	=	____________	mAs
6.	500	mA	1/2	sec	=	____________	mAs
7.	500	mA	2/10	sec	=	____________	mAs
8.	500	mA	35	msec	=	____________	mAs
9.	500	mA	200	msec	=	____________	mAs
10.	500	mA	5	msec	=	____________	mAs

Calculate the mAs with the time listed, which is the same for all problems.

11.	100	mA	.05	sec	=	____________	mAs
12.	50	mA	.05	sec	=	____________	mAs
13.	200	mA	.05	sec	=	____________	mAs
14.	600	mA	.05	sec	=	____________	mAs
15.	1200	mA	.05	sec	=	____________	mAs
16.	300	mA	.05	sec	=	____________	mAs
17.	500	mA	.05	sec	=	____________	mAs
18.	100	mA	.05	sec	=	____________	mAs
19.	400	mA	.05	sec	=	____________	mAs
20.	600	mA	.05	sec	=	____________	mAs

NAME ______________________________

DATE ______________________________

ACTIVITY 5.H

CALCULATION OF THE UNKNOWN FACTOR

Calculate the mAs.

1.	200	mA	.05	sec	=	____________	mAs
2.	500	mA	.15	sec	=	____________	mAs
3.	50	mA	.25	sec	=	____________	mAs
4.	200	mA	1/60	sec	=	____________	mAs
5.	600	mA	1/20	sec	=	____________	mAs
6.	100	mA	3/20	sec	=	____________	mAs
7.	300	mA	1/30	sec	=	____________	mAs
8.	400	mA	50	msec	=	____________	mAs
9.	25	mA	400	msec	=	____________	mAs
10.	500	mA	6	msec	=	____________	mAs

Calculate the mA.

11.	25	mAs	.5	sec	=	____________	mA
12.	5	mAs	.10	sec	=	____________	mA
13.	50	mAs	.25	sec	=	____________	mA
14.	10	mAs	1/30	sec	=	____________	mA
15.	60	mAs	1/10	sec	=	____________	mA
16.	20	mAs	1/20	sec	=	____________	mA
17.	15	mAs	1/40	sec	=	____________	mA
18.	4	mAs	10	msec	=	____________	mA
19.	30	mAs	150	msec	=	____________	mA
20.	6	mAs	5	msec	=	____________	mA

Calculate the time.

21.	15	mAs	500	mA	=	____________	sec
22.	50	mAs	100	mA	=	____________	sec
23.	10	mAs	200	mA	=	____________	sec
24.	15	mAs	600	mA	=	____________	sec
25.	30	mAs	400	mA	=	____________	sec
26.	8	mAs	200	mA	=	____________	sec
27.	40	mAs	400	mA	=	____________	sec
28.	4	mAs	500	mA	=	____________	sec
29.	12	mAs	200	mA	=	____________	sec
30.	60	mAs	600	mA	=	____________	sec

Use the following chart for Activities 5.I, 5.J, and 5.K. This is a sample control panel with mA stations and time stations stated in the three different time values. On an actual control panel there would only be one type of timer, but this is practice. Depending on the type of equipment and manufacturer, the mA and time stations may be different; but if you can do calculations with one type, you can do them with any type of control panel.

mA Stations

Small Focal Spot	Large Focal Spot	
25 mA	300 mA	800 mA
50 mA	400 mA	1000 mA
100 mA	500 mA	1200 mA
200 mA	600 mA	

Time in Fractions

1/120	1/10	1/2	2
1/60	3/20	3/5	3
1/40	1/5	2/3	4
1/30	1/4	3/4	6
1/20	1/3	4/5	
1/15	2/5	1	

Time in Decimals

.005	.03	.20	.70
.007	.035	.25	1
.01	.05	.30	2
.015	.07	.35	3
.02	.10	.40	4
.025	.15	.50	6

Time in Milliseconds

1.0	4.0	16.0	64.0
1.2	5.0	20.0	80.0
1.6	6.4	25.0	100.0
2.0	8.0	32.0	125.0
2.5	10.0	40.0	150.0
3.2	12.5	50.0	

NAME ____________________

DATE ____________________

ACTIVITY 5.I

CONTROL OF MOTION WITH THE RECIPROCITY LAW

Use the sample control panel for this activity. Pretend that you are standing in front of the control panel and can only use the selections that are on the control panel. The trial-and-error method necessary may be a little frustrating. Using the type of timer listed, select the mA and time that will best control motion and achieve the mAs indicated.

DECIMAL

	mA	Time	
1.	________	________	12 mAs
2.	________	________	4 mAs
3.	________	________	20 mAs
4.	________	________	16 mAs
5.	________	________	6 mAs
6.	________	________	30 mAs
7.	________	________	10 mAs
8.	________	________	15 mAs
9.	________	________	5 mAs
10.	________	________	18 mAs

FRACTION

	mA	Time	
11.	________	________	10 mAs
12.	________	________	6.66 mAs
13.	________	________	40 mAs
14.	________	________	30 mAs
15.	________	________	5 mAs
16.	________	________	50 mAs
17.	________	________	15 mAs
18.	________	________	8.3 mAs
19.	________	________	7.5 mAs
20.	________	________	20 mAs

MILLISECOND

	mA	Time		
21.	________	________	5	mAs
22.	________	________	12	mAs
23.	________	________	10	mAs
24.	________	________	4	mAs
25.	________	________	32	mAs
26.	________	________	15	mAs
27.	________	________	3	mAs
28.	________	________	25	mAs
29.	________	________	8	mAs
30.	________	________	16	mAs

NAME ____________________

DATE ____________________

ACTIVITY 5.J

USING THE SMALL FOCAL SPOT WITH THE RECIPROCITY LAW

Use the sample control panel for this activity. Pretend that you are standing at the control panel and can only use the selections that are on the control panel. Using the type of timer listed, select the mA and time that will achieve the mAs indicated. The mA must be within the small focal spot range.

DECIMAL

	mA	Time	
1.	______	______	14 mAs
2.	______	______	4 mAs
3.	______	______	20 mAs
4.	______	______	15 mAs
5.	______	______	6 mAs
6.	______	______	3 mAs
7.	______	______	10 mAs
8.	______	______	75 mAs
9.	______	______	25 mAs
10.	______	______	5 mAs

FRACTION

	mA	Time	
11.	______	______	12.5 mAs
12.	______	______	10 mAs
13.	______	______	2.5 mAs
14.	______	______	5 mAs
15.	______	______	3.3 mAs
16.	______	______	20 mAs
17.	______	______	40 mAs
18.	______	______	50 mAs
19.	______	______	1.66 mAs
20.	______	______	6.66 mAs

MILLISECOND

	mA	Time		
21.	__________	__________	5	mAs
22.	__________	__________	2.5	mAs
23.	__________	__________	10	mAs
24.	__________	__________	4	mAs
25.	__________	__________	2	mAs
26.	__________	__________	15	mAs
27.	__________	__________	5	mAs
28.	__________	__________	.4	mAs
29.	__________	__________	8	mAs
30.	__________	__________	16	mAs

NAME ______________________

DATE ______________________

ACTIVITY 5.K

USING THE BREATHING TECHNIQUE WITH THE RECIPROCITY LAW

Use the sample control panel for this activity. Pretend that you are standing at the control panel and can only use the selections that are on the control panel. Using the type of timer listed, select the mA and time that will be the best breathing technique and achieve the mAs indicated.

DECIMAL

	mA	Time		
1.	______	______	15	mAs
2.	______	______	50	mAs
3.	______	______	10	mAs
4.	______	______	5	mAs
5.	______	______	40	mAs
6.	______	______	12.5	mAs
7.	______	______	25	mAs
8.	______	______	20	mAs
9.	______	______	17.5	mAs
10.	______	______	7.5	mAs

FRACTION

	mA	Time		
11.	______	______	20	mAs
12.	______	______	30	mAs
13.	______	______	15	mAs
14.	______	______	80	mAs
15.	______	______	12.5	mAs
16.	______	______	75	mAs
17.	______	______	25	mAs
18.	______	______	50	mAs
19.	______	______	10	mAs
20.	______	______	40	mAs

The millisecond times on the sample control panel are all short times. When using this type of control panel, the shorter times are in milliseconds and then the control panel switches over to decimals for the longer times. So a breathing technique cannot be achieved with the milliseconds listed on the sample control panel. If you have an x-ray unit available to you with milliseconds, see which time stations are in milliseconds and which are in decimals.

NAME ____________________

DATE ____________________

ACTIVITY 5.K

USING THE BREATHING TECHNIQUE WITH THE RECIPROCITY LAW

Use the sample control panel for this activity. Pretend that you are standing at the control panel and can only use the selections that are on the control panel. Using the type of timer listed, select the mA and time that will be the best breathing technique and achieve the mAs indicated.

DECIMAL

	mA	Time	
1.	______	______	15 mAs
2.	______	______	50 mAs
3.	______	______	10 mAs
4.	______	______	5 mAs
5.	______	______	40 mAs
6.	______	______	12.5 mAs
7.	______	______	25 mAs
8.	______	______	20 mAs
9.	______	______	17.5 mAs
10.	______	______	7.5 mAs

FRACTION

	mA	Time	
11.	______	______	20 mAs
12.	______	______	30 mAs
13.	______	______	15 mAs
14.	______	______	80 mAs
15.	______	______	12.5 mAs
16.	______	______	75 mAs
17.	______	______	25 mAs
18.	______	______	50 mAs
19.	______	______	10 mAs
20.	______	______	40 mAs

The millisecond times on the sample control panel are all short times. When using this type of control panel, the shorter times are in milliseconds and then the control panel switches over to decimals for the longer times. So a breathing technique cannot be achieved with the milliseconds listed on the sample control panel. If you have an x-ray unit available to you with milliseconds, see which time stations are in milliseconds and which are in decimals.

NAME ______________________

DATE ______________________

ACTIVITY 5.L

mAs CHARTS

Use the mAs chart to find the following mAs values.

1. ________	500	mA	.015	sec
2. ________	100	mA	35	msec
3. ________	300	mA	.02	sec
4. ________	25	mA	1/20	sec
5. ________	600	mA	.030	sec
6. ________	400	mA	50	msec
7. ________	300	mA	10	msec
8. ________	50	mA	.015	sec
9. ________	600	mA	1/60	sec
10. ________	100	mA	1/30	sec

Use the mAs chart to find the following mA values.

11. ________	.35	mAs	.007	sec
12. ________	5.0	mAs	25	msec
13. ________	2.0	mAs	.010	sec
14. ________	1.25	mAs	1/20	sec
15. ________	30	mAs	50	msec
16. ________	.70	mAs	.007	sec
17. ________	10.5	mAs	.035	sec
18. ________	12	mAs	30	msec
19. ________	2.5	mAs	1/40	sec
20. ________	25	mAs	1/20	sec

Use the mAs chart to find the following time values. Write it in whatever unit you want to.

21. ________	.70	mAs	100	mA
22. ________	4.5	mAs	300	mA
23. ________	.414	mAs	50	mA
24. ________	3.0	mAs	600	mA
25. ________	12.0	mAs	400	mA
26. ________	.50	mAs	25	mA
27. ________	17.5	mAs	500	mA
28. ________	4.98	mAs	300	mA
29. ________	15.0	mAs	600	mA
30. ________	4.0	mAs	200	mA

NAME ______________________

DATE ______________________

ACTIVITY 5.M

CHAPTER REVIEW

MULTIPLE CHOICE

_____ 1. Density and time have what relationship?
   a. directly proportional
   b. inversely proportional
   c. no relationship

_____ 2. The exposure factor that should be used to control density is:
   a. kVp
   b. SID
   c. mAs
   d. mA

_____ 3. mAs controls or influences which of the following:
      1. density
      2. contrast
      3. recorded detail
      4. distortion
   a. 1 and 4
   b. 2 only
   c. 3 and 4
   d. 1 only

_____ 4. To reduce the chance of motion on a radiograph, the radiographer should choose the lowest:
   a. mA
   b. time
   c. mAs
   d. kVp

_____ 5. The factor that determines the total quantity of x-rays produced in a beam is the:
   a. mA
   b. time
   c. mAs
   d. kVp

_____ 6. The length of the x-ray exposure is determined by the:
   a. mA
   b. time
   c. mAs
   d. all of these

_____ 7. Time controls or influences which of the following?
      1. density
      2. contrast
      3. recorded detail
      4. distortion

a. 1 and 4
b. 2 only
c. 3 and 4
d. 1 only

____ 8. Density and mAs have what relationship?
a. directly proportional
b. inversely proportional
c. no relationship

____ 9. If the mAs is decreased by 50%, the density will be decreased by:
a. 30%
b. 50%
c. 100%
d. 200%

____ 10. Which two sets of mA and time are an example of the reciprocity law?
1. 200 mA 1/20 sec
2. 400 mA .03 sec
3. 500 mA .02 sec
4. 600 mA 50 msec
a. 1 and 3
b. 2 and 4
c. 1 and 4
d. 2 and 3

____ 11. mA controls or influences which of the following?
1. density
2. contrast
3. recorded detail
4. distortion
a. 1 and 4
b. 2 only
c. 3 and 4
d. 1 only

____ 12. Which set of factors would produce a radiograph with the greatest density?
a. 400 mA .10 sec
b. 200 mA .30 sec
c. 500 mA .01 sec
d. 600 mA .025 sec

____ 13. Which set of factors would produce a radiograph with the least density?
a. 200 mA 1/30 sec
b. 400 mA 1/40 sec
c. 300 mA 1/20 sec
d. 100 mA 2/3 sec

____ 14. Which set of factors would produce a radiograph with the greatest density?
a. 50 mA 18 msec
b. 500 mA 3 msec
c. 300 mA 25 msec
d. 200 mA 40 msec

____ 15. Which one of these factors is the amount of current in the x-ray tube at the time of the exposure?
a. mA
b. time

c. mAs
d. none of these

_____ 16. Changing from 200 mA at .05 sec to 200 mA at .10 sec will increase:
a. density
b. contrast
c. recorded detail
d. distortion

_____ 17. Which one of these milliseconds is the same as 1/40 sec?
a. 4
b. 12
c. 25
d. 40

_____ 18. Which one of these techniques would be the best to control motion on a radiograph?
a. 100 mA .05 sec
b. 200 mA 1/40 sec
c. 500 mA 10 msec
d. 50 mA .10 sec

_____ 19. Which one of these techniques would produce the best recorded detail on the radiograph?
a. 50 mA 200 msec
b. 500 mA .02 sec
c. 400 mA 1/40 sec
d. 1000 mA 10 msec

_____ 20. Which one of these techniques would be the best for a breathing technique?
a. 500 mA .05 sec
b. 1000 mA 1/40 sec
c. 50 mA 1/2 sec
d. 25 mA 1 sec

Fill in the unknown factors on this chart.

	mA	Time	mAs
21.	300	.025	_____
22.	500	_____	15
23.	_____	5 msec	5
24.	50	_____	10
25.	200	1/20	_____

	mA	Time	mAs	New mA	New Time	New mAs
26.	100	.10	10	500	_____	10
27	300	1/20	15	_____	1/20	30
28.	400	1/40	_____	200	1/20	_____
29.	200	.20	40	_____	.10	20
30.	500	.05	25	500	_____	50

NAME ______________________

DATE ______________________

ACTIVITY 6.A

The x-ray beam and a light beam have similar characteristics. This activity will help you see the change in the intensity and size of a light beam. The intensity and size of the x-ray beam changes in the same way a light beam does.

MATERIALS

A collimator with a light
A ruler

PROCEDURE

1. Position the x-ray tube over the table top at a 25-inch SID. Do not angle the tube. Shine the light from the collimator onto the x-ray table. Measure the length and width of the light shining on the table and record it.

   length ____________ width ____________

2. Calculate the area of the light used in procedure 1 by multiplying the length by the width and record it.

   area ____________

3. Now move the x-ray tube to a 50-inch SID without adjusting the collimation used on procedure 1. Shine the light from the collimator onto the x-ray table. Measure the length and width of the light shining on the table and record it.

   length ____________ width ____________

4. Calculate the area of the light used in procedure 3 by multiplying the length by the width and record it.

   area ____________

5. Approximately how many times bigger is the area calculated in procedure 2 than the area calculated in procedure 4?

   ____

6. Now move the tube back to the 25-inch source-image distance, and then back to the 50-inch source-image distance. Do you observe any difference in the brightness of the light at the two different distances. What do you conclude about the x-ray beam and the source-image distance from this activity?

   ____

   ____

   ____

NAME ________________

DATE ________________

ACTIVITY 6.B

Calculate the following using the inverse square law.

	I_2	I_1	D_1	D_2
1.	________	90 mR	40 in.	72 in.
2.	________	120 mR	56 in.	68 in.
3.	________	50 mR	36 cm	58 cm
4.	________	5 mR	30 cm	82 cm
5.	________	40 mR	44 in.	72 in.
6.	________	2 mR	72 in.	40 in.
7.	________	25 mR	80 in.	60 in.
8.	________	50 mR	56 in.	40 in.
9.	________	35 mR	62 cm	34 cm
10.	________	250 mR	48 in.	40 in.
11.	100 mR	________	36 in.	72 in.
12.	65 mR	________	64 in.	52 in.
13.	40 mR	________	32 in.	84 in.
14.	5 mR	________	40 in.	50 in.
15.	400 mR	________	72 in.	56 in.

NAME ____________________

DATE ____________________

ACTIVITY 6.C

Calculate the following using the inverse square law. You may not even need to use a calculator.

	I_2	I_1	D_1	D_2
1.	____________	10 mR	36 in.	72 in.
2.	____________	150 mR	34 in.	68 in.
3.	____________	45 mR	29 cm	58 cm
4.	____________	15 mR	41 cm	82 cm
5.	____________	5 mR	44 in.	88 in.
6.	____________	20 mR	72 in.	36 in.
7.	____________	25 mR	80 in.	40 in.
8.	____________	50 mR	56 in.	28 in.
9.	____________	8 mR	62 cm	31 cm
10.	____________	360 mR	80 in.	40 in.
11.	____________	30 mR	36 in.	72 in.
12.	____________	50 mR	38 in.	76 in.
13.	____________	6 mR	30 cm	60 cm
14.	____________	12 mR	35 cm	70 cm
15.	____________	3 mR	48 in.	96 in.
16.	____________	40 mR	72 in.	36 in.
17.	____________	60 mR	80 in.	40 in.
18.	____________	22 mR	66 in.	33 in.
19.	____________	18 mR	76 cm	38 cm
20.	____________	150 mR	80 in.	40 in.

NAME ____________________

DATE ____________________

ACTIVITY 6.C

Calculate the following using the inverse square law. You may not even need to use a calculator.

	I_2	I_1	D_1	D_2
1.	________	10 mR	36 in.	72 in.
2.	________	150 mR	34 in.	68 in.
3.	________	45 mR	29 cm	58 cm
4.	________	15 mR	41 cm	82 cm
5.	________	5 mR	44 in.	88 in.
6.	________	20 mR	72 in.	36 in.
7.	________	25 mR	80 in.	40 in.
8.	________	50 mR	56 in.	28 in.
9.	________	8 mR	62 cm	31 cm
10.	________	360 mR	80 in.	40 in.
11.	________	30 mR	36 in.	72 in.
12.	________	50 mR	38 in.	76 in.
13.	________	6 mR	30 cm	60 cm
14.	________	12 mR	35 cm	70 cm
15.	________	3 mR	48 in.	96 in.
16.	________	40 mR	72 in.	36 in.
17.	________	60 mR	80 in.	40 in.
18.	________	22 mR	66 in.	33 in.
19.	________	18 mR	76 cm	38 cm
20.	________	150 mR	80 in.	40 in.

ACTIVITY 6.D

LAB ASSIGNMENT—MEASURING RADIATION INTENSITY

MATERIALS

A radiographic room
An ionization chamber

PROCEDURE

For all exposures, place the ionization chamber on the x-ray table. Position the x-ray tube directly over the ionization chamber. Do not angle the tube. Adjust the collimation to include all four edges of the ionization chamber. Set the exposure factors at 5 mAs and 80 kVp.

Exposure 1. Place the x-ray tube at a distance of 25 inches from the ionization chamber. Make the exposure and record the reading from the ionization chamber.

____

Exposure 2. Place the x-ray tube at a distance of 50 inches from the ionization chamber. Make the exposure and record the reading from the ionization chamber.

____

Exposure 3. Place the x-ray tube at any distance from the ionization chamber other than 25 and 50 inches. Make the exposure and record the reading from the ionization chamber.

_______________ reading

_______________ distance used

Answer the questions on the lab analysis.

NAME ______________________

DATE ______________________

ACTIVITY 6.D

LAB ANALYSIS—MEASURING RADIATION INTENSITY

1. Record the ionization chamber readings from exposure 1 and 2.

   Exposure 1 ____________ Exposure 2 ____________

2. Calculate the difference between the readings for exposures 1 and 2 and record it.

   ____

3. Is there any relationship between the readings and the distance used for exposures 1 and 2. Explain.

   ____

   ____

4. Using the inverse square law, calculate the new radiation intensity you should have gotten when changing from the 25-inch distance used for exposure 1 and the 50-inch distance used for exposure 2.

   ____

5. Did the answer you calculated in procedure number 4 match the ionization chamber reading you got when you made exposure 2? Explain.

   ____

   ____

6. Record the distance you used for exposure 3 and the ionization chamber reading.

   ____________ ____________

7. Using the inverse square law, calculate the new radiation intensity you should have gotten when changing from the 50-inch distance used for exposure 2 and the distance you used for exposure 3.

   ____

8. Did the answer you calculated in procedure 7 match the ionization chamber reading you got when you made exposure 3? Explain.

   ____

   ____

9. Have you shown any relationship between the distance between the x-ray tube and ionization chamber and the exposure readings?

   ____

   ____

NAME ______________________

DATE ______________________

ACTIVITY 6.E

Calculate the following using the density maintenance formula.

	New mAs	Old mAs	New D	Old D
1.	________	30	40 in.	72 in.
2.	________	12	52 in.	64 in.
3.	________	20	30 in.	56 in.
4.	________	5	36 in.	68 in.
5.	________	40	48 in.	64 in.
6.	________	4	72 in.	40 in.
7.	________	15	80 in.	50 in.
8.	________	150	66 in.	40 in.
9.	________	8	62 in.	38 in.
10.	________	200	48 in.	40 in.
11.	________	30	36 in.	72 in.
12.	________	24	38 in.	78 in.
13.	________	60	30 in.	70 in.
14.	________	12	40 in.	70 in.
15.	________	120	42 in.	56 in.
16.	________	40	64 in.	36 in.
17.	________	60	80 in.	40 in.
18.	________	28	64 in.	38 in.
19.	________	15	72 in.	30 in.
20.	________	150	60 in.	40 in.

ACTIVITY 6.F

LAB ASSIGNMENT—DENSITY MAINTENANCE FORMULA

MATERIALS

A radiographic phantom of a small body part that can be exposed tabletop, a step wedge, or a skeletal bone
Three loaded cassettes big enough to fit an image of the phantom, step wedge, or bone you are using. You may also use a large cassette and divide it into three sections.
A radiographic room
A processor
A densitometer

PROCEDURE

For all exposures, place the cassette on top of the x-ray table. Place the phantom, step wedge, or bone directly on the cassette in the center of the cassette or section of the cassette you are using. Keep the object parallel to the cassette. Position the center of the x-ray beam directly over the center of the object. Do not angle the x-ray tube. Adjust the collimation so that all four edges of the object will be included on the film.

Exposure 1. Make the first exposure using a 40-inch SID. You may need to ask your instructor for the first technique. For a bone, you can usually use about the same technique you would use for a hand exam. For a step wedge, the technique you would use for a foot will usually work. With the phantom, it will depend on the size and type of phantom. Label this image exposure 1. Record the exposure factors used.

Exposure 1 factors mA ____________ time ____________
mAs ____________ kVp ____________

Exposure 2. Move the x-ray tube so that you are using a 50-inch SID. Use the same technique as for exposure 1. Label this image exposure 2.

Exposure 3. Using the density maintenance formula, calculate the new mAs to be used to maintain film density when the x-ray tube is moved from the 40-inch SID used for exposure 1 to the 50-inch SID used for exposure 2. Set this new mAs on the control panel. Try to adjust only the time to get the new mAs. If you can't get the exact mAs you calculated, get as close to it as possible. Make the exposure using these new factors. Label this image exposure 3. Record the exposure factors used.

Exposure 3 factors mA ____________ time ____________
mAs ____________ kVp ____________

NAME ____________________

DATE ____________________

ACTIVITY 6.F

LAB ANALYSIS—DENSITY MAINTENANCE FORMULA

1. What object (phantom, step wedge, or bone) did you use for your experiments?

   ____

2. What exposure factors did you use for the three exposures?

   Exposure 1 mA ________ time ________ mAs ________ kVp ________

   Exposure 2 mA ________ time ________ mAs ________ kVp ________

   Exposure 3 mA ________ time ________ mAs ________ kVp ________

3. Select a medium-gray spot within the image from the first radiograph to measure with a densitometer. Measure this same spot on all three images and record the numeric reading.

   Exposure 1 ____________

   Exposure 2 ____________

   Exposure 3 ____________

4. According to the density maintenance formula, which two of the three exposures should have the same densitometer reading and density appearance? Did they? Explain.

   ____

   ____

   ____

5. Visually compare the density appearance on the radiographs from the three exposures?

   Exposure 1 ____________________________________

   Exposure 2 ____________________________________

   Exposure 3 ____________________________________

NAME ____________________

DATE ____________________

ACTIVITY 6.G

Calculate the new time using the density maintenance formula.

	New Time	Old Time	New D	Old D
1.	________	.05 sec	40 in.	72 in.
2.	________	2/5 sec	51 in.	72 in.
3.	________	20 msec	30 in.	40 in.
4.	________	.2 sec	40 in.	68 in.
5.	________	2/15 sec	44 in.	72 in.
6.	________	4 msec	72 in.	40 in.
7.	________	.15 sec	60 in.	50 in.
8.	________	150 msec	50 in.	40 in.
9.	________	1/20 sec	57 in.	40 in.
10.	________	.025	68 in.	40 in.

NAME ____________________

DATE ____________________

ACTIVITY 6.H

Calculate the new mAs or time using the density maintenance formula. Try it without a calculator.

	New mAs	Old mAs	New D	Old D
1.	________	50	40 in.	80 in.
2.	________	10	50 in.	25 in.
3.	________	8	30 in.	60 in.
4.	________	100	34 in.	68 in.
5.	________	25	44 in.	88 in.
6.	________	16	70 in.	35 in.
7.	________	70	60 in.	30 in.
8.	________	12	28 in.	56 in.
9.	________	4	64 in.	32 in
10.	________	32	72 in.	36 in.
	New Time	**Old Time**	**New D**	**Old D**
11.	________	.10	44 in.	88 in.
12.	________	2/5	23 in.	46 in.
13.	________	20 msec	35 in.	70 in.
14.	________	.025	76 in.	38 in.
15.	________	1/2	40 in.	80 in.
16.	________	240 msec	30 in.	60 in.
17.	________	3/15	32 in.	64 in.
18.	________	.07	58 in.	29 in.
19.	________	.25	72 in.	36 in.
20.	________	36 msec	68 in.	34 in.

NAME ____________________

DATE ____________________

ACTIVITY 6.1

Estimate the new mAs with the distance change using the chart in the book. Then calculate the new mAs using the density maintenance formula and see how close your estimate was.

	Estimate	New mAs	Old mAs	New D	Old D
1.	________	________	15	66 in.	40 in.
2.	________	________	10	48 in.	72 in.
3.	________	________	6	60 in.	40 in.
4.	________	________	120	62 in.	40 in.
5.	________	________	20	54 in.	72 in.
6.	________	________	12	60 in.	72 in.
7.	________	________	30	60 in.	40 in.
8.	________	________	18	44 in.	72 in.
9.	________	________	40	64 in.	72 in.
10.	________	________	24	55 in.	40 in.

NAME ______________________

DATE ______________________

ACTIVITY 6.J

CHAPTER REVIEW

MULTIPLE CHOICE

_____ 1. If the x-ray tube is moved closer to the film, the radiation intensity at the film:
   a. increases
   b. decreases

_____ 2. Which one of these tells the radiographer what new mAs to use when the SID changes to maintain film density?
   a. the reciprocity law
   b. the inverse square law
   c. Coulomb's law
   d. the density maintenance formula

_____ 3. As the x-ray tube is moved farther away from the film, the collimator light will:
   a. cover a smaller area of the film
   b. cover a larger area of the film

_____ 4. The distance between the x-ray tube and the film is called the:
   a. source-object distance
   b. object-image distance
   c. source-image distance
   d. target-image distance

_____ 5. If the SID doubles, the radiation intensity at the film:
   a. doubles
   b. is cut in half
   c. quadruples
   d. is reduced by a factor of 4

_____ 6. If the same exposure factors are used on four different radiographs and all that is changed is the SID, which radiograph would display the greatest density? The one taken at:
   a. 36-inch SID
   b. 44-inch SID
   c. 56-inch SID
   d. 72-inch SID

_____ 7. Which one of these is performed first when calculating the density maintenance formula?
   a. find the old radiation intensity
   b. cross-multiply
   c. find the new mAs
   d. square the distances

_____ 8. Which one of these factors should usually *not* be changed when changing exposure factors using the density maintenance formula:
   a. the exposure time
   b. the mA
   c. the mAs
   d. the SID

_____ 9. If the original mAs is 10 and the SID changes from 36 inches to 72 inches, which one of these mAs values would produce a radiograph with density the same as the original radiograph taken at 10 mAs:
a. 2.5 mAs
b. 10 mAs
c. 20 mAs
d. 40 mAs

Radiograph A	**Radiograph B**
500 mA	500 mA
.02 sec	.08 sec
36-inch SID	72-inch SID

_____ 10. Using the above exposure factors, which one of these statements is true about the two different radiographs:
a. radiograph A would display more density than radiograph B
b. radiograph A would display less density than radiograph B
c. radiograph B would display less density than radiograph A
d. the two radiographs would display the same density

Calculate the new radiation intensity.

	I_2	I_1	D_1	D_2
11.	_____	15 mR	40 in.	72 in.
12.	_____	12 mR	34 in.	58 in.
13.	_____	6 mR	66 in.	44 in.
14.	_____	115 mR	72 in.	50 in.
15.	_____	40 mR	44 in.	72 in.

Calculate the new mAs.

	New mAs	Old mAs	New D	Old D
16.	_____	8	72 in.	40 in.
17.	_____	10	60 in.	50 in.
18.	_____	120	56 in.	40 in.
19.	_____	17	62 in.	38 in.
20.	_____	100	48 in.	40 in.

NAME ____________________

DATE ____________________

ACTIVITY 7.A

Draw two gray-scale charts, one representing your concept of what high contrast would look like, and one representing your concept of what low contrast would look like. Label the two charts high and low contrast and also label the charts short and long scale contrast.

ACTIVITY 7.B

LAB ASSIGNMENT—EFFECT OF WATER ON SCATTERED RADIATION

MATERIALS

Three metal objects with different thicknesses and densities that will not be ruined by immersion in water and will not float in water

A plastic food storage container with sides that are at least 2 inches high. It must be large enough to accommodate all three objects when they are lying flat in the container and not touching each other

Two loaded cassettes large enough to fit an image of all three objects in the food storage container on the same film

A radiographic room

A processor

A densitometer

PROCEDURE

Exposure 1. Arbitrarily assign the numbers 1 through 3 to your objects. Place the three objects flat in the food storage container so that they are not touching each other. Place the cassette on the x-ray tabletop and put the food container on top of the cassette. Position the x-ray tube over the container and the film at a 40-inch SID. Do not angle the x-ray tube. Adjust the collimation so that all four edges of the food container will be included on the film. You may need some help from your instructor with the exposure factors. The exposure you would use for a foot will probably work. Label the radiograph exposure 1.

Exposure 2. Repeat the above procedure but this time fill the food storage container with as much water as you can. Do not change the position of the three objects in the container. Label the radiograph exposure 2.

NAME ________________

DATE ________________

ACTIVITY 7.B

LAB ANALYSIS—EFFECT OF WATER ON SCATTERED RADIATION

1. Describe the objects you used for this experiment.

   Object 1 ________________

   Object 2 ________________

   Object 3 ________________

2. Rank the objects in order according to their density.

   1. ________
   2. ________
   3. ________

3. Rank the objects in order according to their thickness.

   1. ________
   2. ________
   3. ________

4. Using the radiographs from both exposures, measure with a densitometer the same area on the image of each of the three objects and record the measurement. Also measure one other area on each radiograph between the objects. This area should not include the image of any of the three objects.

Exposure 1		**Exposure 2**	
Object 1	________	Object 1	________
Object 2	________	Object 2	________
Object 3	________	Object 3	________
Other area	________	Other area	________

5. How did the measurements of the objects from exposure 1 and exposure 2 vary? Why do you think this happened?

   ____

   ____

   ____

6. How did the measurements of the objects and other area compare between exposures 1 and 2? Why do you think this happened?

   ____

   ____

   ____

7. What do you conclude about subject contrast as a result of this experiment?

   ____

   ____

   ____

ACTIVITY 7.C

LAB ASSIGNMENT—PRODUCTION OF SCATTERED RADIATION

MATERIALS

An abdomen, pelvis, or chest radiographic phantom
Two loaded 10 × 12 cassettes
A radiographic side marker
A radiographic room
A processor
A densitometer

PROCEDURE

Exposure 1. Place the abdomen, pelvis, or chest phantom on the x-ray table. Position the x-ray tube over the phantom and adjust the collimation to include all the edges of the phantom in the beam. You will not have a cassette under the phantom, but you will make an exposure of the phantom as if you did. Prop one of the 10 × 12 cassettes 12 inches from the end of the phantom so that the cassette is perpendicular to the tabletop. Make an exposure using the normal technique for the phantom you are using and develop the film that was propped up next to the phantom. Label it exposure 1.

Exposure 2. Repeat the procedure from exposure 1 but remove the phantom before making the exposure. Develop the film that was propped up next to the absent phantom and label it exposure 2.

NAME ______________________

DATE ______________________

ACTIVITY 7.C

LAB ANALYSIS—PRODUCTION OF SCATTERED RADIATION

1. Make two density measurements from each exposure with the densitometer. Measure the density in the center of each radiograph and record the measurements.

   Exposure 1 __________ Exposure 2 __________

2. If you measured a difference in the density measurements in procedure 1, what do you think caused the difference?

   ____

   ____

   ____

3. What do you conclude about scattered radiation production from this experiment?

   ____

   ____

   ____

NAME ______________________

DATE ______________________

ACTIVITY 7.D

CHAPTER REVIEW

MULTIPLE CHOICE

c 1. Which one of these is the controlling factor for radiographic contrast?
  a. mA
  b. time
  c. kVp
  d. mAs

a 2. Which type of image would be considered high contrast?
  a. black and white and few gray shades
  b. black, white, and many gray shades

a 3. Which contrast scale is also considered high contrast?
  a. short scale
  b. long scale

b 4. Which contrast is produced with a high kVp?
  a. short scale
  b. long scale

d 5. Which one of these has the most tissue density?
  a. air
  b. muscle
  c. fat
  d. bone

a 6. Which one of these body components would display the most radiographic density?
  a. air
  b. muscle
  c. fat
  d. bone

b 7. The degree of difference between adjacent densities on a radiograph defines:
  a. density
  b. contrast
  c. recorded detail
  d. distortion

c 8. The radiographic contrast caused by the differences in the patient's body components is called:
  a. high contrast
  b. differential absorption
  c. subject contrast
  d. attenuation

a 9. Which would absorb more x-ray photons?
  a. a body component with many electrons
  b. a body component with few electrons

____ 10. The ability of a body component to absorb x-rays differently depending on its average atomic number and atom compactness is called:
a. differential absorption
b. attenuation
c. radiographic contrast
d. subject density

____ 11. The reduction in intensity of radiation as it passes through matter is called:
a. differential absorption
b. attenuation
c. subject contrast
d. tissue density

____ 12. If two body components were exactly the same except for their thickness, which component would absorb the most radiation?
a. the thicker body component
b. the thinner body component

____ 13. If two body components received the same amount of radiation, which would display the most radiographic density?
a. the thicker body component
b. the thinner body component

____ 14. Radiographs of which one of these patients would display the highest radiographic contrast?
a. a muscular patient
b. a patient who is retaining water due to disease
c. a patient who has lost minerals in his bones due to disease
d. a patient who has been sick for a very long time

____ 15. Which one of these can a radiographer usually see on a plain radiograph of the abdomen?
a. the pancreas
b. the liver
c. the spleen
d. the stomach

____ 16. The addition of which one of these contrast media to the body will decrease the tissue density of the body part?
a. air
b. iodine
c. barium

____ 17. Which one of these contrast media has the highest atomic number?
a. air
b. iodine
c. barium

____ 18. Which exposure factor gives kinetic energy to electrons as they travel from the filament to the anode of the x-ray tube?
a. mA
b. time
c. kVp
d. mAs

____ 19. An electron that has a lot of kinetic energy as it travels from the filament to the anode of the x-ray tube will probably produce an x-ray photon with:
a. high energy
b. low energy

a 20. Which beam would penetrate through body tissues easily?
a. a beam produced with high kVp
b. a beam produced with low kVp

a 21. Which kVp produces more scattered radiation?
a. a high kVp
b. a low kVp

a 22. Which type of image would be produced on a radiograph produced with low kVp?
a. high contrast
b. low contrast

c 23. Another term for the presence of scattered radiation on the film is:
a. attenuation
b. differential absorption
c. fog
d. exit radiation

Circle the appropriate term in each row to describe the variables in this chart:

kVp	Photon Energy	Radiographic Contrast	Contrast Scale	Penetrating Ability
High	High/Low	High/Low	Short/Long	High/Low
High/Low	High/Low	High/Low	**Short**	High/Low

NAME ______________________

DATE ______________________

ACTIVITY 8.A

List the kVp the radiographers in your clinical assignment usually use for each of the following:

1. ____________ an AP wrist
2. ____________ an AP foot
3. ____________ an AP knee
4. ____________ an AP elbow
5. ____________ an AP hip
6. ____________ an AP pelvis
7. ____________ an AP skull
8. ____________ a KUB
9. ____________ an AP chest performed portable
10. ____________ a PA chest performed in the department
11. ____________ an AP cervical spine
12. ____________ an AP lumbar spine
13. ____________ a PA stomach with barium
14. ____________ a PA colon with barium
15. ____________ a PA colon with barium and air

Refer to Table 8–1, which lists the optimum kVp for commonly radiographed body parts. Note any differences of more than 10 kVp between Table 8–1 and what the radiographers are actually using. Find out why there are any differences, and explain the reason.

____

____

____

NAME ______________________

DATE ______________________

ACTIVITY 8.B

CALCULATION OF THE 15% RULE

Calculate the new kVp with the change in the mAs.

	Original mAs	Original kVp	New mAs	New kVp
1.	10	70	5	______
2.	6	90	12	______
3.	25	75	50	______
4.	100	60	50	______
5.	4	100	8	______
6.	20	40	10	______
7.	150	85	75	______
8.	15	68	30	______
9.	35	72	70	______
10.	24	66	12	______

Calculate the new mAs with the change in the kVp.

	Original mAs	Original kVp	New mAs	New kVp
11.	12	70	______	80
12.	10	90	______	77
13.	15	68	______	78
14.	7	66	______	56
15.	120	100	______	115
16.	30	50	______	57
17.	100	76	______	65
18.	18	82	______	70
19.	40	58	______	67
20.	60	92	______	78

NAME ____________________

DATE ____________________

ACTIVITY 8.C

15% RULE TO CONTROL MOTION AND CONTRAST

Calculate the new kVp and mAs that will increase contrast.

	Original mAs	Original kVp	New mAs	New kVp
1.	15	80	______	______
2.	20	90	______	______
3.	32	85	______	______
4.	120	82	______	______
5.	24	110	______	______

Calculate the new kVp and mAs that will decrease contrast.

	Original mAs	Original kVp	New mAs	New kVp
6.	5	60	______	______
7.	50	75	______	______
8.	12	88	______	______
9.	25	78	______	______
10.	8	66	______	______

Calculate the new mAs and kVp that will decrease motion.

	Original mAs	Original kVp	New mAs	New kVp
11.	10	90	______	______
12.	15	70	______	______
13.	9	68	______	______
14.	50	74	______	______
15.	100	60	______	______
16.	38	55	______	______
17.	26	85	______	______
18.	14	77	______	______
19.	42	66	______	______
20.	40	78	______	______

ACTIVITY 8.D

LAB ASSIGNMENT—15% RULE

MATERIALS

A step wedge or radiographic phantom of a small body part that can be exposed tabletop
Three loaded cassettes large enough to fit an image of the step wedge or phantom.
You may also use a large cassette and divide it into three sections.
A radiographic room
A processor
A densitometer

PROCEDURE

For all exposures, place the cassette on top of the x-ray table. Place the step wedge or phantom directly on the cassette in the center of the cassette or section of the cassette you are using. Keep the object parallel to the cassette. Use a 40-inch SID and position the center of the x-ray beam directly over the center of the object. Do not angle the x-ray tube. Adjust the collimation so that all four edges of the object will be included on the film.

Exposure 1. Make the first exposure using a good technique with the optimum kVp. For the step wedge, the technique used for a foot will probably work. For the phantom, use the ordinary technique for the body part you are using. Label this image exposure 1. Record the exposure factors used.

mA ______________ time ______________ mAs ______________

kVp ______________

Exposure 2. Using the 15% rule, calculate the new mAs and kVp if the kVp is decreased and the mAs is increased. Repeat all the conditions for exposure 1, but use the new exposure factors you calculated. Label this image exposure 2. Record the exposure factors used.

mA ______________ time ______________ mAs ______________

kVp ______________

Exposure 3. Starting back with the exposure factors used for exposure 1, use the 15% rule and calculate the new mAs and kVp if the kVp is increased and the mAs is decreased. Repeat all the conditions for exposure 1, but use the new exposure factors you calculated. Label this image exposure 3. Record the exposure factors used.

mA ______________ time ______________ mAs ______________

kVp ______________

NAME ______________________________

DATE ______________________________

ACTIVITY 8.D

LAB ANALYSIS—15% RULE

1. Record the mAs and kVp used for each of the exposures.

	Exposure 1	**Exposure 2**	**Exposure 3**
mAs	____________	____________	____________
kVp	____________	____________	____________

2. Measure the density of four different areas within the images and record the measurements. Measure the same four areas on each of the three images.

	Exposure 1	**Exposure 2**	**Exposure 3**
1.	____________	____________	____________
2.	____________	____________	____________
3.	____________	____________	____________
4.	____________	____________	____________

3. Are there any differences in the measurements among the three exposures? Explain.

____

____

____

4. Can you see any contrast or density differences among the three exposures? Explain.

____

____

____

5. Did the 15% rule work on the radiographs like it is supposed to? Explain.

____

____

____

NAME ______________________

DATE ______________________

ACTIVITY 8.E

CALCULATION OF THE 15% RULE WITH THE 60- TO 90-kVp RANGE

Calculate the new kVp with the change in the mAs.

	Original mAs	Original kVp	New mAs	New kVp
1.	5	70	10	________
2.	7	90	14	________
3.	60	75	30	________
4.	100	60	50	________
5.	14	85	28	________
6.	70	70	35	________
7.	130	80	65	________
8.	20	78	40	________
9.	3	72	6	________
10.	16	76	32	________

Calculate the new mAs with the change in the kVp.

	Original mAs	Original kVp	New mAs	New kVp
11.	10	70	________	80
12.	15	90	________	80
13.	7	60	________	70
14.	40	66	________	56
15.	110	75	________	65
16.	25	68	________	78
17.	90	76	________	66
18.	8	80	________	70
19.	14	86	________	76
20.	24	62	________	72

NAME ______________________

DATE ______________________

ACTIVITY 8.F

CHAPTER REVIEW

MULTIPLE CHOICE

_____ 1. kVp is the controlling factor for:
  a. density
  b. contrast
  c. recorded detail
  d. distortion

_____ 2. mAs is the controlling factor for:
  a. density
  b. contrast
  c. recorded detail
  d. distortion

_____ 3. If the original radiograph is of good quality and the kVp is increased, which of these statements is true?
    1. density increases
    2. contrast increases
    3. density decreases
    4. contrast decreases
    5. density stays the same
    6. contrast stays the same
  a. 1 and 2
  b. 3 and 4
  c. 2 and 5
  d. 2 and 3
  e. 1 and 4
  f. 1 and 6

_____ 4. If the original radiograph is of good quality and the mAs is increased, which of these statements is true?
    1. density increases
    2. contrast increases
    3. density decreases
    4. contrast decreases
    5. density stays the same
    6. contrast stays the same
  a. 1 and 2
  b. 3 and 4
  c. 3 and 6
  d. 2 only
  e. 1 only
  f. 2 and 5

_____ 5. If the original radiograph is of good quality and the mAs is increased and the kVp is decreased according to the 15% rule, which of these statements is true?

1. density increases
2. contrast increases
3. density decreases
4. contrast decreases
5. density stays the same
6. contrast stays the same

a. 1 and 2
b. 3 and 4
c. 2 and 5
d. 2 only
e. 1 only
f. 3 and 6

_____ 6. Which one of these is the optimum kVp for an exposure of the pelvis?
a. 60
b. 70
c. 80
d. 110

_____ 7. Which one of these is the optimum kVp for an abdomen with barium?
a. 60
b. 70
c. 80
d. 110

_____ 8. Which one of these is the optimum kVp for skull radiography?
a. 60
b. 70
c. 80
d. 110

_____ 9. Increasing the kVp has what effect on the average energy of the photons in the x-ray beam?
a. it increases the average energy
b. it decreases the average energy

_____ 10. Which one of these statements is *not* true about optimum kVp?
a. it will always penetrate the part
b. it produces sufficient contrast
c. it produces an acceptable amount of scattered radiation
d. it determines the quantity of radiation in the x-ray beam

_____ 11. Which kVp selection would produce the most scattered radiation?
a. a high kVp
b. a low kVp
c. the optimum kVp

_____ 12. Which one of these factors determines the quality of the x-ray beam?
a. mAs
b. kVp

_____ 13. Which one of these factors determines the quantity of the x-ray beam?
a. mAs
b. kVp

_____ 14. Which one of these statements is *not* true?
a. mAs controls density
b. kVp controls contrast

c. kVp affects density
d. mAs affects contrast

_____ 15. When using the 15% rule, if the mAs is increased, the kVp must be:
a. increased
b. decreased

_____ 16. When using the 15% rule, if the kVp is increased by 15%, the mAs should be:
a. cut in half
b. doubled

_____ 17. When the 15% rule is used to control contrast:
a. the kVp should be increased and the mAs decreased
b. the kVp should be decreased and the mAs increased

_____ 18. When the 15% rule is used to control motion:
a. the kVp should be increased and the mAs decreased
b. the kVp should be decreased and the mAs increased

_____ 19. The 15% rule should *not* be used in which one of the following circumstances?
a. when the optimum kVp is used for the original radiograph
b. when the contrast is too low
c. when the contrast is too high
d. when the kVp is already at the upper or lower end of the acceptable kVp

_____ 20. Ten kVp is considered a 15% change in which one of these kVp ranges?
a. 50–80
b. 60–90
c. 70–100
d. 40–110

Using the 15% rule, calculate the new kVp with the change in the mAs.

	Original mAs	Original kVp	New mAs	New kVp
21.	15	60	7	_____
22.	10	90	20	_____
23.	40	50	20	_____
24.	100	60	50	_____
25.	3	100	6	_____

Using the 15% rule, calculate the new mAs with the change in the kVp.

	Original mAs	Original kVp	New mAs	New kVp
26.	15	70	_____	80
27.	6	90	_____	80
28.	20	100	_____	115
29.	17	86	_____	76
30.	25	90	_____	70

NAME ____________________

DATE ____________________

ACTIVITY 8.G

REVIEW OF PRIMARY EXPOSURE FACTORS

MULTIPLE CHOICE

_____ 1. The quantity of current passing through the x-ray tube at the time of the exposure is the:
a. exposure time
b. milliamperage
c. kilovoltage
d. density

_____ 2. The relationship between mA and density is:
a. direct
b. inverse

_____ 3. A radiograph with very black and white tones and few gray tones would have:
a. high contrast
b. low contrast

_____ 4. 20 milliseconds is equal to which one of these decimals?
a. .002
b. .02
c. .20
d. 2.0

_____ 5. The total quantity of x-rays produced in an x-ray beam is determined by the:
a. mA
b. time
c. mAs
d. kVp

_____ 6. If the mAs is increased, density will:
a. increase
b. decrease
c. stay the same

Use these mA and time stations to answer questions 7–11.

1. 25 mA × .80 seconds = 20 mAs
2. 500 mA × .04 seconds = 20 mAs

_____ 7. These two sets of factors express the:
a. inverse square law
b. density maintenance law
c. reciprocity law
d. 15% rule

_____ 8. Which one of these two techniques would be the best to control motion?
a. technique 1
b. technique 2
c. neither technique 1 or 2

_____ 9. Which one of these two techniques would produce the best recorded detail because of the use of a small focal spot?
a. technique 1
b. technique 2
c. neither technique 1 or 2

_____ 10. Which one of these two techniques would be the best breathing technique?
a. technique 1
b. technique 2
c. neither technique 1 or 2

_____ 11. Which one of these two techniques would produce the lowest radiographic contrast?
a. technique 1
b. technique 2
c. neither technique 1 or 2

_____ 12. The distance between the x-ray tube and film is called the:
a. source-image distance
b. source-object distance
c. object-image distance
d. focus-object distance

_____ 13. The radiographic contrast caused by the patient's body is called:
a. high contrast
b. long scale contrast
c. subject contrast
d. optimum contrast

_____ 14. If the distance between the x-ray tube and the film is doubled, the intensity of radiation at the film:
a. doubles
b. is cut in half
c. quadruples
d. is reduced by a factor of 4

_____ 15. The intensity of radiation can be measured with a device called:
a. a densitometer
b. an intensitometer
c. a penetrometer
d. an ionization chamber

_____ 16. If a radiograph produced at 72-inch SID is of good quality and the SID is decreased to 56 inches, what change must be made to keep the original radiographic quality?
a. increase the exposure time
b. decrease the OID
c. decrease the mAs
d. increase the mA

_____ 17. What must be done first when calculating either the inverse square law or density maintenance formula?
a. cross-multiply
b. square the distances
c. solve the equation
d. convert the milliseconds to a decimal

_____ 18. In clinical situations, which one of these is best to use:
a. the highest mA station

b. the highest kVp station
c. the highest time station
d. the highest SID

_____ 19. The difference between adjacent densities on a radiograph is the definition of:
a. density
b. contrast
c. recorded detail
d. distortion

_____ 20. The relationship between time and density is:
a. direct
b. inverse

_____ 21. Low radiographic contrast is also called:
a. optimum contrast
b. short scale contrast
c. long scale contrast
d. high scale contrast

_____ 22. If the x-ray beam is moved closer to the object, the intensity of the beam at the object:
a. increases
b. decreases
c. stays the same

_____ 23. If the x-ray photons enter a part of the body that has compact atoms with a high atomic number, it is likely they will:
a. pass through the part
b. be absorbed in the part
c. produce scattered radiation
d. bounce back toward the x-ray tube

_____ 24. The difference in the ability of body parts to absorb x-rays differently is called:
a. attenuation
b. differential absorption
c. reciprocity
d. ionization

_____ 25. If time is decreased, which one of these statements is correct?
a. density increases
b. contrast decreases
c. the chance of motion decreases
d. the gray-scale image changes

_____ 26. The relationship between mAs and density is:
a. direct
b. inverse

_____ 27. If the same amount of radiation is sent through two tissues of the same type but different thicknesses, the most radiation will emerge from the:
a. thicker tissue
b. thinner tissue

_____ 28. Which one of these people would display the most subject contrast?
a. a patient with a high fat content
b. a muscular patient
c. a patient who is retaining a lot of water
d. a patient who has been bedridden for several years

_____ 29. Adding air to a body part changes its tissue density by:
a. increasing it
b. decreasing it

_____ 30. Which one of these is *not* a common contrast medium?
a. air
b. iodine
c. barium
d. tungsten

_____ 31. Which one of these is the controlling factor for contrast?
a. mA
b. time
c. mAs
d. kVp

_____ 32. Increasing the kVp does what to the average photon energy:
a. it increases it
b. it decreases it

_____ 33. The "p" in kVp stands for:
a. penetrating
b. polyenergetic
c. power
d. peak

_____ 34. Which type of x-ray photons are scattered more easily?
a. those produced by a high kVp
b. those produced by a low kVp

_____ 35. Scattered radiation has what effect on radiographic contrast?
a. it increases it
b. it decreases it

_____ 36. Which one of these determines the quality of the x-ray beam?
a. mA
b. time
c. mAs
d. kVp

_____ 37. Which one of these kVp selections would be the most penetrating?
a. 60 kVp
b. 70 kVp
c. 80 kVp
d. 90 kVp

_____ 38. When using the 15% rule, if the kVp is decreased, the mAs should be:
a. increased
b. decreased

_____ 39. When using the 15% rule, if the kVp is increased by 15%, the mAs should be:
a. doubled
b. cut in half
c. reduced by 15%
d. quadrupled

_____ 40. When using the 15% rule, if the kVp is decreased, which one of these statements is true:
a. density increases
b. contrast increases

c. recorded detail increases
d. photon energy increases

Calculate the following unknown factors:

	mA	Time	mAs
41.	500	.10	________
42.	200	________	30
43.	________	.40	20
44.	600	1/15	________
45.	400	________	40

	I_1	I_2	D_1^2	D_2^2
46.	50	________	72	56
47.	26	________	45	65
48.	14	________	80	40
49.	8	________	60	40
50.	15	________	36	72

	New mAs	Old mAs	New SID	Old SID
51.	________	18	72	48
52.	________	30	56	42
53.	________	3	62	72
54.	________	12	80	60
55.	________	100	72	36

	Old mAs	Old kVp	New mAs	New kVp
56.	17	70	________	80
57.	55	90	________	80
58.	6	100	12	________
59.	28	75	14	________
60.	2	60	1	________

ACTIVITY 8.H

H G I H H A L F R L T
V M K V P F I V E O W
Y O N G R A Y S C W E
A T T E N U A T I O N
H I I E T E O O P Y T
K O R T R Y D F R T Y
B N T C N I T A O R N
Q O E H N A M R C O A
F D N E G I U N I F M
F T C E R I D Q T H A
D N I P K X E I Y X T

See questions on following page.

NAME ____________________

DATE ____________________

ACTIVITY 8.H

WORD SEARCH—THE PRIMARY EXPOSURE FACTORS

Decide which word best matches the definition or completes the sentence. Write the word on the line, and then find it in the word search puzzle and circle it.

____________ 1. An mA of 400 and a time of 20 milliseconds equals this mAs.

____________ 2. mAs has this relationship to density.

____________ 3. At 80 kVp with the 15% rule, if the mAs is cut in half, the kVp should be increased by how much?

____________ 4. A contrast medium with the atomic number of 53.

____________ 5. Doubling the SID requires the mAs to be increased by this many times.

____________ 6. Short scale contrast is also this type of contrast.

____________ 7. This body component would absorb many photons

____________ 8. An mA of 600 and a time of 1/20 equals this mAs.

____________ 9. 500 mA × .02 = 10 mAs and 50 mA × .20 = 10 mAs. This describes what law.

____________ 10. At 10 mAs, if the kVp is changed from 70 to 80, what should the new mAs be?

____________ 11. If the original exposure is 10 mR at an 80-inch distance from the source, what is the new exposure if a 40-inch distance is used?

____________ 12. The exposure factor that should be changed when the density needs to be adjusted.

____________ 13. The reduction in intensity as radiation passes through matter.

____________ 14. This exposure factor affects density but controls contrast.

____________ 15. A high kVp will produce long scale and ____________ contrast.

____________ 16. A high mA and low time help to control this problem.

____________ 17. A change from 80 to 90 kVp will cause contrast to ____________ .

____________ 18. The radiation that emerges from the x-ray tube.

____________ 19. mAs controls the ____________ of photons in the x-ray beam.

____________ 20. If the kVp is increased by 15%, the mAs should be cut in ____________ .

ACTIVITY 8.1

See clues on following page.

Across Clues

2. In a low contrast image, adjacent shades of gray would be ____________.
4. An increase in kVp increases the energy of the ____________.
6. A change in kVp will ____________ density.
9. A high kVp beam is more ____________ than a low kVp beam.
10. At 28 mAs, if the SID is decreased from 72 to 36 inches, the new mAs should be ____________.
11. A mostly black-and-white image has this contrast scale.
14. This exposure factor is directly proportional to density.
16. An mA of 100 and a time of.01 second equals this mAs.
17. Decreasing the mAs will produce ____________ density.
19. A primary photon that hits something in the patient's body and changes direction is ____________.
21. This kVp should be used most of the time.
22. If the kVp is decreased, the image will have ____________ contrast.
25. This exposure factor determines how long thermionic emission takes place.
26. A tissue is dense if its atoms are this.
27. The difference between adjacent densities defines this radiographic quality.
29. kVp determines the ____________ of the x-ray photons.
31. If this distance is increased, density decreases.
32. The overall blackness of the radiograph.

Down Clues

1. The amount of radiographic contrast is determined by the number of gray ____________.
3. Decreasing the time will produce a ____________ density.
4. A radiographic contrast medium.
5. At 22 mAs, if the SID is changed from 56 inches to 40 inches, what should be the new mAs.
7. kVp is used to ____________ contrast.
8. A low contrast image is also this contrast scale.
10. Tissue density determines this type of contrast.
12. To maintain density after a change from 10 to 20 mAs, this should be decreased.
13. If the SID is decreased, the beam will have more ____________ at the film.
14. This type of time should be changed to a fraction or decimal before calculating the mAs.
15. This exposure factor controls density.
18. An mA of 200 and a time of .05 would produce the ____________ density as 500 mA and .02 second.
20. A long time and a low mA produces this type of technique.
23. This is the controlling factor for contrast.
24. When using the 15% rule, if the mAs goes up, the kVp has to go ____________.
28. At 36 mAs, if the SID is decreased from 72 to 36 inches, what new mAs is required.
30. A low contrast image has many shades of ____________.

NAME ______________________________

DATE ______________________________

ACTIVITY 9.A

Draw the grid line pattern for each of the grids listed as it would look from the edge and the face of the grid.

FOCUSED GRID

Edge Face

PARALLEL GRID

Edge Face

CROSSED GRID

Edge Face

ACTIVITY 9.B

LAB ASSIGNMENT—SID AND GRID CUT-OFF

MATERIALS

A phantom that would normally require grid use, such as a pelvis or abdomen
Two loaded cassettes large enough to fit an image of the phantom
A stationary focused grid the same size as the cassettes
A radiographic room
A processor
A densitometer

PROCEDURE

Exposure 1. Place the stationary grid on one of the cassettes and put the grid and cassette on the x-ray tabletop. Place the phantom on top of the grid and cassette and center it on the grid and cassette. Use a 40-inch SID and position the x-ray tube so that it is over the phantom. Center the central ray to the center line of the grid, and do not angle the tube. Adjust the collimation to include all the edges of the phantom. Make the exposure using the normal technique for the phantom in use. Label this image exposure 1.

Exposure 2. Repeat the same conditions for exposure 1, but reduce the SID to 28 inches. Adjust the collimation to include all the edges of the phantom. Cut the mAs used for exposure 1 in half, and make the exposure. Label this image exposure 2.

Answer the lab analysis questions.

NAME ______________________

DATE ______________________

ACTIVITY 9.B

LAB ANALYSIS—SID AND GRID CUT-OFF

1. With the densitometer, measure the same two areas in the center of the image for each exposure and record the measurements. Calculate any differences between the measurements from the areas on exposure 1 and exposure 2.

	Exposure 1	Exposure 2	Measurement Difference
Area 1	______	______	______
Area 2	______	______	______

2. Measure the same four areas, one on each edge within the image for each exposure and record the measurements. Calculate any differences between the measurements from exposure 1 and 2 for each area.

	Exposure 1	Exposure 2	Measurement Difference
Area 1	______	______	______
Area 2	______	______	______
Area 3	______	______	______
Area 4	______	______	______

3. Measure the same 4 areas, one on each edge of the film for each exposure and record the measurements. This time the areas selected should not be within the image. Calculate any differences between the measurements from exposure 1 and 2 for each area.

	Exposure 1	Exposure 2	Measurement Difference
Area 1	______	______	______
Area 2	______	______	______
Area 3	______	______	______
Area 4	______	______	______

4. Where on the radiographs did the measurements differ the most? Why do you think this occurred?

____

____

____

5. Can you see any differences in the images without even measuring the differences? Describe the differences.

____

____

____

ACTIVITY 9.C

LAB ASSIGNMENT—TUBE ANGLE AND GRID CUT-OFF

MATERIALS

A phantom that would normally require grid use such as a pelvis or abdomen
Two loaded cassettes large enough to fit an image of the phantom
A stationary focused grid the same size as the cassettes
A radiographic room
A processor
A densitometer

PROCEDURE

Exposure 1. Place the stationary grid on one of the cassettes and put the grid and cassette on the x-ray tabletop. Place the phantom on top of the grid and cassette and center it on the grid and cassette. Use a 40-inch SID and position the x-ray tube so that it is over the phantom. Center the central ray to the center line of the grid, and do not angle the tube. Adjust the collimation to include all the edges of the phantom. Make the exposure using the normal technique for the phantom in use. Label this image exposure 1.

Exposure 2. Repeat the same conditions for exposure 1 but use a 37-inch SID and angle the x-ray tube across the grid lines at an angle of 15 degrees. Center the central ray to the center line of the grid. Adjust the collimation to include all the edges of the phantom. Make the exposure using the same technique used for exposure 1. Label this image exposure 2.

Answer the lab analysis questions.

NAME ______________________

DATE ______________________

ACTIVITY 9.C

LAB ANALYSIS—TUBE ANGLE AND GRID CUT-OFF

1. With the densitometer, measure the same two areas in the center of the image for each exposure and record the measurements. Calculate any difference between the measurements from the areas on exposure 1 and exposure 2.

	Exposure 1	Exposure 2	Measurement Difference
Area 1	________	________	________
Area 2	________	________	________

2. Measure the same four areas, one on each edge within the image for each exposure and record the measurements. Calculate any differences between the measurements from the areas on each of the four exposures.

	Exposure 1	Exposure 2	Measurement Difference
Area 1	________	________	________
Area 2	________	________	________
Area 3	________	________	________
Area 4	________	________	________

3. Measure the same four areas, one on each edge of the film for each exposure and record the measurements. This time the areas selected should not be within the image. Calculate any differences between the measurements from exposures 1 and 2 for each area.

	Exposure 1	Exposure 2	Measurement Difference
Area 1	________	________	________
Area 2	________	________	________
Area 3	________	________	________
Area 4	________	________	________

4. Where on the radiographs did the measurements differ the most? Why do you think this occurred?

____

____

____

5. Can you see any differences in the images without even measuring the differences? Describe the differences.

____

____

____

ACTIVITY 9.D

LAB ASSIGNMENT—GRID ANGLE AND GRID CUT-OFF

MATERIALS

A phantom that would normally require grid use, such as a pelvis or abdomen
Two loaded cassettes large enough to fit an image of the phantom
A stationary focused grid the same size as the cassettes
A radiographic room
A processor
A densitometer
An angled radiographic sponge

PROCEDURE

Exposure 1. Place the stationary grid on one of the cassettes and put the grid and cassette on the x-ray tabletop. Place the phantom on top of the grid and cassette and center it on the grid and cassette. Use a 40-inch SID and position the x-ray tube so that it is over the phantom. Center the central ray to the center line of the grid, and do not angle the tube. Adjust the collimation to include all the edges of the phantom. Make the exposure using the normal technique for the phantom in use. Label this image exposure 1.

Exposure 2. Repeat the same conditions for exposure 1, but prop the grid and phantom up on a radiographic sponge at a 15 degree angle. Center the central ray to the center line of the grid. Adjust the collimation to include all the edges of the phantom. Make the exposure using the same technique used for exposure 1. Label this image exposure 2.

Answer the lab analysis questions.

NAME ____________________

DATE ____________________

ACTIVITY 9.D

LAB ANALYSIS—GRID ANGLE AND GRID CUT-OFF

1. With the densitometer, measure the same two areas in the center of the image for each exposure and record the measurements. Calculate any differences between the measurements from the areas on exposure 1 and exposure 2.

	Exposure 1	Exposure 2	Measurement Difference
Area 1	________	________	________
Area 2	________	________	________

2. Measure the same four areas, one on each edge within the image for each exposure and record the measurements. Calculate any differences between the measurements from the areas on each of the four exposures.

	Exposure 1	Exposure 2	Measurement Difference
Area 1	________	________	________
Area 2	________	________	________
Area 3	________	________	________
Area 4	________	________	________

3. Measure the same four areas, one on each edge of the film for each exposure and record the measurements. This time the areas selected should not be within the image. Calculate any differences between the measurements from exposures 1 and 2 for each area.

	Exposure 1	Exposure 2	Measurement Difference
Area 1	________	________	________
Area 2	________	________	________
Area 3	________	________	________
Area 4	________	________	________

4. Where on the radiographs did the measurements differ the most? Why do you think this occurred?

____

____

____

5. Can you see any differences in the images without even measuring the differences? Describe the differences.

____

____

____

ACTIVITY 9.E

LAB ASSIGNMENT—OFF-CENTERING AND GRID CUT-OFF

MATERIALS

A phantom that would normally require grid use such as a pelvis or abdomen
Two loaded cassettes large enough to fit the image of the phantom
A stationary focused grid the same size as the cassettes
A radiographic room
A processor
A densitometer

PROCEDURE

Exposure 1. Place the stationary grid on one of the cassettes and put the grid and cassette on the x-ray tabletop. Place the phantom on top of the grid and cassette and center it on the grid and cassette. Use a 40-inch SID and position the x-ray tube so that it is over the phantom. Center the central ray to the center line of the grid, and do not angle the tube. Adjust the collimation to include all the edges of the phantom. Make the exposure using the normal technique for the phantom in use. Label this image exposure 1.

Exposure 2. Repeat the same conditions for exposure 1, but move the x-ray tube so that the central ray is not centered to the center line of the grid. It should be moved off center about 3 inches. Adjust the collimation to include all the edges of the phantom. Make the exposure using the same technique used for exposure 1. Label this image exposure 2.

Answer the lab analysis questions.

NAME ____________________

DATE ____________________

ACTIVITY 9.E

LAB ANALYSIS—OFF-CENTERING AND GRID CUT-OFF

1. With the densitometer, measure the same two areas in the center of the image for each exposure and record the measurements. Calculate any differences between the measurements from the areas on exposure 1 and exposure 2.

	Exposure 1	**Exposure 2**	**Measurement Difference**
Area 1	______	______	______
Area 2	______	______	______

2. Measure the same four areas, one on each edge within the image for each exposure and record the measurements. Calculate any differences between the measurements from the areas on each of the four exposures.

	Exposure 1	**Exposure 2**	**Measurement Difference**
Area 1	______	______	______
Area 2	______	______	______
Area 3	______	______	______
Area 4	______	______	______

3. Measure the same four areas, one on each edge of the film for each exposure and record the measurements. This time the areas selected should not be within the image. Calculate any differences between the measurements from exposures 1 and 2 for each area.

	Exposure 1	**Exposure 2**	**Measurement Difference**
Area 1	______	______	______
Area 2	______	______	______
Area 3	______	______	______
Area 4	______	______	______

4. Where on the radiographs did the measurements differ the most? Why do you think this occurred?

____

____

____

5. Can you see any differences in the images without even measuring the differences? Describe the differences.

____

____

____

ACTIVITY 9.F

LAB ASSIGNMENT—UPSIDE-DOWN GRID AND GRID CUT-OFF

MATERIALS

A phantom that would normally require grid use such as a pelvis or abdomen
Two loaded cassettes large enough to fit an image of the phantom
A stationary focused grid the same size as the cassettes
A radiographic room
A processor
A densitometer

PROCEDURE

Exposure 1. Place the stationary grid on one of the cassettes and put the grid and cassette on the x-ray tabletop. Place the phantom on top of the grid and cassette and center it on the grid and cassette. Use a 40-inch SID and position the x-ray tube so that it is over the phantom. Center the central ray to the center line of the grid, and do not angle the tube. Adjust the collimation to include all the edges of the phantom. Make the exposure using the normal technique for the phantom in use. Label this image exposure 1.

Exposure 2. Repeat the same conditions for exposure 1, but turn the stationary grid upside down. The center line of the grid should be pointing toward the film instead of the phantom. Make the exposure using the same technique used for exposure 1. Label this image exposure 2.

Answer the lab analysis questions.

NAME ______________________

DATE ______________________

ACTIVITY 9.F

LAB ANALYSIS—UPSIDE-DOWN GRID AND GRID CUT-OFF

1. With the densitometer, measure two areas in the center of the image for each exposure and record the measurements. Calculate any differences between the measurements from the areas on exposure 1 and exposure 2.

	Exposure 1	Exposure 2	Measurement Difference
Area 1	________	________	________
Area 2	________	________	________

2. Measure the same four areas, one on each edge within the image for each exposure and record the measurements. Calculate any differences between the measurements from the areas on each of the four exposures.

	Exposure 1	Exposure 2	Measurement Difference
Area 1	________	________	________
Area 2	________	________	________
Area 3	________	________	________
Area 4	________	________	________

3. Measure the same four areas, one on each edge of the film for each exposure and record the measurements. This time the areas selected should not be within the image. Calculate any differences between the measurements from exposures 1 and 2 for each area.

	Exposure 1	Exposure 2	Measurement Difference
Area 1	________	________	________
Area 2	________	________	________
Area 3	________	________	________
Area 4	________	________	________

4. Where on the radiographs did the measurements differ the most? Why do you think this occurred?

____

____

____

5. Can you see any differences in the images without even measuring the differences? Describe the differences.

____

____

____

NAME ______________________

DATE ______________________

ACTIVITY 9.G

List what the radiographers in your clinical assignment usually use for each of the following. Write yes or no under grid/bucky to indicate whether a grid or bucky is used. List the average part size. You may find this information on a technique chart or you might have to measure some volunteers with a caliper. List the average kVp used.

Exam	Grid/Bucky	Grid Ratio	Part Size	kVp
PA hand				
AP forearm				
AP lower leg				
AP knee				
AP shoulder				
AP hip				
KUB				
AP skull				
AP port chest				
PA chest done in the dept.				
AP cervical				
AP lumbar				
PA stomach with barium				
PA colon with barium				
AP ribs				

Refer to the information under grid selection in the text. Note any differences between what is on your list and what the text says. Find out why if there are any differences, and explain the reason.

____

____

____

ACTIVITY 9.1

LAB ASSIGNMENT—GRID RATIO

MATERIALS

A phantom that would normally require grid use, such as a pelvis or abdomen
Two loaded cassettes large enough to fit an image of the phantom
Two stationary focused grids the same size as the cassette each a different grid ratio
A radiographic room
A processor
A densitometer

PROCEDURE

Exposure 1. Place one of the stationary grids on one of the cassettes and put the grid and cassette on the x-ray tabletop. Place the phantom on top of the grid and cassette and center it on the grid and cassette. Use a 40-inch SID and position the x-ray tube so that it is over the phantom. Center the central ray to the center line of the grid, and do not angle the tube. Adjust the collimation to include all the edges of the phantom. Make the exposure using the normal technique for the phantom in use. Label this image exposure 1.

Exposure 2. Repeat the same conditions for exposure 1, but change to the other grid ratio. Use the same technique used for exposure 1. Label this image exposure 2.

Exposure 3. Repeat the same conditions for exposure 2. This time calculate the new mAs to be used because of the grid ratio change between exposure 1 and 2. Use this new mAs and expose the film. Label this image exposure 3.

NAME ______________________

DATE ______________________

ACTIVITY 9.1

LAB ANALYSIS—GRID RATIO

1. List the grid ratio, mAs, and kVp used for each exposure.

	Grid Ratio	mAs	kVp
Exposure 1	________	________	________
Exposure 2	________	________	________
Exposure 3	________	________	________

2. Measure the same four areas with the densitometer on each of the three radiographs. One of the areas should be in the dense area not within the image. The other three areas must be within the image and must be the same area on each of the three images. Record the measurements.

	Exposure 1	Exposure 2	Exposure 3
Area 1	________	________	________
Area 2	________	________	________
Area 3	________	________	________
Area 4	________	________	________

3. Where did the measurements differ the most? Why do you think this occurred?

____

____

____

4. Can you see any differences in the images without even measuring the differences? What are they?

____

____

____

NAME ____________________

DATE ____________________

ACTIVITY 9.J

CHAPTER REVIEW

MULTIPLE CHOICE

_____ 1. Which of these statements is true about scattered radiation?
1. Scattered radiation has less energy than primary radiation.
2. Scattered radiation is produced in the x-ray tube.
3. Scattered radiation puts density on the film.
4. Scattered radiation travels in a different direction from primary radiation.
5. Scattered radiation increases radiographic contrast.

a. 1 and 3
b. 1, 2, and 4
c. 1, 3, 4
d. 2, 4, 5

_____ 2. The spaces between the lead strips of a grid are called:
a. interspaces
b. gaps
c. lucencies
d. grid lines

_____ 3. Which one of these grid patterns will clean up the most scattered radiation?
a. focused grid
b. parallel grid
c. crossed grid

_____ 4. When the grid is assembled, the grid strips are always placed:
a. parallel to each other
b. perpendicular to each other
c. parallel to the center line of the grid
d. on edge, next to one another

_____ 5. The most common type of grid pattern is the:
a. focused grid
b. parallel grid
c. crossed grid

_____ 6. Unwanted absorption of primary radiation by the grid is the definition of:
a. grid ratio
b. grid focusing distance
c. grid frequency
d. grid cut-off

_____ 7. Which one of these grid patterns most closely matches the way the x-ray beam emerges from the tube?
a. focused grid
b. parallel grid
c. crossed grid

_____ 8. The purpose of moving the grid with the Bucky is:
a. to image the grid lines on the film
b. to blur the grid lines
c. so the grid will be captured
d. to change the grid ratio

_____ 9. Which of these is the purpose of the grid?
1. absorb scattered radiation
2. allow scattered radiation to pass through it
3. allow primary radiation to pass through it
4. absorb primary radiation
a. 1 and 2
b. 3 and 4
c. 2 and 4
d. 1 and 3

_____ 10. The center line of the grid is drawn:
a. perpendicular to the direction of the grid lines
b. in the same direction as the grid lines
c. the same thickness as the interspaces
d. on the grid focusing distance

_____ 11. Which one of these grid patterns is the most restrictive for angling the central ray?
a. focused grid
b. parallel grid
c. crossed grid

_____ 12. The height of the lead strips compared to the distance between the lead strips is the definition of:
a. grid ratio
b. grid focusing distance
c. interspacing
d. grid frequency

_____ 13. The minimum kVp that requires the use of a grid is:
a. 50
b. 60
c. 70
d. 80

_____ 14. Which one of these grid ratios will absorb the most scattered radiation?
a. 5:1
b. 6:1
c. 8:1
d. 12:1

_____ 15. Which one of these maneuvers would produce grid cut-off?
a. using a SID below the focal range
b. angling the central ray in the direction of the center line of the grid
c. moving the central ray along the direction of the center line of the grid
d. placing the grid so that the center line points toward the x-ray tube

_____ 16. The number of grid lines per inch is the definition of:
a. grid ratio
b. grid focusing distance
c. grid frequency
d. grid cut-off

_____ 17. The presence of a large amount of scattered radiation on the radiograph has what effect on contrast?
a. it increases it
b. it decreases it

_____ 18. Which one of these maneuvers would produce grid cut-off?
a. using the SID within the focal range
b. angling the central ray against the grid lines
c. moving the central ray along the direction of the center line of the grid
d. placing the grid so that the center line points toward the x-ray tube

_____ 19. The tolerance range of acceptable source-image distances that can be used with a focused grid is the:
a. grid focusing distance
b. focusing point
c. focal range
d. focal film distance

_____ 20. The name of the man who invented the grid is:
a. Gustave Bucky
b. Hollis Potter
c. Wilhelm Conrad Roentgen
d. Albert Einstein

_____ 21. A grid should be used if the body part measures more than:
a. 80 cm
b. 50 cm
c. 30 cm
d. 10 cm

_____ 22. The use of a grid on a radiograph has what effect on contrast?
a. it increases it
b. it decreases it

_____ 23. A grid that has strips that are .120 inch high and interspaces that are .010 inch wide has a:
a. 120:1 grid ratio
b. 12:1 grid ratio
c. 24:1 grid ratio
d. .120:1 grid ratio

_____ 24. A kVp above 90 requires at least a ratio of:
a. 5:1
b. 6:1
c. 8:1
d. 12:1

_____ 25. Which one of these maneuvers would produce grid cut-off?
a. using a SID within the focal range
b. angling the central ray perpendicular to the center line of the grid
c. moving the central ray along the direction of the center line of the grid
d. placing the grid so that the center line points toward the front of the cassette

Calculate the new mAs to be used with the following grid ratio changes.

	Original mAs	Original grid	New grid	New mAs
26.	20	6:1	12:1	________
27.	7	16:1	5:1	________
28.	12	12:1	None	________
29.	40	5:1	8:1	________
30.	15	16:1	6:1	________

NAME ____________________

DATE ____________________

ACTIVITY 10.A

TECHNIQUE COMPENSATION FOR COLLIMATION

Calculate the new mAs with the following changes in collimation field size:

	Original mAs	Original collimation	New collimation	New mAs
1.	15	14 × 17	10 × 12	______
2.	4.6	14 × 17	8 × 10	______
3.	12	10 × 12	14 × 17	______
4.	100	8 × 10	14 × 17	______
5.	8	10 × 12	8 × 10	______
6.	10	8 × 10	10 × 12	______
7.	2	14 × 17	8 × 10	______
8.	17	10 × 12	14 × 17	______
9.	2.5	8 × 10	10 × 12	______
10.	5	8 × 10	14 × 17	______

11. You exposed an AP lumbar spine on a 14 × 17 inch film using 15 mAs and 80 kVp. The radiologist requests a coned-down view of L-2 on an 8 × 10 inch film because of a possible bone lesion. What new mAs would you use for this film?

12. You exposed an AP sacrum on a 10 × 12 inch film using 20 mAs and 80 kVp. Now you need to take an AP pelvis on a 14 × 17 inch film. What new mAs would you use for this film?

13. You exposed a lateral skull on a 10 × 12 inch film using 5 mAs and 80 kVp. The radiologist requests a coned-down view of the sella turcica on an 8 × 10 inch film. What new mAs would you use for this film?

ACTIVITY 10.B

LAB ASSIGNMENT—COLLIMATION

MATERIALS

An abdomen, pelvis, or chest radiographic phantom
Three loaded cassettes—one 14 × 17 and two 8 × 10
A radiographic room
A processor
A densitometer

PROCEDURE

Exposure 1. Place the phantom on the center of the x-ray tabletop. Detent the x-ray tube if necessary. Use a 40-inch SID and position the x-ray tube so that it is centered over the phantom. Do not angle the x-ray tube. Place a 14 × 17 inch cassette in the Bucky tray and center the cassette to the x-ray tube and phantom. Adjust the collimation size to 14 × 17 inches or use automatic collimation. Make the exposure using the normal technique for the phantom in use. Label this image exposure 1.

Exposure 2. Use the same conditions used for exposure 1, but use one of the 8 × 10 inch cassettes. Adjust the collimation size to an 8 × 10 inch or use automatic collimation. Make the exposure using the same technique used for exposure 1. Label this image exposure 2.

Exposure 3. Use the same conditions used for exposure 1, but use one of the 8 × 10 inch cassettes. Adjust the collimation size to 8 × 10 inches or use automatic collimation. Calculate the new mAs, which should be used when changing from the technique you used for exposure 1 on the 14 × 17 to what should be used for the change to an 8 × 10 inch collimation. Expose the film using the technique you calculated. Label this image exposure 3. Answer the lab analysis questions.

NAME ______________________

DATE ______________________

ACTIVITY 10.B

LAB ANALYSIS—COLLIMATION

1. Using the densitometer, measure three areas within the image for each exposure and record the measurements. Measure the same three areas on each radiograph.

	Exposure 1	**Exposure 2**	**Exposure 3**
Area 1	________	________	________
Area 2	________	________	________
Area 3	________	________	________

2. Where did the measurements differ the most? Why do you think this occurred?

____

____

____

3. Where were the measurements the most similar? Why do you think this occurred?

____

____

____

ACTIVITY 10.C

LAB ASSIGNMENT — COMPENSATORY FILTERS

MATERIALS

An abdomen or chest radiographic phantom
Three loaded 14 × 17 inch cassettes
A radiographic room
A processor
A densitometer
A wedge compensatory filter

PROCEDURE

Exposure 1. Place the phantom on the center of the x-ray tabletop. Detent the x-ray tube if necessary. Use a 40-inch SID and position the x-ray tube so that it is centered over the phantom. Do not angle the tube. Place a 14 × 17 inch cassette in the Bucky tray and center the cassette to the x-ray tube and phantom. Adjust the collimation size to 14 × 17 inches or use automatic collimation. Make the exposure using the normal technique for the phantom in use. Label this image exposure 1.

Exposure 2. Use the same conditions used for exposure 1, but place a wedge compensatory filter in the track under the collimator. Position the filter so that the thick end of the filter is over the superior end of the phantom. Make the exposure using the same technique used for exposure 1. Label this image exposure 2.

Exposure 3. Use the same conditions used for exposure 1, but place a wedge compensatory filter in the track under the collimator. Position the filter so that the thin end of the filter is over the superior end of the phantom. Make the exposure using the same technique used for exposure 1. Label this image exposure 3.

Answer the lab analysis questions.

NAME ______________________

DATE ______________________

ACTIVITY 10.C

LAB ANALYSIS—COMPENSATORY FILTERS

1. Using the densitometer, measure two areas on the superior end of the radiograph within the image for each exposure and record the measurements. Measure the same two areas on each radiograph.

	Exposure 1	**Exposure 2**	**Exposure 3**
Area 1	________	________	________
Area 2	________	________	________

2. Using the densitometer, measure two areas on the inferior end of the radiograph within the image for each exposure and record the measurements. Measure the same two areas on each radiograph.

	Exposure 1	**Exposure 2**	**Exposure 3**
Area 1	________	________	________
Area 2	________	________	________

3. Did you record a difference in the measurements between the superior end and inferior end of the images? Why do you think this occurred?

____

____

____

4. Can you see a difference in the images without measuring density? Describe.

____

____

____

ACTIVITY 10.D

LAB ASSIGNMENT—AIR-GAP TECHNIQUE

MATERIALS

An abdomen, pelvis, or chest radiographic phantom
Two loaded 14 × 17 inch cassettes
A radiographic room
A processor
A densitometer
Several large square or rectangle radiographic sponges

PROCEDURE

Exposure 1. Place the phantom on the center of the x-ray tabletop. Detent the x-ray tube if necessary. Use a 40-inch SID and position the x-ray tube so that it is centered over the phantom. Do not angle the tube. Place a 14 × 17 inch cassette in the Bucky tray and center the cassette to the x-ray tube and phantom. Adjust the collimation size to 14 × 17 inches or use automatic collimation. Make the exposure using the normal technique for the phantom in use. Label this image exposure 1.

Exposure 2. Use the same conditions used for exposure 1, but prop the phantom up with the radiographic sponges so that there is a 10-inch OID. Keep the phantom parallel to the film. Make the exposure using the same technique used for exposure 1. Label this image exposure 2.

Answer the lab analysis questions.

NAME ______________________

DATE ______________________

ACTIVITY 10.D

LAB ANALYSIS—AIR-GAP TECHNIQUE

1. Using the densitometer, measure four areas within the image for each exposure and record the measurements. Measure the same four areas on each radiograph. Calculate the difference between the measurements for exposure 1 and 2 and record the difference.

	Exposure 1	**Exposure 2**	**Measurement Difference**
Area 1	________	________	________
Area 2	________	________	________
Area 3	________	________	________
Area 4	________	________	________

2. Where did the measurements differ the most? Why do you think this occurred?

____

____

____

3. Can you see a difference in the two images without measuring density? Describe.

____

____

____

ACTIVITY 10.E

LAB ASSIGNMENT—LEAD BLOCKERS

MATERIALS

An abdomen or pelvis radiographic phantom
Two loaded 10 × 12 inch cassettes
A radiographic room
A processor
A densitometer
A lead apron

PROCEDURE

Exposure 1. Place the phantom on the center of the x-ray tabletop in the lateral position. Detent the x-ray tube if necessary. Use a 40-inch SID and position the x-ray tube so that it is centered over the sacrum area of the phantom. Do not angle the x-ray tube. Place a 10 × 12 inch cassette in the Bucky tray lengthwise and center it to the x-ray tube and phantom. Adjust the collimation size to 10 × 12 inches or use automatic collimation. Make the exposure using the normal technique for the phantom in use. Label this image exposure 1.

Exposure 2. Use the same conditions as for exposure 1, but place a folded lead apron on the posterior edge of the sacrum. Do not allow the apron to touch the phantom or extend under the edge of the phantom. Position the lead apron so that it will be in the unabsorbed primary beam only. Make the exposure using the same technique as for exposure 1. Label this image exposure 2.

Answer the lab analysis questions.

NAME ______________________

DATE ______________________

ACTIVITY 10.E

LAB ANALYSIS—LEAD BLOCKERS

1. Using the densitometer, measure two areas on the anterior portion of the radiograph within the image of the sacrum and two areas on the posterior portion of the radiograph within the image of the sacrum for each exposure and record the measurements. Measure the same areas on each exposure. Calculate the difference between the measurements for exposure 1 and 2 and record the difference.

	Exposure 1	**Exposure 2**	**Difference**
Anterior portion			
Area 1	________	________	________
Area 2	________	________	________
Posterior portion			
Area 3	________	________	________
Area 4	________	________	________

2. If you recorded any measurement differences, why do you think these occurred?

____

____

____

3. Can you see a difference in the two images without measuring density? Describe.

____

____

____

NAME ______________________

DATE ______________________

ACTIVITY 10.F

CHAPTER REVIEW

MULTIPLE CHOICE

_____ 1. Which would produce the most scattered radiation?
   a. a patient with a small abdomen
   b. a patient with a large abdomen

_____ 2. What part of the collimator absorbs the edges of the x-ray beam?
   a. the mirror that also produces the collimation light
   b. the lead shutters
   c. the cathode and anode
   d. the window

_____ 3. Which one of these types of filters is sometimes shaped like a wedge?
   a. inherent filtration
   b. added filtration
   c. total filtration
   d. compensatory filtration

_____ 4. A decrease in the collimation field size has what effect on contrast?
   a. it increases it
   b. it increases it

_____ 5. An increase in filtration has what effect on density:
   a. it increases it
   b. it decreases it

_____ 6. If 15 mAs and 80 kVp were used on an 8 × 10 inch film of the spine using automatic collimation, what technique will maintain film density if a 14 × 17 inch film is used for a second exposure?
   a. 30 mAs and 70 kVp
   b. 8.9 mAs and 80 kVp
   c. 10.7 mAs and 80 kVp
   d. 18.4 mAs and 80 kVp

_____ 7. Which one of these can be used during radiography of a body part where there will be a lot of unabsorbed primary radiation on the film?
   a. the air-gap technique
   b. lead blockers
   c. compression
   d. the back of the cassette

_____ 8. Which would produce the most scattered radiation?
   a. a small area of radiation
   b. a large area of radiation

_____ 9. The main purpose of filtration is to:
   a. increase contrast
   b. decrease the patient's radiation dose
   c. decrease contrast
   d. decrease density

_____ 10. Filtration absorbs more:
a. low energy photons
b. high energy photons

_____ 11. Which would best protect the patient's body from excess radiation?
a. a small area of radiation
b. a large area of radiation

_____ 12. An increase in filtration has what effect on contrast?
a. it increases it
b. it decreases it

_____ 13. Which one of these types of filtration is a result of the design of the x-ray tube?
a. inherent filtration
b. added filtration
c. total filtration
d. compensatory filtration

_____ 14. The air-gap technique uses:
a. a large SID and small OID
b. a large OID and small SID
c. a large SID and large OID
d. a small SID and small OID

_____ 15. The glass envelope of the x-ray tube provides which type of filtration?
a. inherent
b. added
c. compensatory

_____ 16. If an AP thoracic spine is performed with a wedge compensatory filter, the thick end of the filter should be placed over the:
a. superior end of the spine
b. inferior end of the spine

_____ 17. Which one of these types of filtration is removable?
a. inherent filtration
b. added filtration
c. total filtration
d. compensatory filtration

_____ 18. The trough compensatory filter is used most often on:
a. spines
b. abdomens
c. skulls
d. chests

_____ 19. If 10 mAs and 80 kVp were used on a 14 × 17 inch film of the abdomen using automatic collimation, what technique will maintain film density if a 10 × 12 inch film is used for a second exposure?
a. 5 mAs and 90 kVp
b. 7.5 mAs and 80 kVp
c. 12.5 mAs and 80 kVp
d. 14 mAs and 80 kVp

_____ 20. A decrease in the area of radiation at the patient's body has what effect on density?
a. it increases it
b. it decreases it

_____ 21. The purpose of a compensatory filter is to:
a. make the density more uniform
b. decrease the contrast
c. decrease the density
d. protect the patient from excess radiation

_____ 22. Which one of these acts like a filter?
a. the air-gap technique
b. lead blockers
c. compression
d. the back of the cassette

_____ 23. Which one of these would be the best method for the radiographer to use to control scattered radiation?
a. increase the filtration
b. reduce the area of radiation
c. use lead blockers
d. increase inherent filtration

_____ 24. Compression to reduce the production of scattered radiation can be used best on which one of these exams?
a. abdomen
b. chest
c. elbow
d. skull

_____ 25. Adding more filtration would have what effect on the average energy of the photons in the x-ray beam?
a. it would decrease the average energy
b. it would increase the average energy

NAME ______________________

DATE ______________________

ACTIVITY 10.G

REVIEW OF CONTROL OF SCATTERED RADIATION

MULTIPLE CHOICE

_____ 1. Most scattered radiation is produced in the:
  a. cassette
  b. film
  c. x-ray tube
  d. patient

_____ 2. Scattered radiation compared to primary radiation:
  a. has more energy
  b. has less energy

_____ 3. Scattered radiation that hits the x-ray film produces:
  a. decreased recorded detail and density
  b. increased distortion and lower contrast
  c. increased density and lower contrast
  d. higher contrast and decreased density

_____ 4. Which one of these devices reduces the *production* of scattered radiation?
  a. using a grid
  b. decreasing the collimation field size
  c. using the air-gap technique
  d. decreasing the amount of filtration

_____ 5. Which type of contrast does a large amount of scattered radiation produce?
  a. long scale
  b. short scale

_____ 6. Which is the most common type of grid pattern in use?
  a. focused
  b. parallel
  c. crossed

_____ 7. Which one of these grid patterns best matches the pattern of the primary beam?
  a. focused
  b. parallel
  c. crossed

_____ 8. Which statement defines grid ratio?
  a. the total amount of lead in the grid
  b. the number of grid lines per inch
  c. the height of the grid strips compared to the distance between the grid strips
  d. the grid efficiency divided by the grid frequency

_____ 9. Which one of these grid ratios will absorb the most scattered radiation?
  a. 5:1
  b. 6:1
  c. 8:1
  d. 12:1

_____ 10. Unwanted absorption of primary radiation by the grid is called?
a. grid cut-off
b. grid frequency
c. grid ratio
d. capturing the grid

_____ 11. The range of acceptable source-image distances that can be used on a grid is called the:
a. focal range
b. grid focusing distance
c. grid ratio
d. grid pattern

_____ 12. Grid cut-off is more likely to occur during which of these conditions?
a. using the grid on the tabletop
b. using the grid in an upright Bucky
c. using the grid during portable radiography
d. using the Bucky in the tabletop

_____ 13. Which one of these maneuvers will produce grid cut-off?
a. angling the beam along the grid lines
b. positioning the central ray at the center line of the grid
c. angling the grid so the central ray will not be perpendicular to the grid
d. using a SID within the focal range

_____ 14. Which one of these maneuvers will produce grid cut-off?
a. angling the beam across the grid lines
b. positioning the central ray at the center line of the grid
c. positioning the grid so the center line faces the x-ray tube
d. using a SID within the focal range

_____ 15. Which one of these maneuvers will produce grid cut-off?
a. angling the beam along the grid lines
b. positioning the central ray at the center line of the grid
c. positioning the grid so that the center line faces the film
d. using a SID within the focal range

_____ 16. Which one of these maneuvers will produce grid cut-off?
a. angling the beam along the grid lines
b. positioning the central ray at the center line of the grid
c. positioning the grid so the center line faces the x-ray tube
d. using a SID that is out of the focal range

_____ 17. Which one of these maneuvers will produce grid cut-off?
a. angling the beam along the grid lines
b. positioning the central ray 3 inches to the left of the center line of the grid
c. positioning the grid so that the center line faces the x-ray tube
d. using a SID that is within the focal range

_____ 18. At 15 mAs and 80 kVp, what new technique would be best to maintain film density with a change from nongrid to a 6:1 ratio grid?
a. 30 mAs and 80 kVp
b. 15 mAs and 90 kVp
c. 45 mAs and 80 kVp
d. 15 mAs and 70 kVp

_____ 19. At 8 mAs and 75 kVp, what new technique would be best to maintain film density with a change from an 8:1 ratio grid to a 16:1 ratio grid?

a. 12 mAs and 75 kVp
b. 8 mAs and 85 kVp
c. 10 mAs and 75 kVp
d. 16 mAs and 65 kVp

_____ 20. At 12 mAs and 70 kVp, what new technique would be best to maintain film density with a change from 14 × 17 collimation to 8 × 10 collimation?
a. 12 mAs and 80 kVp
b. 8.2 mAs and 80 kVp
c. 15 mAs and 70 kVp
d. 16.8 mAs and 70 kVp

_____ 21. At 20 mAs and 80 kVp, what new technique would be best to maintain film density with a change from 10 × 12 collimation to 14 × 17 collimation?
a. 14 mAs and 80 kVp
b. 10 mAs and 80 kVp
c. 16 mAs and 80 kVp
d. 12 mAs and 70 kVp

_____ 22. Which one of these collimator field sizes would produce the most scattered radiation?
a. 5 × 7
b. 8 × 10
c. 10 × 12
d. 14 × 17

_____ 23. Which one of these collimator field sizes would be the best to protect the patient's body from radiation?
a. 5 × 7
b. 8 × 10
c. 10 × 12
d. 14 × 17

_____ 24. Which one of these collimator field sizes would produce the longest scale of contrast?
a. 5 × 7
b. 8 × 10
c. 10 × 12
d. 14 × 17

_____ 25. Adding more filtration does what to the x-ray beam?
a. it increases the average energy of the photons
b. it decreases the average energy of the photons

_____ 26. Adding more filtration does what to contrast?
a. it increases it
b. it decreases it

_____ 27. Adding more filtration does what to density?
a. it increases it
b. it decreases it

_____ 28. Which one of these types of filtration results from the design of the x-ray tube?
a. inherent
b. added
c. total
d. compensatory

_____ 29. The thick end of the wedge compensatory filter should be placed over which end of the body?
a. the thick end
b. the thin end

_____ 30. The air-gap technique uses a large OID and a:
a. small SID
b. large SID

_____ 31. When using a lead blocker, it should be placed:
a. on the patient's gonads
b. under the patient's body
c. on the table in the unabsorbed radiation
d. in the track under the x-ray tube

_____ 32. When using a trough filter, it should be placed:
a. on the patient's gonads
b. under the patient's body
c. on the table in the unabsorbed radiation
d. in the track under the x-ray tube

_____ 33. Which one of these would produce the least scattered radiation?
a. an AP abdomen
b. a lateral abdomen
c. an oblique abdomen
d. a PA abdomen

_____ 34. Which one of these does not require technique compensation?
a. changing to the air-gap technique
b. changing the grid ratio
c. compensatory filtration
d. adjusting the collimation

_____ 35. What is the main purpose of filtration?
a. reduce the contrast
b. increase the density
c. protect the patient
d. change the amount of radiation reaching the film

ACTIVITY 10.H

See clues on following page.

Across Clues

1. The SID used with a grid should be within the __________ range.
3. This technique uses a long OID and a long SID.
5. A light bulb and a __________ produce the collimator light.
6. A filter usually absorbs __________ energy photons.
9. At 16 mAs a switch from an 8:1 ratio grid to a 5:1 ratio grid would require this new mAs.
10. A grid absorbs this type of radiation.
11. The movement of the Bucky __________ the grid lines on the radiograph.
15. Using a grid will __________ contrast.
19. The unwanted absorption of primary radiation by the grid.
20. The scale of contrast produced by using a 16:1 grid ratio instead of a 6:1.
21. This device moves the grid.
23. The type of filter that can be used to produce even density on an AP thoracic spine radiograph.
24. A grid ratio with a multiplier of 5 is a __________ to one ratio grid.
25. The thick end of a wedge filter should be placed over the __________ part of the body.
26. Using compression increases this quality factor.
28. At 8.8 mAs, a change from a 14 × 17 to a 10 × 12 would require this new mAs.
30. At 9 mAs, a change from a 6:1 grid to no grid would require this new mAs.
31. A __________ :1 ratio grid requires the mAs to be doubled when changing from a nongrid exposure.
32. The use of a grid reduces this quality factor.

Down Clues

2. The tube cannot be angled __________ the grid lines.
4. A piece of metal placed under the x-ray tube window is __________ filtration.
6. This is what grid strips are made of.
7. The __________ side of a wedge filter is placed over the larger part of the body.
8. This type of radiation usually gets through a grid.
12. Using a 16:1 ratio grid would produce __________ contrast.
13. Increasing the amount of filtration causes both contrast and density to __________.
14. These devices in the collimator adjust the size of the beam.
16. The height of the lead strips compared to the interspaces defines grid __________.
17. The grid strips are not parallel to each other in this type of grid.
18. This device produces less scatter and also less radiation dose to the patient.
20. More matter = more __________.
22. To avoid cut-off the central ray must be __________ to the center line of the grid.
27. At 2 mAs, a switch from non grid to a 12:1 grid would require this new mAs.
29. At 6 mAs, a change from an 8:1 grid ratio to a 16:1 grid ratio would require this new mAs.

ACTIVITY 11.A

LAB ASSIGNMENT—RECORDED DETAIL AND THE FOCAL SPOT SIZE

MATERIALS

A skeletal bone or a radiographic phantom of a small body part that can be exposed tabletop
Two loaded cassettes large enough to fit an image of the bone or phantom. You may also use a large cassette and divide it into two sections
A radiographic room with small and large focal spots
A processor

PROCEDURE

Exposure 1. Place the cassette on top of the x-ray table. Place the phantom or bone directly on the cassette in the center of the cassette or section of the cassette you are using. Keep the object parallel to the cassette. Use a 40-inch source-image distance and position the center of the x-ray beam directly over the center of the object. Do not angle the x-ray tube. Adjust the collimation so that all four edges of the phantom or bone will be included on the film. For the bone, the technique used for a hand should work. For the phantom, use the technique you would ordinarily use for that body part. Adjust the mA and time according to the reciprocity law (Chapter 5) to achieve the required mAs, with the mA falling in the large focal spot range. Label this image exposure 1.

Exposure 2. Use the same conditions used for exposure 1. Adjust the mA and time according to the reciprocity law to achieve the required mAs, but this time with the mA falling in the small focal spot range. Label this image exposure 2.

Answer the lab analysis questions. Save the radiographs and lab analysis for use with Activity 11.E.

NAME ____________________

DATE ____________________

ACTIVITY 11.A

LAB ANALYSIS—RECORDED DETAIL AND THE FOCAL SPOT SIZE

1. Do you see any recorded detail differences between the two exposures? Explain.

____

____

____

2. If you saw recorded detail differences, which image displays the best recorded detail? Explain.

____

____

____

3. If you saw recorded detail differences, were they easy to see? Where were they seen the easiest?

____

____

____

4. Do you see changes in any of the other radiographic qualities of density, contrast, or distortion? Explain.

____

____

____

ACTIVITY 11.B

LAB ASSIGNMENT—RECORDED DETAIL AND OBJECT-IMAGE DISTANCE

MATERIALS

A skeletal bone or a radiographic phantom of a small body part that can be exposed tabletop
Three loaded cassettes large enough to fit an image of the bone or phantom. You may also use a large cassette and divide it into three sections.
Two square or rectangular radiographic sponges about 2 to 3 inches thick
A radiographic room
A processor

PROCEDURE

Exposure 1. Place the cassette on top of the x-ray table. Place the phantom or bone directly on the cassette in the center of the cassette or section of the cassette you are using. Keep the object parallel to the cassette. Use a 40-inch source-image distance and position the center of the x-ray beam directly over the center of the object. Do not angle the tube. Adjust the collimation so that all four edges of the phantom or bone will be included on the film. For the bone, the technique used for a hand should work. For the phantom, use the technique you would ordinarily use for that body part. Label this image exposure 1.

Exposure 2. Use the same conditions as for exposure 1, but place one of the radiographic sponges between the phantom or bone and the cassette. Keep the phantom or bone parallel to the cassette. Label this image exposure 2.

Exposure 3. Use the same conditions as for exposure 1, but place 2 radiographic sponges between the phantom or bone and the cassette. The sponges should be stacked on top of each other so that the object-image distance is double what was used for exposure 2. Keep the phantom or bone parallel to the cassette. Label this image exposure 3.

Answer the lab analysis questions. Save the radiographs and lab analysis for use with Activity 11.E.

NAME ______________________

DATE ______________________

ACTIVITY 11.B

LAB ANALYSIS—RECORDED DETAIL AND OBJECT-IMAGE DISTANCE

1. Do you see any recorded detail differences between the three exposures? Explain.

____

____

____

2. If you saw recorded detail differences, which image displays the best and which displays the worst recorded detail?

____

____

____

3. If you saw recorded detail differences, were they easy to see? Where were they seen the easiest?

____

____

____

4. Do you see changes in any of the other radiographic qualities of density, contrast, or distortion? Explain.

____

____

____

ACTIVITY 11.C

LAB ASSIGNMENT—RECORDED DETAIL AND SOURCE-IMAGE DISTANCE

MATERIALS

A skeletal bone or a radiographic phantom of a small body part that can be exposed tabletop
Three loaded cassettes large enough to fit an image of the phantom or bone. You may also use a large cassette and divide it into three sections.
A radiographic room
A processor

PROCEDURE

Exposure 1. Place the cassette on top of the x-ray table. Place the phantom or bone directly on the cassette in the center of the cassette or section of the cassette you are using. Keep the object parallel to the cassette. Use a 40-inch source-image distance, and position the center of the x-ray beam directly over the center of the object. Do not angle the x-ray tube. Adjust the collimation so that all four edges of the phantom or bone will be included on the film. For the bone, the technique used for a hand should work. For the phantom, use the technique you would ordinarily use for that body part. Label this image exposure 1.

Exposure 2. Use the same conditions used for exposure 1. Change the source-image distance to 28 inches. Cut the exposure time used for exposure 1 in half. Label this image exposure 2.

Exposure 3. Use the same conditions used for exposure 1. Change the source-image distance to 56 inches. Double the exposure time used for exposure 1. Label this image exposure 3.

Answer the lab analysis questions. Save the radiographs and lab analysis for use with Activity 11.E.

NAME ______________________

DATE ______________________

ACTIVITY 11.C

LAB ANALYSIS—RECORDED DETAIL AND SOURCE-IMAGE DISTANCE

1. Do you see any recorded detail differences between the three exposures? Explain.

____

____

____

2. If you saw recorded detail differences, which image displays the best and which displays the worst recorded detail?

____

____

____

3. If you saw recorded detail differences, were they easy to see? Where were they seen the easiest?

____

____

____

4. Do you see changes in any of the other radiographic qualities of density, contrast, or distortion? Explain.

____

____

____

NAME ____________________

DATE ____________________

ACTIVITY 11.D

14G 14H 14I 11F

CALCULATION OF UNSHARPNESS

Assume a radiograph was taken with the following conditions:

.6 mm focal spot
.6 inch object-image distance (OID)
34 inch source-object distance (SOD)

.01 ____________ 1. Calculate the amount of unsharpness

Calculate the amount of unsharpness with the changes listed below. Each problem refers to the original conditions. Indicate whether the unsharpness increased or decreased and whether the recorded detail increased or decreased for each change by placing a + for an increase and a − for a decrease on the lines next to the changes.

	Amount of unsharpness	Effect on unsharpness	Effect on recorded detail
2. .3-mm focal spot	0.05	−	+
3. 2-inch OID	.035	−	+
4. 38-inch SOD	.009	−	+
5. 46-inch SID 6-inch OID	.09		
6. 2.0-mm focal spot	.35	+	−
7. 56-inch SOD	.064		
8. 12-inch OID	.21		
9. 72-inch SID 6-inch OID	.054		
10. 1.6-mm focal spot	.28		
11. 3-inch OID	.05		
12. 30-inch SOD	.12		
13. 60-inch SID 6-inch OID	.06		
14. 8-inch OID	.14		
15. 1.2-mm focal spot	.21		

NAME ______________________

DATE ______________________

ACTIVITY 11.E

CALCULATION OF UNSHARPNESS WITH LAB ASSIGNMENTS

Use the factors you used to produce the images for Activities 11.A, 11.B, and 11.C. Calculate the amount of unsharpness for the exposures listed.

Activity 11.A

______________________ exposure 1

______________________ exposure 2

Activity 11.B

______________________ exposure 2

______________________ exposure 3

Activity 11.C

______________________ exposure 2

______________________ exposure 3

Did the unsharpness you calculated correspond with the recorded detail changes you saw on the radiographs? Explain.

____

____

____

NAME ______________________

DATE ______________________

ACTIVITY 11.F

CHAPTER REVIEW

1. List the seven factors that affect recorded detail.
   1.
   2.
   3.
   4.
   5.
   6.
   7.
2. List the three geometric factors that affect recorded detail.
   1.
   2.
   3.

Indicate the effect on unsharpness and recorded detail for each of these changes.

+ = increase

− = decrease

0 = no change

	Unsharpness	Recorded detail
3. Focal spot size increases	________	________
4. OID decreases	________	________
5. mAs increases	________	________
6. SOD decreases; OID unchanged	________	________
7. kVp decreases	________	________
8. SID decreases	________	________
9. Focal spot size decreases	________	________
10. OID increases	________	________
11. SOD increases; OID unchanged	________	________
12. SID increases	________	________

MULTIPLE CHOICE

_____ 13. an increase in the focal spot size causes recorded detail to:
   a. decrease
   b. increase

_____ 14. The ability of an imaging system to record two adjacent structures as separate structures is called:
   a. definition
   b. recorded detail
   c. visibility of detail
   d. resolution

_____ 15. An increase in source-image distance causes recorded detail to:
   a. decrease
   b. increase

_____ 16. As resolution increases:
   a. recorded detail decreases
   b. recorded detail increases

_____ 17. The sharpness of the lines of the image is called:
   a. density
   b. visibility of detail
   c. recorded detail
   d. unsharpness

_____ 18. A decrease in object-image distance causes recorded detail to:
   a. decrease
   b. increase

_____ 19. A line pair of a resolution grid is:
   a. the number of pairs that can fit into a millimeter
   b. a metal line and the space next to it
   c. a pair of two metal lines
   d. two metal lines and the space between them

_____ 20. An increase in size distortion causes recorded detail to:
   a. decrease
   b. increase

Use the factors listed below to answer questions 21–25. Calculate the amount of unsharpness with the changes listed.

focal spot = .6 mm

object-image distance = 4 inches

source-object distance = 68 inches

_____ 21. the object-image distance changes to 1 inch

_____ 22. the source-object distance changes to 58 inches

_____ 23. the focal spot changes to 1.2 mm

_____ 24. the object-image distance changes to 10 inches

_____ 25. the source-object distance changes to 40 inches

ACTIVITY 12.A

MATERIALS

Double-emulsion film
Single-emulsion film
A densitometer
A darkroom

PROCEDURE

Go into the darkroom, shut the door, and turn out all the lights but the safelights. Take two sheets of double-emulsion film and 1 sheet of single-emulsion film out of the film drawers. Don't forget to shut the drawer. Run one of the double-emulsion films through the processor. Observe the colors of both sides of the remaining single- and double-emulsion films under the safelights. Now turn on the white lights. Observe the colors of both sides of the single- and double-emulsion films under the white light. Run both the single- and double-emulsion films through the processor.

Answer the lab analysis questions.

NAME ______________________

DATE ______________________

ACTIVITY 12.A

LAB ANALYSIS

1. What color were both sides of the single- and double-emulsion film under the safelights?

   Single-emulsion film ____________

   Double-emulsion film ____________

2. What color were both sides of the single- and double-emulsion film under the white light?

   Single-emulsion film ____________

   Double-emulsion film ____________

3. Hang the first double-emulsion film that you put in the processor on a view box. What color is it?

   ____

4. Hang the second double-emulsion film and the single-emulsion film that you exposed to white light and put in the processor on a view box. What color are they?

   Single-emulsion film ____________

   Double-emulsion film ____________

5. Measure the density on all three films with a densitometer and record the readings.

   Double-emulsion film 1 ____________

   Double-emulsion film 2 ____________

   Single-emulsion film ____________

6. If you recorded differences in the densitometer readings, what do you think caused the differences?

   ____

   ____

7. Record any other differences you observe between the three films.

   ____

   ____

NAME ______________________

DATE ______________________

ACTIVITY 12.B

Fill in the blanks with the answer to the statement.

1. ____________ Two components of film

   ____

2. ____________ The base of film is made of this
3. ____________ Will modern x-ray film burn?
4. ____________ The thickness of the film base
5. ____________ The thickness of one film emulsion
6. ____________ The thickness of one sheet of single-emulsion film
7. ____________ The thickness of one sheet of double-emulsion film
8. ____________ Which is thicker, the base or emulsion?
9. ____________ The blue tint lets how much light through when hung on a view box?
10. ____________ The property that causes the film to maintain its size
11. ____________ What the crystals in the emulsion are made of
12. ____________ The term that means the film can be used in an acid and an alkali
13. ____________ The name of the protective layer
14. ____________ Gelatin property that suspends crystals
15. Write the names of the layers of a double-emulsion film in order from front to back.

16. Write the names of the layers of a single-emulsion film in order from front to back.

NAME ______________________________

DATE ______________________________

ACTIVITY 12.C

Find out all the types of film that are available in your clinical education assignment. List the name of the film, describe what it is used for, indicate whether it is single- or double-emulsion film, and list anything special or different about the film type.

NAME ____________________

DATE ____________________

ACTIVITY 12.D

Fill in the blanks with the answer to the statement.

1. ____________ The section of the processor where the exposed silver bromide crystals are reduced to metallic silver
2. ____________ The image on the film after exposure and before development
3. ____________ The preservative used in both the fixer and developer
4. ____________ The approximate range of time for a processor to fully develop a film
5. ____________ The usual temperature range for developer
6. ____________ The hardener used in the developer
7. ____________ The section of the processor where the unexposed and undeveloped silver bromide crystals are removed
8. ____________ The chemical that develops the gray tones of the image
9. ____________ The agent that clears the film
10. ____________ The section of the processor from which silver is retrieved
11. ____________ The name of the excess density caused by the developer temperature being too high
12. ____________ The chemical that develops the black areas of the image
13. ____________ The chemical used as a restrainer
14. ____________ This section of the processor has an alkali solution
15. ____________ The section of the processor that washes away any chemicals remaining on the film
16. ____________ The agent that makes the fixer an acid
17. ____________ The chemical used as a fixing agent
18. ____________ The section of the processor where the film gets dried
19. ____________ The agent that controls film fog
20. ____________ The chemical used as a hardener in the fixer

ACTIVITY 12.E

This activity must be performed with adherence to the safety standards at the institution.

MATERIALS

Four clear glasses (you must be able to see through them)
Developer replenisher
Fixer replenisher
An occlusal film
A small heavy metal object that will fit on an occlusal film
A hemostat
A pair of protective gloves
Protective eye glasses
A fluid-barrier protective gown
Some paper towels
A teaspoon
A radiographic room
A dark room

PROCEDURE

Place the occlusal film on the x-ray tabletop with the metal object on top of the film. Use a 40-inch SID and place the center of the x-ray beam directly over the center of the metal object and film. Adjust the collimation to include all four edges of the film. Expose the film using 300 mAs and 54 kVp.

Put on the protective gloves, gown, and eye glasses. Dip a glass into the developer replenisher tank filling it with about 5 inches of developer. Fill another glass the same way with fixer. Wipe the sides and bottoms of the glasses with paper towels. Smell both the developer and fixer. Observe their colors. Put 4 spoonfuls of developer into the third glass, then put 1 spoonful of fixer into it. Mix it and smell the mixture.

Fill the fourth glass with cool water. In the darkroom under safelights, open the exposed occlusal film. There are two films in an occlusal package. Holding the edge of one film with the hemostat, place the film in the glass of developer, and observe what happens to the film through the glass. After 1 minute, place the film in the glass of water for 5 seconds and then in the glass of fixer. Leave it there for 3 minutes. While the first film is in the fixer, place the second film in the developer for 1 minute and then remove it and place it on a paper towel. When the 3 minutes are up, remove the first film from the fixer and place it alongside the film you took from the developer. Now turn on the white lights and note any differences between the two films.

Take care of the chemicals, paper towels, spoon, glasses, protective gloves, gown, and eyeglasses according to policy at the institution.

Answer the questions on the lab analysis.

NAME ______________________

DATE ______________________

ACTIVITY 12.E

1. What is the color of the chemicals in the glasses?
   Developer ____________ Fixer ____________
2. Can you describe the smell of the chemicals?
   Developer ____________ Fixer ____________
3. What happened when you mixed the fixer into the developer?
   ____
4. What happened when you placed the occlusal films in the developer?
   ____
   ____
5. What happened after you left the film in the fixer for 3 minutes?
   ____
   ____
6. Describe the difference in the appearance of the two occlusal films under the white light.
   ____
   ____

ACTIVITY 12.F

CHARACTERISTIC CURVE

MATERIALS

A step wedge
A densitometer
Three loaded cassettes large enough to fit an image of the step wedge
The blank graph on page 480.
A pencil
A radiographic room
A processor

PROCEDURE

Exposure 1. Place the cassette on the x-ray tabletop. Put the step wedge directly on the cassette in the center of the cassette. Use a 40-inch SID and place the center of the x-ray beam directly over the center of the step wedge and cassette. Adjust the collimation to include all four edges of the cassette. Make the exposure and develop the film. The technique usually used for a foot should work. Evaluate exposure 1 for adequate density and contrast. You may need your instructor's input on this. The radiograph should show an adequate gray scale, with several steps on the one end of the film being light, and several steps on the other end of the film being dark. The steps in between should show increasing shades of gray. Label the image exposure 1.

Exposure 2. Use the same conditions for exposure 1. The only thing you need to change is to increase the density on the radiograph by multiplying the mAs used for exposure 1 by 1.5. Use this new mAs on exposure 2. Label the image exposure 2.

Exposure 3. Use the same conditions for exposure 1. The only thing you need to change is to divide the mAs used for exposure 1 in half and increase the kVp used for exposure 1 by 10. Use these new technique factors on exposure 3. Label the image exposure 3.

Plotting the Curve. Using the radiograph from exposure 1, measure the lightest density step on the radiograph. Plot this density reading on the graph above the number corresponding to 0 relative log exposure. Then measure the next step up from the lightest density step. If you are using a 21-step penetrometer, plot this density reading on the graph above the number corresponding to .15 relative log exposure. If you are using an 11-step penetrometer, plot this density reading on the graph above the number corresponding to .30 relative log exposure. Continue by measuring the next step on the radiograph and plotting the density readings on the graph in increments of .15 for a 21-step penetrometer or .30 for an 11-step penetrometer. After plotting the last (most dense) reading, connect all the dots. This should produce a continuous curve that appears the same shape as a characteristic curve.

Plot a characteristic curve in the same manner for the radiographs produced from exposure 2 and exposure 3. Plot all 3 curves on the same piece of paper. Label the curves 1, 2, and 3 corresponding to the exposures.

Answer the questions on the lab analysis.

NAME ____________________

DATE ____________________

ACTIVITY 12.F

LAB ANALYSIS—CHARACTERISTIC CURVE

1. Do you see evidence of speed changes between the curves? If so, how is it demonstrated? Why do you think this occurred?

____

____

____

2. Do you see evidence of contrast changes between the curves? If so, how is it demonstrated? Why do you think this occurred?

____

____

____

3. Do you see evidence of exposure latitude differences between the curves? If so, how is it demonstrated? Why do you think this occurred?

____

____

____

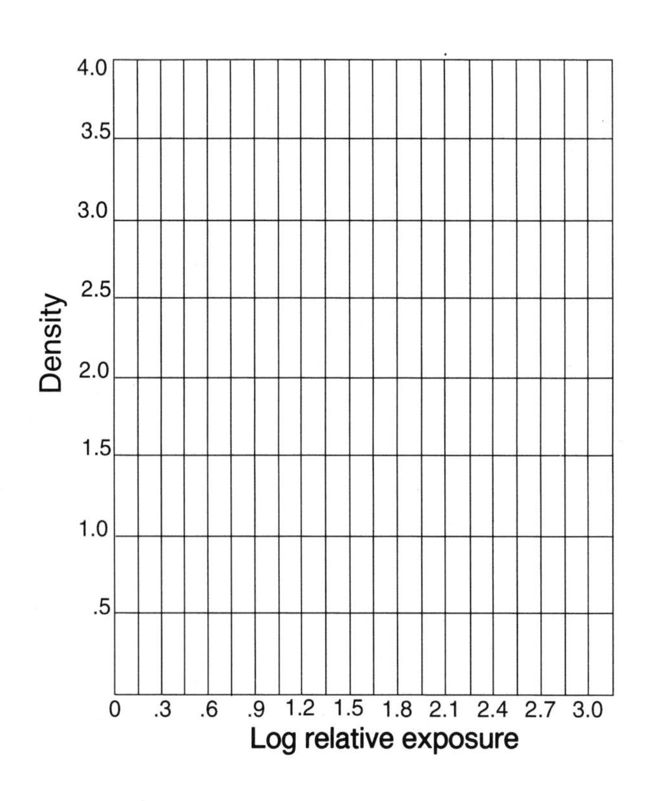

NAME ______________________

DATE ______________________

ACTIVITY 12.G

CHAPTER REVIEW

MATCHING

_____ 1. glutaraldehyde
_____ 2. potassium bromide
_____ 3. ammonium thiosulfate
_____ 4. hydroquinone
_____ 5. preservative
_____ 6. sodium carbonate
_____ 7. phenidone
_____ 8. acetic acid
_____ 9. sodium sulfite
_____ 10. potassium alum

a. chemical used as a preservative
b. chemical which maintains the Ph of the developer
c. hardener used in developer
d. develops the gray areas
e. chemical used as a restrainer
f. develops the black areas
g. hardener used in fixer
h. chemical used as a fixing agent
i. chemical that makes the fixer an acid
j. agent that prolongs the life of the developer and fixer

MULTIPLE CHOICE

_____ 11. The image on the film before development and after exposure is called a:
a. visible image
b. latent image
c. manifest image
d. developed image

_____ 12. Which one of these is the right order for a film going through the automatic processor?
a. developer, rinse, fixer, wash, dryer
b. fixer, developer, wash, dryer
c. developer, fixer, wash, dryer
d. developer, wash, fixer, dryer

_____ 13. The base of modern x-ray film is composed of:
a. cardboard
b. Formica
c. rubber
d. polyester

_____ 14. The type of film used for teeth radiography is:
a. subtraction
b. duplicating
c. periapical
d. cinefluorography

_____ 15. Base-plus-fog is measured:
a. on any blank area of the film
b. on a high density step
c. on a medium density step
d. on a low density step

_____ 16. The emulsion of film consists of:
a. sodium carbonate and potassium bromide
b. acetic acid and sodium sulfite
c. glutaraldehyde and potassium alum
d. silver bromide and gelatin

_____ 17. The area of underexposure of a characteristic curve is called the:
a. threshold
b. toe
c. average gradient
d. gamma

_____ 18. Replenishment is controlled by which rollers of the automatic processor?
a. the turnarounds
b. the crossovers
c. the fixer rollers
d. the entrance rollers

Use this figure for questions 19, 20, and 21.

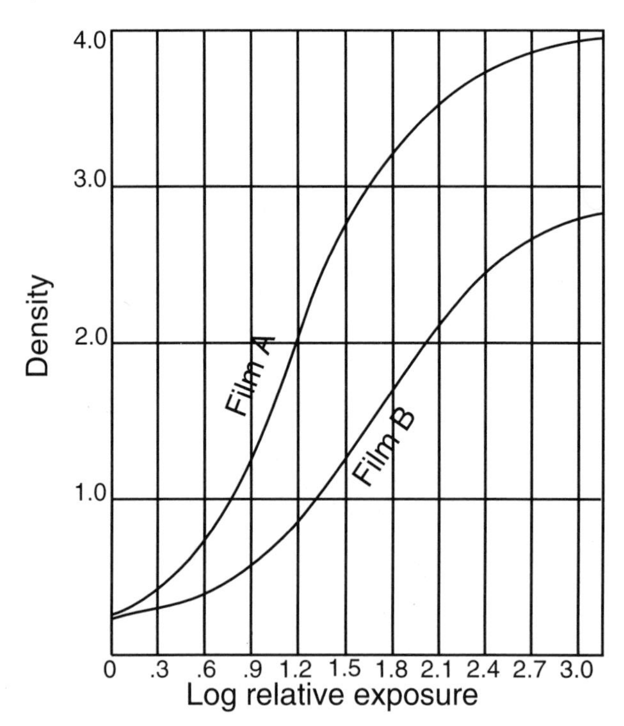

_____ 19. Which film has the highest speed?
a. film A
b. film B

_____ 20. Which film will display long scale contrast?
a. film A
b. film B

_____ 21. Which film will give the radiographer the most room for error?
a. film A
b. film B

_____ 22. Which one of these is the right order for a single emulsion film?
a. adhesive, emulsion, supercoating, base
b. emulsion, adhesive, base, supercoating
c. supercoating, emulsion, adhesive, base
d. base, supercoating, emulsion, adhesive

_____ 23. The usual range for developer temperature is:
a. 30–50 degrees
b. 70–80 degrees
c. 93–98 degrees
d. 105–115 degrees

_____ 24. The processor chemicals can become contaminated by splashing:
a. fixer into developer
b. water into fixer
c. developer into fixer
d. developer into water

_____ 25. The average gradient ranges from densities:
a. .20 to .25 above base-plus-fog
b. .5 to 2.5 above base-plus-fog
c. .1 to .3 above base-plus-fog
d. .25 to 2.0 above base-plus-fog

ACTIVITY 13.A

LAB ASSIGNMENT—POOR SCREEN CONTACT

MATERIALS

A wire mesh for testing poor screen contact
Two loaded 14 × 17 inch cassettes
A tissue
A radiographic room
A processor

PROCEDURE

Exposure 1. Place the cassette on top of the x-ray table. Place the wire mesh directly on the cassette in the center of the cassette. Use a 40-inch SID and position the center of the x-ray beam directly over the center of the wire mesh and cassette. Adjust the collimation so that all four edges of the cassette are within the collimation. Make an exposure of the wire mesh and develop the film. The technique you would use for a foot will probably work. Label this image exposure 1.

Exposure 2. Tear off a piece of the tissue and wad it up into a ball about 2-mm thick. Go into the dark room, open the 14 × 17 inch cassette and place the ball of tissue in the center of the cassette on top of the film. Close the cassette sandwiching the tissue inside the cassette with the film. Make another exposure of the wire mesh using the cassette with the piece of tissue in it. Use the same conditions used for exposure 1. Label this image exposure 2.

Answer the questions on the lab analysis.

NAME ______________________________

DATE ______________________________

ACTIVITY 13.A

LAB ANALYSIS—POOR SCREEN CONTACT

1. Analyze the recorded detail of the wire mesh lines on the radiograph from exposure 1. Do you see any areas on the radiograph where the recorded detail looks poor? Explain.

____

____

____

2. Analyze the recorded detail of the wire mesh lines on the radiograph from exposure 2. Do you see any areas on the radiograph where the recorded detail looks poor? Explain.

____

____

____

3. If you saw any areas of poor recorded detail on either exposure, why do you think this occurred?

____

____

____

ACTIVITY 13.B

LAB ASSIGNMENT—INTENSIFYING SCREEN LIGHT

MATERIALS

An unloaded cassette containing rare earth intensifying screens
An unloaded cassette containing calcium tungstate intensifying screens
A radiographic room

PROCEDURE

Exposure 1. Open the cassette with rare earth intensifying screens and lay it flat on the x-ray table. Use a 40-inch SID and position the center of the x-ray beam directly over the center of one half of the open cassette. Adjust the collimation to include all four edges of the half of the cassette in the x-ray beam. Set this technique on the control panel: 200 mA, 1 second, 60 kVp. Turn off all the lights in the radiographic room. From the control panel observe the cassette through the leaded-glass window while you make the exposure.

Exposure 2. Repeat the same conditions used for exposure 1, but this time use the cassette containing the calcium tungstate intensifying screens.

Answer the questions on the lab analysis.

NAME ______________________

DATE ______________________

ACTIVITY 13.B

LAB ANALYSIS—INTENSIFYING SCREEN LIGHT

1. What did you observe when you made the exposure using the cassette containing the rare earth intensifying screens?

____

____

____

2. What did you observe when you made the exposure using the cassette containing the calcium tungstate intensifying screens?

____

____

____

3. Did you observe any differences between exposure 1 and exposure 2? Explain.

____

____

____

NAME ______________________

DATE ______________________

ACTIVITY 13.C

CALCULATION OF TECHNIQUE COMPENSATION WITH SCREEN USE

Calculate the multiplication factor for the screen speed listed.

1. 400 speed ____________
2. 600 speed ____________
3. 50 speed ____________
4. 100 speed ____________
5. 200 speed ____________
6. 500 speed ____________
7. 800 speed ____________
8. 300 speed ____________
9. 700 speed ____________
10. 250 speed ____________

Calculate the new mAs to be used when changing to the screen speed listed.

	Old mAs	Old screen	New screen	New mAs
11.	10	100	200	____________
12.	4	200	400	____________
13.	25	800	300	____________
14.	12	500	250	____________
15.	4	50	400	____________
16.	3	600	300	____________
17.	15	100	500	____________
18.	6	200	800	____________
19.	1.25	100	50	____________
20.	.7	200	50	____________

ACTIVITY 13.D

LAB ASSIGNMENT—INTENSIFYING SCREEN SPEED

MATERIALS

A step wedge or a radiographic phantom of a small body part that is exposed tabletop
Two loaded cassettes containing intensifying screens with different speeds; they must be large enough to fit an image of the step wedge or radiographic phantom
A densitometer
A radiographic room
A processor

PROCEDURE

Exposure 1. Place one of the cassettes on top of the x-ray table. Place the step wedge or phantom directly on the cassette in the center of the cassette. Keep the object parallel to the cassette. Use a 40-inch SID and position the center of the x-ray beam directly over the center of the object. Do not angle the x-ray tube. Adjust the collimation so that all four edges of the object will be included on the film. For the step wedge, the technique used for a foot for the speed of intensifying screen being used will probably work. For the phantom, use the technique ordinarily used for that body part for the speed of intensifying screen being used. Label this image exposure 1.

Exposure 2. Use the same conditions for exposure 1, but change to the other cassette that contains an intensifying screen of a different speed. Use the same technique factors used for exposure 1. Label this image exposure 2.

Exposure 3. Use the same conditions for exposure 2. Calculate the new mAs to be used with the change from the speed of intensifying screen used for exposure 1 to the speed of intensifying screen used for exposure 2. Use this new mAs for exposure 3. Label this image exposure 3.

Answer the questions on the lab analysis.

NAME ______________________

DATE ______________________

ACTIVITY 13.D

LAB ANALYSIS—INTENSIFYING SCREEN SPEED

1. What object did you use for the lab assignment?

   ____

2. What technique did you use for each exposure?

	mAs	**kVp**
Exposure 1	____________	____________
Exposure 2	____________	____________
Exposure 3	____________	____________

3. Measure three areas with a densitometer within the image for each exposure. Measure the same areas on each image. Record the measurements.

	Exposure 1	**Exposure 2**	**Exposure 3**
Area 1	____________	____________	____________
Area 2	____________	____________	____________
Area 3	____________	____________	____________

4. Where did the measurements differ the most? Why do you think this occurred? Explain.

   ____

   ____

   ____

5. Can you see a difference in recorded detail between the three exposures? Why do you think this occurred? Explain.

   ____

   ____

   ____

NAME ____________________

DATE ____________________

ACTIVITY 13.E

CHAPTER REVIEW

MULTIPLE CHOICE

____ 1. The layers of an intensifying screen in order are:
a. base, white reflecting surface, emulsion, protective coating
b. white reflecting surface, protective coating, active layer, base
c. base, white reflecting surface, active layer, protective coating
d. active layer, base, white reflecting surface, protective coating

____ 2. A material that gives off light when struck by x-ray photons is called:
a. silver bromide
b. a phosphor
c. an active layer
d. an intensifier

____ 3. In places where a large amount of radiation got through the patient's body, the intensifying screen would give off ____________ of light, and this area on the radiograph would be developed as ____________.
a. a large amount, black
b. a small amount, white

____ 4. Which are the two main parts of an intensifying screen?
a. base and emulsion
b. base and active layer
c. emulsion and active layer
d. active and protective layer

____ 5. Delayed light emission of an intensifying screen after the x-ray photons have been turned off is called:
a. afterburn
b. luminescence
c. fluorescence
d. phosphorescence

____ 6. Which one of these is the phenomenon that causes a loss of recorded detail with intensifying screens?
a. afterglow
b. light diffusion
c. phosphorescence
d. fluorescence

____ 7. Fast screens emit ____________ light than slow screens.
a. more
b. less

____ 8. Changing from a slower screen to a faster screen will have what effect on the patient's radiation dose?
a. it will increase the dose
b. it will decrease the dose

_____ 9. The part of the active layer of an intensifying screen that produces light is the:
a. white reflecting surface
b. protective coat
c. silver bromide
d. phosphor

_____ 10. An area of poor screen contact occurs:
a. when there is a decreased distance between the screen and film inside the cassette
b. when there is an increased distance between the screen and film inside the cassette

_____ 11. Changing from a slower screen to a faster screen will have what effect on density?
a. it will increase it
b. it will decrease it

_____ 12. A relative speed value of 100 corresponds to a:
a. detail screen
b. slow speed screen
c. medium speed screen
d. high speed screen

_____ 13. The ability of a material to give off light when struck by x-rays is called:
a. afterglow
b. screen lag
c. fluorescence
d. phosphorescence

_____ 14. Increasing the speed of an intensifying screen also increases:
a. the patient's dose
b. light diffusion
c. contrast
d. recorded detail

_____ 15. A test for poor screen contact is performed with which one of these devices?
a. a resolution grid
b. a radiographic phantom
c. a wire mesh
d. a penetrometer

_____ 16. Changing from a slower screen to a faster screen will have what effect on recorded detail?
a. it will increase it
b. it will decrease it

_____ 17. Which one of these systems would require the highest mAs to produce the image?
a. direct exposure
b. calcium tungstate screen system
c. computed radiography
d. rare earth screen system

_____ 18. The color of light given off by a rare earth intensifying screen is:
a. yellow green
b. blue violet

_____ 19. Which one of these systems is usually better for producing a low radiation dose to the patient?
a. calcium tungstate

b. rare earth
c. direct exposure

____ 20. The type of film used with an intensifying screen and the safelight used must be matched with the type of screen. This is called:
a. light diffusion
b. resolution
c. spectral matching
d. fluorescence

____ 21. The brightness of a computed radiography image is similar to the film/screen system quality of:
a. density
b. contrast
c. recorded detail
d. distortion

____ 22. The two different intensifying screen systems in use today are:
a. calcium tungstate and silver bromide
b. rare earth and calcium tungstate
c. silver bromide and rare earth
d. direct exposure and rare earth

____ 23. Conversion efficiency is the ability to convert:
a. light energy to x-ray energy
b. x-ray energy to light energy

____ 24. Direct exposure systems produce good recorded detail because:
a. no film is used to record the image
b. no radiation is used to record the image
c. no light is used to record the image
d. a computer is used to record the image

____ 25. The recorded detail of a computed radiography system is determined by:
a. the numbers assigned to the pixels
b. the number of pixels used in the matrix
c. the gray scale used
d. the brightness of the image

Calculate the following:

____________ 26. The multiplication factor for a 400-speed screen.

____________ 27. The new mAs to be used when changing from a 100-speed screen to a 500-speed screen. The original mAs was 12.

____________ 28. The multiplication factor for a 600-speed screen.

____________ 29. The new mAs to be used when changing from a 200-speed screen to a 50-speed screen. The original mAs was 5.

____________ 30. The new mAs to be used when changing from a 300-speed screen to an 800-speed screen. The original mAs was 8.

NAME ______________________________

DATE ______________________________

ACTIVITY 13.F

REVIEW OF RECORDED DETAIL

1. List the seven factors that affect recorded detail:
   1.
   2.
   3.
   4.
   5.
   6.
   7.
2. Will recorded detail increase, decrease, or not change as each of these factors is increased?

	Increase	Decrease	No change
a. screen speed	________	________	________
b. motion	________	________	________
c. OID	________	________	________
d. mAs	________	________	________
e. film speed	________	________	________
f. focal spot size	________	________	________
g. SID	________	________	________
h. kVp	________	________	________

_____ 3. Which one of these help the film travel from one processing section to the next?
   a. turnarounds
   b. crossovers
   c. guide shoes
   d. entrance rollers

_____ 4. The layer of film that touches the protective coating of the intensifying screen in a closed cassette is the:
   a. base
   b. emulsion
   c. supercoating
   d. adhesive layer

_____ 5. One type of film used to record an image from a computer screen is:
   a. periapical film
   b. occlusal film
   c. roll film
   d. laser film

_____ 6. The device used to test the resolution of a film/screen imaging system is a:
a. wire mesh
b. resolution grid
c. penetrometer
d. radiographic phantom

_____ 7. If the OID is decreased, unsharpness __________ and recorded detail __________:
a. increases, decreases
b. increases, increases
c. decreases, increases
d. decreases, decreases

_____ 8. What is the amount of unsharpness if the focal spot size is a .6, the OID is 7 inches, and the SID is 40 inches:
a. .06
b. .10
c. .13
d. .50

_____ 9. What new mAs should be used when changing from a 100-speed screen to a 400-speed screen if 5 mAs was used originally:
a. .25
b. .50
c. 1.25
d. 2.50

_____ 10. Film emulsion is composed of
a. phosphors and gelatin
b. silver bromide and gelatin
c. polyester and calcium tungstate
d. yttrium and lanthanum

_____ 11. If the SID is increased, unsharpness __________, and recorded detail __________:
a. increases, decreases
b. increases, increases
c. decreases, increases
d. decreases, decreases

_____ 12. Which one of these chemicals is the hardener used in the developer?
a. sodium sulfite
b. glutaraldehyde
c. potassium bromide
d. hydroquinone

_____ 13. Which one of these processor sections clears the film of unexposed and undeveloped silver bromide?
a. wash
b. dryer
c. developer
d. fixer

_____ 14. If the focal spot size is decreased, unsharpness __________ and recorded detail __________.
a. increases, decreases
b. increases, increases
c. decreases, increases
d. decreases, decreases

_____ 15. Which one of these intensifying screen systems gives off a yellow-green light?
a. rare earth
b. calcium tungstate

_____ 16. Poor screen contact is tested with a:
a. resolution grid
b. penetrometer
c. radiographic phantom
d. wire mesh

_____ 17. Which one of these agents stops developer action?
a. hardener
b. restrainer
c. activator
d. preservative

_____ 18. Which one of these agents reduces the exposed silver bromide crystals to metallic silver?
a. fixing
b. developing
c. hardener
d. preservative

_____ 19. If the intensifying screen speed is increased, unsharpness _____________ and recorded detail _____________:
a. increases, decreases
b. increases, increases
c. decreases, increases
d. decreases, decreases

Using this diagram, place an A or B on the answer line for questions 20–22.

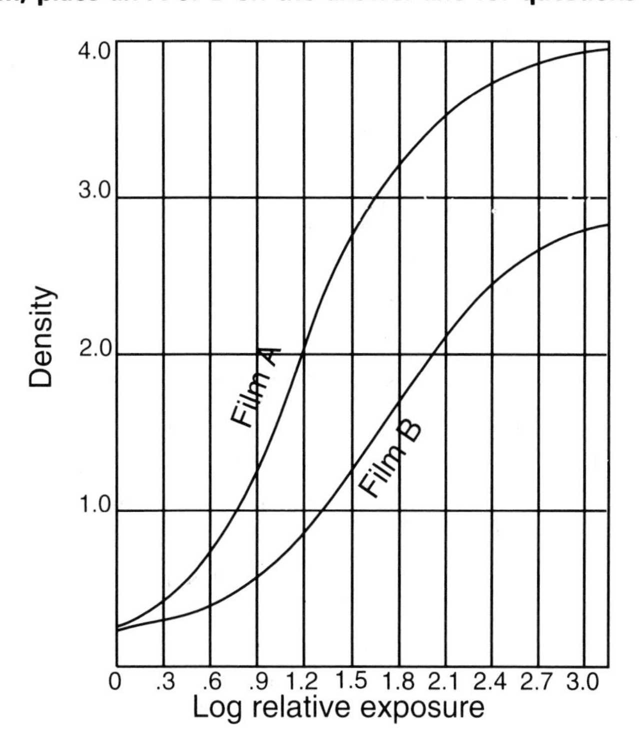

_____ 20. This film will display the most density.

_____ 21. This film will display long scale contrast.

_____ 22. This film will give the most exposure latitude.

_____ 23. Which chemical is responsible for producing the gray tones of the image?
a. acetic acid
b. hydroquinone
c. phenidone
d. sodium sulfite

_____ 24. Which one of these has the least effect on recorded detail?
a. SID
b. OID
c. screen speed
d. film speed

_____ 25. Where is base-plus-fog measured?
a. on a high-density step
b. on a medium-density step
c. on a low-density step
d. on any blank area of the film

_____ 26. The ability of an imaging system to record two adjacent structures as separate structures is:
a. recorded detail
b. visibility of detail
c. resolution
d. unsharpness

_____ 27. If magnification increases:
a. recorded detail decreases
b. recorded detail increases

_____ 28. The blue tint of the film base stops how much light from getting through it?
a. 10%
b. 15%
c. 50%
d. 85%

_____ 29. Which is the correct order for film travel through the processor?
a. developer, fixer, wash, dryer
b. fixer, developer, wash, dryer
c. wash, developer, dryer, fixer
d. dryer, fixer, developer, wash

_____ 30. The latent image is on the film:
a. after development
b. after exposure and before development
c. before exposure
d. after exposure and development

_____ 31. A developer temperature that is too high may:
a. increase distortion
b. increase contrast
c. increase recorded detail
d. increase density

_____ 32. Light diffusion is caused by:
a. an increased object-image distance
b. the space between the phosphor and film
c. x-rays striking the front of the cassette
d. x-rays striking the patient

_____ 33. Which one of these intensifying screen speeds would produce the best recorded detail?
a. 100 speed
b. 200 speed
c. 300 speed
d. 400 speed

_____ 34. Which one of these systems has the best conversion efficiency?
a. direct exposure
b. calcium tungstate
c. rare earth
d. computed radiography

_____ 35. Calculate the amount of unsharpness with these conditions: 20 mAs, 70 kVp, 1.5-mm focal spot, 2.5mm Al filtration, 94 degree developer temperature, 2 inch OID, 72 inch SID. Write your answer on the answer line.

_____ 36. Calculate the new mAs to be used when changing from a 200-speed screen to a 600-speed screen when the original exposure factors were: 500 mA, .05 sec, 80 kVp, 12:1 grid. Write your answer on the answer line.

_____ 37. Which term is the same as density in a computed radiography system?
a. brightness
b. gray scale
c. resolution
d. matrix

_____ 38. A quality control system for an automatic processor measures:
a. speed, accuracy, contrast
b. brightness, contrast, and base-plus-fog
c. contrast, slope, and resolution
d. speed, contrast, and base-plus-fog

_____ 39. Which gets replenished in an automatic processor?
a. wash, developer, and fixer
b. dryer, developer, and fixer
c. fixer and developer
d. developer and wash

_____ 40. What controls the film feeding rate and the replenishment rate?
a. the fixer and developer
b. the entrance rollers
c. the turnarounds and crossovers
d. the offset rollers

ACTIVITY 13.G

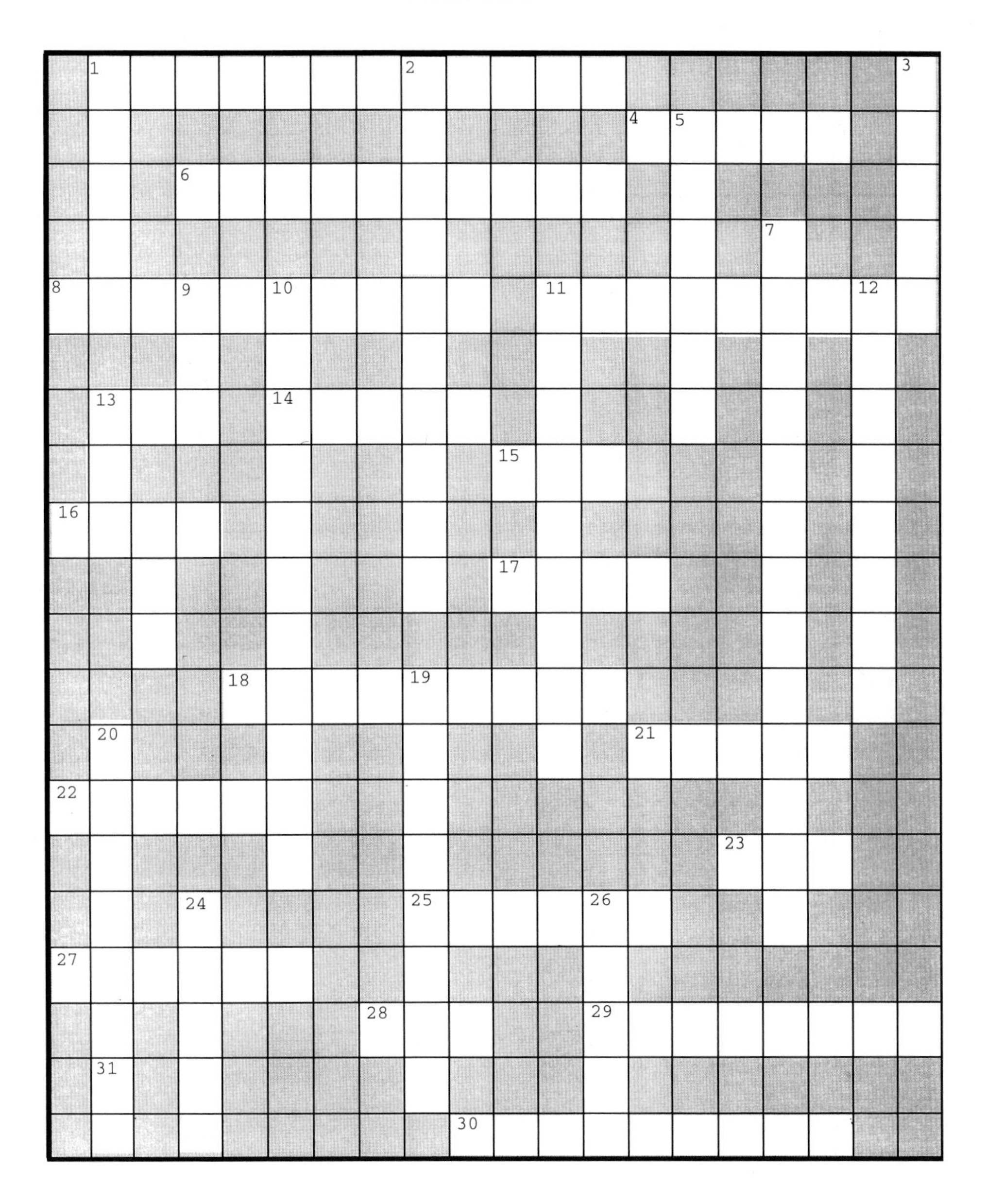

Across Clues

1. This film layer protects the emulsion from being scratched.
4. Hydroquinone develops the _____________ areas of the film.
6. This is the type of film used to produce an image of teeth.
8. This is good when a large number of line pairs per millimeter are imaged.
11. Silver bromide is reduced to metallic silver in this section of the processor.
13. Increasing this distance reduces unsharpness and increases recorded detail.
14. Another name for film sensitivity.
15. A computed radiography image may be seen on this device.
16. This part of the film is made of polyester.

Clues continued on following page.

Across Clues

17. This section of the processor removes all the developing chemicals.
18. Recorded detail decreases if OID ______________.
21. If an area of a screen receives little radiation, the area of the film will be developed ______________?
22. One way of increasing screen speed is to increase the ______________ of phosphor crystals.
23. The area of underexposure of a characteristic curve.
25. A ______________ emulsion film has emulsion on only one side of the base.
27. A descriptive term for a 100-speed screen.
28. A high developer temperature may produce this increased film density.
29. Another name for the developing agent.
30. The part of the characteristic curve where the film is beginning to respond to the radiation.

Down Clues

1. The contrast of a film is read on this part of the characteristic curve.
2. This characteristic of a film allows it to be placed in an alkali and acid solution.
3. The unexposed and undeveloped silver bromide crystals are removed by this agent.
5. The image on the film after exposure and before development.
7. Putting fixer in the developer will result in ______________ of the processing chemicals.
9. Recorded detail decreases if this distance is increased.
10. A large focal spot increases this.
11. If the screen speed is changed from 100 to 600, recorded detail ______________.
12. These processor rollers control the replenishment rate.
13. Recorded detail increases with a ______________ focal spot.
19. This part of the film contains silver bromide and gelatin.
20. This agent is in both the fixer and developer.
24. A small element of a computer matrix
26. The film will be developed black if it receives a ______________ amount of light from the screen.

NAME ______________________________

DATE ______________________________

ACTIVITY 13.H

H K P A D H E S I V E F M S H P M

G L U T A R A L D E H Y D E F E A

F J M W S E O K R P M Z A A H M T

T N O I R T A T R S D A O T U M R

T Y D R O E L E A W E Q R I Y J I

S P U E H M V Q Y R V A N E D F X

A X B M P O U P M T E I L D I R R

R Y I E S T W G I E L L L X R E X

T J F S O I G T R O O A E E U S E

N P O H H S B A D W P R R C S T Z

O R T O P N R A G F E I Q G C R U

C Q Q P G E G R J U R X S O E A M

E C N E C S E R O U L F P O M I W

V I N C R E A S E S C E M A D N H

D O K E N O D I N E H P S T E E P

U L J L Y Q V P O L Y E S T E R J

See questions on following page.

ACTIVITY 13.H

WORD SEARCH—RECORDED DETAIL

Decide which word best matches the definition or completes the sentence. Write the word on the appropriate answer line, then circle the word in the puzzle.

_______________ 1. The chemical that develops the gray tones of the image

_______________ 2. A rare earth phosphor

_______________ 3. The hardener used in developer

_______________ 4. This controls the resolution of a computed radiography system

_______________ 5. The ability of a phosphor to give off light when struck by x-rays

_______________ 6. What new mAs should be used when changing from a 200-speed screen to a 400-speed screen when the original mAs was 12?

_______________ 7. This device is used to test a cassette for poor screen contact (2 words)

_______________ 8. The agent that contains the chemical potassium bromide

_______________ 9. The developing agent that makes the solution an alkali

_______________ 10. This radiographic quality is read on the slope of a characteristic curve

_______________ 11. The color of light given off by rare earth screens (2 words)

_______________ 12. This device is used to produce a step wedge image for processor quality control

_______________ 13. A film that gives little exposure latitude would have this type of slope

_______________ 14. This film layer is between the base and the emulsion

_______________ 15. These rollers guide the film as it travels from one automatic processor section to another

_______________ 16. The multiplication factor for an intensifying screen with a relative speed value of 50

_______________ 17. This processor chemical is an acid solution

_______________ 18. If SID increases, recorded detail _______________

_______________ 19. Film base is made of this material

_______________ 20. Recorded detail decreases with a _______________ focal spot

_______________ 21. This has the ability to give off light when struck by x-rays

_______________ 22. The film emulsion swells in this processor section

_______________ 23. This distance is directly proportional to recorded detail

_______________ 24. This type of intensifying screen was developed in the 1970s

_______________ 25. If this distance increases, unsharpness increases and recorded detail decreases

NAME ______________________

DATE ______________________

ACTIVITY 14.A

DENSITY

A good radiograph was produced using the factors listed. Each change is made independently. Indicate the effect on density after each change.

+ for increase — for decrease 0 for no change

Good Radiograph:

600 mA	60 kVp	2.0-mm focal spot	2.0-mm filtration
1/10 sec	48″ SID	16:1 grid ratio	300-speed screen
60 mAs	6″ OID	8 × 10 collimation field size	92° developer temperature

Factors Changed	Effect on Density
200 mA	
1/15 sec	
30 mAs	
70 kVp	
68″ SID	
4″ OID	
1.5-mm focal spot	
6:1 grid ratio	
10 × 12 collimation field size	
2.5-mm filtration	
100-speed screen	
96° developer temperature	

NAME ____________________

DATE ____________________

ACTIVITY 14.B

DENSITY

A good radiograph was produced using the factors listed. Each change is made independently. Indicate the effect on density after each change.

+ for increase — for decrease 0 for no change

Good Radiograph:

400 mA	70 kVp	1.2-mm focal spot	3.0-mm filtration
15 msec	36″ SID	5:1 grid ratio	400-speed screen
6 mAs	2″ OID	10 × 12 collimation field size	96° developer temperature

Factors Changed	Effect on Density
600 mA	
25 msec	
3 mAs	
80 kVp	
56″ SID	
10″ OID	
2.0-mm focal spot	
12:1 grid ratio	
8 × 10 collimation field size	
2.0-mm filtration	
50-speed screen	
88° developer temperature	

NAME ____________________

DATE ____________________

ACTIVITY 14.C

DENSITY

A good radiograph was produced using the factors listed. Each change is made independently. Indicate the effect on density after each change.

+ for increase — for decrease 0 for no change

Good Radiograph:

300 mA	75 kVp	1.2-mm focal spot	2.5-mm filtration
.03 sec	44″ SID	16:1 grid ratio	200-speed screen
9 mAs	6″ OID	8 × 10 collimation field size	94° developer temperature

Factors Changed	Effect on Density
100 mA	
.04 sec	
12 mAs	
85 kVp	
56″ SID	
2″ OID	
.6-mm focal spot	
12:1 grid ratio	
14 × 17 collimation field size	
3.5-mm filtration	
100-speed screen	
89° developer temperature	

NAME ______________________________

DATE ______________________________

ACTIVITY 14.D

CONTRAST

A good radiograph was produced using the factors listed. Each change is made independently. Indicate the effect on contrast after each change.

+ for increase — for decrease 0 for no change

Good Radiograph:

600	mA	90	kVp	2.0-mm	focal spot	2.5-mm	filtration
1/20	sec	68″	SID	6:1	grid ratio	100-speed	screen
30	mAs	2″	OID	14 × 17	collimation field size	93°	developer temperature

Factors Changed	Effect on Contrast
200 mA	none
1/40 sec	none
40 mAs	none
70 kVp	increase contrast (short scale
62″ SID	none
6″ OID	increase / air gap
1.2-mm focal spot	none
12:1 grid ratio	increase
8 × 10 collimation field size	increase
3.5-mm filtration	decrease
200-speed screen	none
96° developer temperature	decrease

NAME ______________________

DATE ______________________

ACTIVITY 14.E

CONTRAST

A good radiograph was produced using the factors listed. Each change is made independently. Indicate the effect on contrast after each change.

+ for increase — for decrease 0 for no change

Good Radiograph:

600 mA	82 kVp	.6-mm	focal spot	3.0-mm filtration
2/5 sec	72″ SID	No grid		50-speed screen
240 mAs	2″ OID	14 × 17	collimation field size	96° developer temperature

Factors Changed	Effect on Contrast
400 mA	~~None~~ 0
3/5 sec	0
140 mAs	0
70 kVp	+
40″ SID	0
6″ OID	+
1.2-mm focal spot	0
6 : 1 grid ratio	+
8 × 10 collimation field size	+
2.5-mm filtration	+
100-speed screen	⊕
88° developer temperature	0 —

NAME ____________________

DATE ____________________

ACTIVITY 14.F

CONTRAST

A good radiograph was produced using the factors listed. Each change is made independently. Indicate the effect on contrast after each change.

+ for increase — for decrease 0 for no change

Good Radiograph:

50	mA	60	kVp	1.5-mm	focal spot	2.0-mm	filtration
.2	sec	72″	SID	12:1	grid ratio	100-speed	screen
10	mAs	3″	OID	10 × 12	collimation field size	94°	developer temperature

Factors Changed	Effect on Contrast
400 mA	0
.4 sec	0
15 mAs	0
75 kVp	—
60″ SID	0
9″ OID	+
.3-mm focal spot	0
6:1 grid ratio	—
14 × 17 collimation field size	—
3.0-mm filtration	—
300-speed screen	0
100° developer temperature	decrease —

NAME ______________________

DATE ______________________

ACTIVITY 14.G

RECORDED DETAIL

A good radiograph was produced using the factors listed. Each change is made independently. Indicate the effect on recorded detail after each change.

+ for increase — for decrease 0 for no change

Good Radiograph:

800	mA	78	kVp	1.5-mm	focal spot	2.5-mm filtration
25	msec	72″	SID	16:1	grid ratio	200-speed screen
20	mAs	4″	OID	10 × 12	collimation field size	93° developer temperature

Factors Changed	**Effect on Recorded Detail**
500 mA	0
45 msec	—
40 mAs	0
74 kVp	0
40″ SID	—
1″ OID	+
.6-mm focal spot	+
12:1 grid ratio	0
8 × 10 collimation field size	0
3.5-mm filtration	0
400-speed screen	+
95° developer temperature	0

NAME ______________________

DATE ______________________

ACTIVITY 14.H

RECORDED DETAIL

A good radiograph was produced using the factors listed. Each change is made independently. Indicate the effect on recorded detail after each change.

+ for increase   − for decrease   0 for no change

Good Radiograph:

100	mA	50	kVp	.6 mm	focal spot	2.5-mm filtration	
1/20	sec	40″	SID	8:1	grid ratio	50-speed screen	
5	mAs	2″	OID	8 × 10	collimation field size	90° developer temperature	

Factors Changed	Effect on Recorded Detail
200 mA	0
1/60 sec	+
4 mAs	0
60 kVp	0
72″ SID	+
6″ OID	−
1.2-mm focal spot	−
12:1 grid ratio	0
10 × 12 collimation field size	0
3.0-mm filtration	0
100-speed screen	+
92° developer temperature	0

NAME ______________________

DATE ______________________

ACTIVITY 14.I

RECORDED DETAIL

A good radiograph was produced using the factors listed. Each change is made independently. Indicate the effect on recorded detail after each change.

+ for increase — for decrease 0 for no change

Good Radiograph:

400	mA	85	kVp	1.5-mm	focal spot	3.0-mm filtration	
.01	sec	56″	SID	16:1	grid ratio	400-speed screen	
4	mAs	10″	OID	14 × 17	collimation field size	95° developer temperature	

Factors Changed	Effect on Recorded Detail
100 mA	0
.035 sec	
7 mAs	0
72 kVp	0
40″ SID	
3″ OID	
.6-mm focal spot	
8:1 grid ratio	
10 × 12 collimation field size	
2.0-mm filtration	
200-speed screen	
92° developer temperature	

NAME ______________________

DATE ______________________

ACTIVITY 14.J

DISTORTION

A good radiograph was produced using the factors listed. Each change is made independently. Indicate the effect on distortion after each change.

+ for increase − for decrease 0 for no change

Good Radiograph:

500 mA	72 kVp	1.5-mm focal spot	3.0-mm filtration
.015 sec	50″ SID	12:1 grid ratio	100-speed screen
7.5 mAs	8″ OID	10 × 12 collimation field size	94° developer temperature

Factors Changed	Effect on Distortion
200 mA	
.02 sec	
5.8 mAs	
68 kVp	
68″ SID	
4″ OID	
1.0-mm focal spot	
16:1 grid ratio	
14 × 17 collimation field size	
2.5-mm filtration	
200-speed screen	
92° developer temperature	

NAME ____________________

DATE ____________________

ACTIVITY 14.K

DISTORTION

A good radiograph was produced using the factors listed. Each change is made independently. Indicate the effect on distortion after each change.

+ for increase — for decrease 0 for no change

Good Radiograph:

600 mA	60 kVp	.6-mm focal spot	2.5-mm filtration
.2 sec	40″ SID	5:1 grid ratio	400-speed screen
120 mAs	10″ OID	8 × 10 collimation field size	90° developer temperature

Factors Changed	Effect on Distortion
500 mA	
.15 sec	
16 mAs	
70 kVp	
32″ SID	
6″ OID	
.3-mm focal spot	
6:1 grid ratio	
10 × 12 collimation field size	
2.0-mm filtration	
800-speed screen	
96° developer temperature	

NAME ______________________

DATE ______________________

ACTIVITY 14.L

RELATIONSHIP OF ALL FACTORS

A good radiograph was produced using the factors listed. Each change is made independently. Indicate the effect on all of the radiographic qualities after each change.

+ for increase — for decrease 0 for no change

Good Radiograph:

300	mA	70	kVp	1.2-mm	focal spot	3.0-mm filtration
.05	sec	72″	SID	6:1	grid ratio	200-speed screen
15	mAs	2″	OID	10 × 12	collimation field size	94° developer temperature

Factors	Density	Contrast	Recorded Detail	Distortion
200 mA				
.07 sec				
10 mAs				
80 kVp				
40″ SID				
7″ OID				
.3-mm focal spot				
12:1 grid ratio				
8 × 10 field size				
2.5-mm filtration				
100-speed screen				
88° developer temperature				

NAME ____________________

DATE ____________________

ACTIVITY 14.M

RELATIONSHIP OF ALL FACTORS

A good radiograph was produced using the factors listed. Each change is made independently. Indicate the effect on all of the radiographic qualities after each change.

+ for increase — for decrease 0 for no change

Good Radiograph:

600	mA	90	kVp	.6-mm	focal spot	2.5-mm filtration
1/20	sec	48″	SID	12:1	grid ratio	400-speed screen
30	mAs	8″	OID	8 × 10	collimation field size	93° developer temperature

Factors	Density	Contrast	Recorded Detail	Distortion
500 mA				
1/40 sec				
40 mAs				
75 kVp				
60″ SID				
4″ OID				
1.2-mm focal spot				
5:1 grid ratio				
14 × 17 field size				
3.0-mm filtration				
200-speed screen				
98° developer temperature				

NAME ____________________

DATE ____________________

ACTIVITY 14.N

RELATIONSHIP OF ALL FACTORS

A good radiograph was produced using the factors listed. Each change is made independently. Indicate the effect on all of the radiographic qualities after each change.

+ for increase — for decrease 0 for no change

Good Radiograph:

50	mA	80	kVp	1.2-mm	focal spot		2.5-mm filtration
15	msec	60″	SID	5:1	grid ratio		300-speed screen
.75	mAs	2″	OID	8 × 10	collimation field size		95° developer temperature

Factors	Density	Contrast	Recorded Detail	Distortion
100 mA				
25 msec				
1 mAs				
60 kVp				
40″ SID				
9″ OID				
.6-mm focal spot				
12:1 grid ratio				
10 × 12 field size				
2.0-mm filtration				
500-speed screen				
98° developer temperature				

NAME ____________________

DATE ____________________

ACTIVITY 14.0

RELATIONSHIP OF ALL FACTORS

A good radiograph was produced using the factors listed. Each change is made independently. Indicate the effect on all of the radiographic qualities after each change.

+ for increase — for decrease 0 for no change

Good Radiograph:

300 mA	80 kVp	1.2-mm focal spot	2.0-mm filtration
.01 sec	48″ SID	6:1 grid ratio	50-speed screen
3 mAs	6″ OID	10 × 12 collimation field size	94° developer temperature

Factors	Density	Contrast	Recorded Detail	Distortion
200 mA				
.04 sec				
2 mAs				
60 kVp				
56″ SID				
3″ OID				
2.0-mm focal spot				
12:1 grid ratio				
8 × 10 field size				
1.2-mm filtration				
100-speed screen				
87° developer temperature				

NAME ______________________

DATE ______________________

ACTIVITY 15.A

Calculate the following:

mAs

1. 200 mA and .05 sec = __________
2. 600 mA and 1/5 sec = __________
3. 400 mA and 30 sec = __________

mA

4. 30 mAs and .2 sec = __________
5. 10 mAs and 1/40 sec = __________
6. 8 mAs and 20 msec = __________

Time

7. 12 mAs and 200 mA = __________
8. 8 mAs and 500 mA = __________
9. 15 mAs and 300 mA = __________

Reciprocity

10. 200 mA and .12 sec = __________
11. Calculate another mA and time that will equal the same mAs calculated in problem 10.

    mA __________ time __________

12. 500 mA and 1/20 sec = __________
13. Calculate another mA and time that will equal the same mAs calculated in problem 12.

    mA __________ time __________

The Density Maintenance Formula

	New mAs	Old mAs	New distance	Old distance
14.	__________	6	72	40
15.	__________	14	56	48
16.	__________	22	40	66

The 15% Rule

	New kVp	New mAs	Old mAs	Old kVp
17.	__________	15	30	68
18.	__________	40	20	75
19.	65	__________	12	75
20.	90	__________	6	80

Grid Ratio

	New mAs	Old mAs	Old grid ratio	New grid ratio
21.	______________	20	6:1	16:1
22.	______________	14	12:1	5:1
23.	______________	8	16:1	8:1
24.	______________	24	5:1	8:1

Collimation Field Size

	New mAs	Old mAs	Old field size	New field size
25.	______________	10	8 × 10	10 × 12
26.	______________	6	14 × 17	8 × 10
27.	______________	22	10 × 12	14 × 17

Intensifying Screen Speed

	Multiplication factor	Screen speed
28.	______________	500
29.	______________	300
30.	______________	800

	New mAs	Old mAs	Old screen	New screen
31.	______________	5	200	400
32.	______________	16	500	300
33.	______________	22	600	100

X-Ray Generation

	New mAs	Old mAs	Old generator	New generator
34.	______________	6	Single phase	Three phase
35.	______________	4.5	Three phase	Single phase

NAME ______________________

DATE ______________________

ACTIVITY 15.B

Calculate the following:

mAs

1. 500 mA and .02 sec = ____________
2. 300 mA and 1/15 sec = ____________
3. What mAs is achieved with an mA of 400 and a time of .025 sec?

mA

4. 30 mAs and .15 sec = ____________
5. 40 mAs and 1/20 sec = ____________
6. If a mAs of 15 is desired at a time station of .025 sec, what mA station would be necessary?

Time

7. 6 mAs and 300 mA = ____________
8. 24 mAs and 600 mA = ____________
9. If 200 mA is used to produce 10 mAs, what time station must be used?

Use these mA and time stations for problems 10–13.

mA	Time	
25 small focal spot	.01	.30
50	.02	.40
100	.025	.50
200	.03	.70
300 large focal spot	.05	1.0
400	.10	2.0
500	.15	3.0
600	.20	4.0

Reciprocity

10. List three sets of mA and time settings that would produce 10 mAs.

    mA ____________ time ____________

    mA ____________ time ____________

    mA ____________ time ____________

11. The original exposure factors are 500 mA and .15 sec. Change this to a breathing technique.

    mA ____________ time ____________

12. The original exposure factors are 100 mA and .25 sec. Change this to a better technique to control motion.

    mA ____________ time ____________

13. The original exposure factors are 600 mA and .05 sec. Change this to a technique which would produce better recorded detail.

    mA ____________ time ____________

The Density Maintenance Formula

	New mAs	Old mAs	New distance	Old distance
14.	____________	12	72	40
15.	____________	5	56	48

16. The SID is changed from 72 inches to 50 inches. The original mAs was 15. What new mAs is required to maintain film density at the new SID?

The 15% Rule

	New kVp	New mAs	Old mAs	Old kVp
17.	____________	10	20	70
18.	80	____________	7.5	90

19. The original exposure factors are 5 mAs at 90 kVp. Change this to a technique that would produce higher contrast.
20. The original exposure factors are 500 mA, .5 sec, at 70 kVp. Change this to a technique that would control motion better.

Grid Ratio

	New mAs	Old mAs	Old grid ratio	New grid ratio
21.	____________	10	5:1	16:1
22.	____________	6	8:1	6:1
23.	____________	2.5	16:1	8:1

24. The original mAs of 20 was used with a 5:1 grid ratio. If the grid ratio is changed to a 12:1, what new mAs would be required to maintain the original radiographic density?

Collimation Field Size

	New mAs	Old mAs	Old field size	New field size
25.	____________	15	14 × 17	10 × 12
26.	____________	4	8 × 10	10 × 12

27. A KUB was taken on a 14 × 17 using 7.5 mAs at 70 kVp. The radiologist wants a "coned down" view of the right upper quadrant on a 10 × 12. What new mAs would be required?

Intensifying Screen Speed

	Multiplication factor	Screen speed
28.	____________	600
29.	____________	200

	New mAs	Old mAs	Old screen	New screen
30.	____________	15	300	800
31.	____________	6	500	200

32. The ordinary technique for an AP skull is 500 mA, .02 sec., and 80 kVp on a 200-speed intensifying screen. Motion is likely to be a problem on an emergency patient, so a 400-speed intensifying screen is used. What new exposure factors are required?

33. An AP knee is performed at 1.25 mAs and 70 kVp using a 400-speed screen. The radiologist suspects a bony lesion at the medial malleolus and needs a film with good recorded detail. It is decided to change to a screen with a speed of 50. What new mAs is required?

X-Ray Generation

	New mAs	Old mAs	Old generator	New generator
34.	____________	5	Three phase	Single phase
35.	____________	7	Single phase	Three phase

NAME ____________________

DATE ____________________

ACTIVITY 15.C

Use this control panel for the problems in this activity.

mA	Time		kVp
25 small focal spot	.01	.30	50
50	.02	.40	60
100	.025	.50	70
200	.03	.70	80
300 large focal spot	.05	1.0	90
400	.10	2.0	100
500	.15	3.0	110
600	.20	4.0	120

1. An exposure of 2.5 mAs at 70 kVp is required on a lower leg. The radiologist wants to see very good recorded detail. What mA and time should be used?

   mA ____________ time ____________

2. The non-breathing technique for a lateral thoracic spine is 50 mAs at 70 kVp. Change this to a breathing technique.

   mA ____________ time ____________ kVp ____________

3. A lateral skull technique calls for 5 mAs at 80 kVp. Choose an mA and time to best control motion.

   mA ____________ time ____________

4. A KUB taken at 400 mA, .1 sec, and 80 kVp on a large patient shows poor contrast. What exposure factors would improve the contrast?

   mA ____________ time ____________ kVp ____________

5. A lateral skull taken at a 40-inch SID, 500 mA, .01 sec, and 80 kVp shows a possible enlarged sella turcica. The radiologist would like another lateral skull taken with a 72-inch SID to show the true size of the sella turcica. What exposure factors should be used?

   mA ____________ time ____________ kVp ____________

6. Internal and external rotation views of the shoulder taken at 400 mA, .01 sec, 75 kVp, with a 6:1 grid ratio show poor contrast. A switch is made to a 16:1 grid ratio to improve the contrast. What new exposure factors should be used?

   mA ____________ time ____________ kVp ____________

7. An AP lumbar spine is taken on a 14 × 17 at 500 mA, .1 sec, 80 kVp. The radiologist suspects a bony lesion on L-2 and would like a coned-down view taken on an 8 × 10. What new exposure factors should be used?

   mA ____________ time ____________ kVp ____________

8. An oblique wrist is taken on a 400-speed intensifying screen at 50 mA, .025 sec, and 60 kVp. The radiologist suspects a fracture of the navicular and would like another film taken on a 50-speed intensifying screen. What new exposure factors should be used?

   mA ____________time ____________ kVp ____________

9. The ordinary technique for an AP skull is 500 mA, .02 sec, at 80 kVp. Use the 15% rule to derive new exposure factors that will reduce the chance of motion on an uncooperative patient.

   mA ____________ time ____________ kVp ____________

10. The ordinary technique for an AP shoulder is 500 mA, .01 sec, at 70 kVp on a 12:1 Bucky. A patient from the emergency room cannot move from a stretcher onto the x-ray table. A cassette can be slipped gently underneath the sheet between the stretcher pad and the patient's arm, and the exposure can be made without moving the patient. Since lining up the beam and grid may be a problem, it is decided not to use a grid. What new exposure factors should be used?

   mA ____________ time ____________ kVp ____________

NAME ______________________________

DATE ______________________________

ACTIVITY 16.A

Calculate the new mAs, mA, or time required for column B.

	A		B	
1.	200	mA	500	mA
	1/2	sec	__________	sec
	6:1	grid	12:1	grid
	30″	SID	40″	SID
2.	400	mA	__________	mA
	.04	sec	.02	sec
	64	kVp	74	kVp
	100	RSV	200	RSV
3.	400	mA	200	mA
	.02	sec	__________	sec
	65″	SID	45″	SID
	200	RSV	100	RSV
	Single	phase	Three	phase
4.	600	mA	__________	mA
	1/15	sec	1/20	sec
	75	kVp	85	kVp
	56″	SID	40″	SID
	6:1	grid	16:1	grid
5.	20	mAs	__________	mAs
	40″	SID	48″	SID
	80	kVp	90	kVp
	8:1	grid	12:1	grid
	8 × 10	collimation	10 × 12	collimation
6.	400	mA	500	mA
	1/4	sec	__________	sec
	80	kVp	70	kVp
	16:1	grid	6:1	grid
	100	RSV	400	RSV
7.	100	mAs	__________	mAs
	70	kVp	80	kVp
	14 × 17	collimation	10 × 12	collimation
	72″	SID	44″	SID
	Three	phase	Single	phase
8.	100	mAs	__________	mAs
	8:1	grid	12:1	grid
	200	RSV	500	RSV
	40″	SID	72″	SID

	A		B	
	00	mA	400	mA
	3	sec	______	sec
	40″	SID	72″	SID
	60	kVp	70	kVp
	12:1	grid	6:1	grid
10.	500	mA	______	mA
	.10	sec	.4	sec
	54	kVp	62	kVp
	400	RSV	50	RSV
	14 × 17	collimation	8 × 10	collimation
11.	100	mA	______	mA
	1/2	sec	1/5	sec
	12:1	grid	5:1	grid
	500	RSV	100	RSV
12.	200	mA	200	mA
	1/4	sec	______	sec
	16:1	grid	12:1	grid
	40″	SID	50″	SID
13.	500	mA	200	mA
	50	msec	______	msec
	70	kVp	80	kVp
	400	RSV	100	RSV
14.	200	mAs	______	mAs
	600	RSV	200	RSV
	72″	SID	48″	SID
	8 × 10	collimation	14 × 17	collimation
	Three	phase	Single	phase
15.	15	mAs	______	mAs
	36″	SID	50″	SID
	90	kVp	80	kVp
	12:1	grid	6:1	grid
	50	RSV	200	RSV
	8 × 10	collimation	10 × 12	collimation

NAME ______________________

DATE ______________________

ACTIVITY 16.B

Use the following control panel for the problems in this activity.

mA	Time		kVp
25 small focal spot	.01	.30	50
50	.02	.40	60
100	.025	.50	70
200	.03	.70	80
300 large focal spot	.05	1.0	90
400	.10	2.0	100
500	.15	3.0	110
600	.20	4.0	120

1. A technique of 200 mA, .25 sec, and 80 kVp, was used for an abdomen on a very large patient. A 6:1 grid was also used. The density was OK, but the contrast was too low. It was decided to switch to a 16:1 grid and 70 kVp. The original radiograph was taken using single-phase equipment and the repeat radiograph has to be taken using three-phase equipment. What new exposure factors should be used for the repeat film?

   mA ____________ time ____________ kVp____________

2. The ordinary technique for an AP skull is 100 mA, .20 sec, at 80 kVp on a 200-speed screen. On an uncooperative patient, it is decided to increase the kVp using the 15% rule and also increase the screen speed to 400 in order to control motion. What exposure factors should be used for this film?

   mA ____________ time ____________ kVp ____________

3. The ordinary technique for a lateral thoracic spine is 40 mAs at 70 kVp. This would be performed on a 500-speed screen on a 14 × 17 size film. A spot of the lower thoracic area is required with very good recorded detail and a breathing technique. It is decided to change to a 200-speed screen to improve the recorded detail, and also to use an 8 × 10 inch film. What exposure factors should be used for this film?

   mA ____________ time ____________ kVp ____________

4. The technique in the department for a patient of average size for a lateral femur is 600 mA, .02 sec, at 70 kVp. This is exposed using a 8:1 grid. A patient in the emergency room requires a portable lateral femur. It is decided to do this non-grid, and the highest mA available on the portable machine is 200. The patient is also an emaciated elderly lady. What exposure factors should be used for this film?

   mA ____________ time ____________ kVp ____________

5. The ordinary technique in the department for an AP hip on a patient of average size is 600 mA, .05 sec, at 70 kVp. This is exposed using a 12:1 grid at a 40-inch SID. A portable AP hip is requested on a very large patient. The stationary grids are 6:1 ratio. The patient is in traction and the maximum SID that can be achieved is 34 inches. The highest mA station on the portable machine is 200. What exposure factors should be used for this film?

   mA ____________ time ____________ kVp ____________

NAME ______________________

DATE ______________________

ACTIVITY 16.B

Use the following control panel for the problems in this activity.

mA	Time		kVp
25 small focal spot	.01	.30	50
50	.02	.40	60
100	.025	.50	70
200	.03	.70	80
300 large focal spot	.05	1.0	90
400	.10	2.0	100
500	.15	3.0	110
600	.20	4.0	120

1. A technique of 200 mA, .25 sec, and 80 kVp, was used for an abdomen on a very large patient. A 6:1 grid was also used. The density was OK, but the contrast was too low. It was decided to switch to a 16:1 grid and 70 kVp. The original radiograph was taken using single-phase equipment and the repeat radiograph has to be taken using three-phase equipment. What new exposure factors should be used for the repeat film?

   mA ____________ time ____________ kVp____________

2. The ordinary technique for an AP skull is 100 mA, .20 sec, at 80 kVp on a 200-speed screen. On an uncooperative patient, it is decided to increase the kVp using the 15% rule and also increase the screen speed to 400 in order to control motion. What exposure factors should be used for this film?

   mA ____________ time ____________ kVp ____________

3. The ordinary technique for a lateral thoracic spine is 40 mAs at 70 kVp. This would be performed on a 500-speed screen on a 14 × 17 size film. A spot of the lower thoracic area is required with very good recorded detail and a breathing technique. It is decided to change to a 200-speed screen to improve the recorded detail, and also to use an 8 × 10 inch film. What exposure factors should be used for this film?

   mA ____________ time ____________ kVp ____________

4. The technique in the department for a patient of average size for a lateral femur is 600 mA, .02 sec, at 70 kVp. This is exposed using a 8:1 grid. A patient in the emergency room requires a portable lateral femur. It is decided to do this non-grid, and the highest mA available on the portable machine is 200. The patient is also an emaciated elderly lady. What exposure factors should be used for this film?

   mA ____________ time ____________ kVp ____________

5. The ordinary technique in the department for an AP hip on a patient of average size is 600 mA, .05 sec, at 70 kVp. This is exposed using a 12:1 grid at a 40-inch SID. A portable AP hip is requested on a very large patient. The stationary grids are 6:1 ratio. The patient is in traction and the maximum SID that can be achieved is 34 inches. The highest mA station on the portable machine is 200. What exposure factors should be used for this film?

   mA ____________ time ____________ kVp ____________

NAME ________________________

DATE ________________________

ACTIVITY 16.C

1. Which one of these exposures would produce the *greatest* density?

A	B	C	D
100 mA	200 mA	200 mA	300 mA
3/4 sec	2 sec	1/2 sec	1 sec
80 kVp	70 kVp	80 kVp	70 kVp
40″ SID	72″ SID	42″ SID	36″ SID

2. Which one of these exposures would produce the *greatest* density?

A	B	C	D
200 mA	500 mA	500 mA	400 mA
.4 sec	.12 sec	.25 sec	.3 sec
72″ SID	60″ SID	72″ SID	64″ SID
6:1 grid	8:1 grid	16:1 grid	12:1 grid

3. Which one of these exposures would produce the *least* density?

A	B	C	D
300 mA	400 mA	1000 mA	800 mA
40 msec	30 msec	10 msec	20 msec
70 kVp	80 kVp	80 kVp	60 kVp
50 RSV	100 RSV	200 RSV	100 RSV
Three phase	Single phase	Three phase	Single phase

4. Which one of these exposures would produce the *greatest* density?

A	B	C	D
200 mA	100 mA	500 mA	600 mA
3/10 sec	1/2 sec	3/10 sec	2/10 sec
80 kVp	90 kVp	80 kVp	105 kVp
8:1 grid	6:1 grid	16:1 grid	8:1 grid
40″ SID	50″ SID	36″ SID	72″ SID

5. Which one of these exposures would produce the *greatest* density?

A	B	C	D
400 mA	300 mA	600 mA	500 mA
.05 sec	.07 sec	.02 sec	.03 sec
70 kVp	90 kVp	80 kVp	70 kVp
5:1 grid	12:1 grid	8:1 grid	16:1 grid
14 × 17 coll.	10 × 12 coll.	14 × 17 coll.	10 × 12 coll.

6. Which one of these exposures would produce the *greatest* density?

A	B	C	D
200 mA	100 mA	300 mA	100 mA
1/2 sec	2/10 sec	2/15 sec	3/5 sec
70 kVp	80 kVp	90 kVp	70 kVp
40″ SID	72″ SID	54″ SID	62″ SID
100 RSV	50 RSV	200 RSV	400 RSV

NAME ______________________

DATE ______________________

ACTIVITY 16.D

1. Which one of these exposures would produce the *greatest* density?

A		B		C		D	
500	mA	500	mA	100	mA	200	mAs
.2	sec	.1	sec	1	sec	1	sec
90	kVp	80	kVp	80	kVp	90	kVp
12:1	grid	16:1	grid	16:1	grid	8:1	grid
40″	SID	48″	SID	36″	SID	72″	SID

2. Which one of these exposures would produce the *greatest* density?

A		B		C		D	
100	mA	200	mA	400	mA	500	mA
1/2	sec	1/4	sec	1/8	sec	1/10	sec
48″	SID	36″	SID	40″	SID	62″	SID
80	kVp	80	kVp	70	kVp	80	kVp
12:1	grid	12:1	grid	16:1	grid	8:1	grid
100	RSV	100	RSV	50	RSV	200	RSV

3. Which one of these exposures would produce the *least* density?

A		B		C		D	
400	mA	300	mA	200	mA	500	mA
40	msec	60	msec	30	msec	10	msec
70	kVp	80	kVp	90	kVp	80	kVp
36″	SID	54″	SID	48″	SID	68″	SID
100	RSV	500	RSV	100	RSV	400	RSV

4. Which one of these exposures would produce the *least* density?

A		B		C		D	
200	mA	300	mA	50	mA	200	mA
1/2	sec	1/6	sec	1	sec	1/8	sec
70	kVp	80	kVp	70	kVp	80	kVp
40″	SID	50″	SID	40″	SID	60″	SID
Single	phase	Three	phase	Single	phase	Three	phase

5. Which one of these exposures would produce the *greatest* density?

A		B		C		D	
1000	mA	100	mA	800	ma	400	mA
.1	sec	.5	sec	.1	sec	.25	sec
90	kVp	104	kVp	80	kVp	80	kVp
12:1	grid	16:1	grid	8:1	grid	8:1	grid
14 × 17	coll.	8 × 10	coll.	10 × 12	coll.	14 × 17	coll.

6. Which one of these exposures would produce the *greatest* density?

A		B		C		D	
500	mA	600	mA	400	mA	500	mA
.05	sec	.03	sec	.015	sec	.01	sec
70	kVp	80	kVp	90	kVp	80	kVp
40″	SID	50″	SID	48″	SID	72″	SID
100	RSV	200	RSV	600	RSV	400	RSV

NAME ____________________

DATE ____________________

ACTIVITY 17.A

CHAPTER REVIEW

MULTIPLE CHOICE

_____ 1. It would be easier to decide whether to use a grid with which type of chart?
a. variable kVp
b. fixed kVp

_____ 2. Technique charts that list techniques by body part measurement usually vary the techniques for each measurement group by:
a. 10%
b. 20%
c. 30%
d. 50%

_____ 3. Which type of technique would produce the least radiation dose to the patient:
a. a high-kVp technique
b. a low-kVp technique

_____ 4. For a variable kVp chart, a difference of 1 cm in part measurement usually requires a kVp change of:
a. 1
b. 2
c. 4
d. 10

_____ 5. The kVp chosen for a fixed kVp chart should be?
a. any kVp as long as it is kept constant
b. 2 times the mAs
c. the optimum kVp for the body part
d. 80 kVp

_____ 6. In general, it takes more radiation exposure to produce a radiograph of a:
a. large patient
b. small patient

_____ 7. If the kVp is dropped very low when using a variable kVp chart it is possible to:
a. overpenetrate the body part
b. underpenetrate the body part

_____ 8. Which one of these radiographic qualities besides density is also changed when a variable kVp chart is used?
a. contrast
b. recorded detail
c. distortion

_____ 9. For a variable kVp chart, which factor is held constant?
a. kVp
b. mAs

_____ 10. An emaciated patient measures 18 cm for an AP lumbar spine. The technique chart calls for 30 mAs at 80 kVp. Which technique would be the best?
a. 25 mAs at 80 kVp
b. 30 mAs at 80 kVp
c. 40 mAs at 80 kVp
d. 50 mAs at 80 kVp

_____ 11. To calculate a correction for a new technique chart, divide:
a. the corrected mAs by the suggested mAs
b. the suggested mAs by the corrected mAs

_____ 12. A correctly formulated technique chart will work as listed about:
a. 10% of the time
b. 50% of the time
c. 85% of the time
d. 100% of the time

_____ 13. Which type of technique chart gives the radiographer the most exposure latitude?
a. variable kVp
b. fixed kVp

For questions 14–20, place an I before the pathology if the radiographer should increase the technique as listed on the chart because of the pathology, and a D before the pathology if the radiographer should decrease the technique as listed on the chart because of the pathology.

_____ 14. pneumonia
_____ 15. emphysema
_____ 16. congestive heart failure
_____ 17. ascites
_____ 18. a bowel obstruction with trapped air in the bowel
_____ 19. osteoporosis
_____ 20. multiple myeloma

ACTIVITY 18.A

LAB ASSIGNMENT—PHOTOCELL ARRANGEMENT

MATERIALS

A radiographic phantom that can be exposed using the Bucky (abdomen, chest, pelvis, skull)
Two loaded cassettes big enough to fit an image of the phantom you are using
A radiographic room equipped with automatic exposure control (phototiming)
A processor
A densitometer

PROCEDURE

For all exposures, place the phantom on the center of the x-ray tabletop. Detent the x-ray tube or center the x-ray tube to the Bucky tray. Use a 40″ SID and position the x-ray tube so that it is centered over the phantom. Do not angle the x-ray tube. Place the cassette in the Bucky tray and center the cassette to the x-ray tube and phantom. Adjust the collimation size to the size of the cassette or use automatic collimation. Activate the automatic exposure control on the control panel. Use a high mA station, the optimum kVp for the type of phantom, and set the backup time to .5 second. Set the phototimer density to the normal setting.

Exposure 1. Make the first exposure with the two outside photocells activated. Label this image exposure 1.

Exposure 2. Make the second exposure with the center photocell activated. Label this image exposure 2.

Answer the lab analysis questions.

NAME ______________________

DATE ______________________

ACTIVITY 18.A

LAB ANALYSIS—PHOTOCELL ARRANGEMENT

1. What type of phantom did you use for your experiment?

   ____

2. Using the densitometer, measure five spots within the image from both exposures. Measure one spot in the center of the image, and one spot on each of the four edges. Measure the same spots on each of the images. Record the readings.

	Exposure 1			Exposure 2	
	Edges	Center		Edges	Center
1.	____________	____________	1.	____________	____________
2.	____________		2.	____________	
3.	____________		3.	____________	
4.	____________		4.	____________	

3. Did the measurements from the two images differ? Explain.

   ____

   ____

   ____

4. Can you see a difference between the two images?

   ____

   ____

5. What do you conclude about the photocell arrangement from this activity?

   ____

   ____

   ____

ACTIVITY 18.B

LAB ASSIGNMENT—COVERING THE PHOTOCELL WITH THE BODY PART

MATERIALS

A small radiographic phantom that can be exposed using the Bucky (skull, knee)
Two loaded cassettes big enough to fit an image of the phantom you are using
A radiographic room equipped with automatic exposure control (phototiming)
A processor
A densitometer

PROCEDURE

For all exposures, place the phantom on the center of the x-ray tabletop. Detent the x-ray tube or center the x-ray tube to the Bucky tray. Use a 40-inch SID and position the x-ray tube so that it is centered over the phantom. Do not angle the x-ray tube. Place the cassette in the Bucky tray and center the cassette to the x-ray tube and phantom. Adjust the collimation size to the size of the cassette or use automatic collimation. Activate the automatic exposure control on the control panel. Use a high mA station, the optimum kVp for the type of phantom, and set the backup time to .5 second. Set the phototimer density to the normal setting. Activate the center photocell.

Exposure 1. Make the first exposure with the phantom centered as directed above. This should place the center of the phantom directly over the center photocell. Label this image exposure 1.

Exposure 2. Make the second exposure with the phantom placed so that the central ray is at the edge of the phantom. This should place the edge of the phantom directly over the center photocell. Label this image exposure 2. Answer the lab analysis questions.

NAME ______________________

DATE ______________________

ACTIVITY 18.B

LAB ANALYSIS—COVERING THE PHOTOCELL WITH THE BODY PART

1. What type of phantom did you use for your experiment?

   ____

2. Using the densitometer, measure five spots within the image from both exposures. Measure one spot in the center of the image, and one spot on each of the four edges. Measure the same spots on each of the images. Record the readings.

Exposure 1		Exposure 2	
Edges	Center	Edges	Center
1. ______	______	1. ______	______
2. ______		2. ______	
3. ______		3. ______	
4. ______		4. ______	

3. Did the measurements from the two images differ? Explain.

   ____

   ____

   ____

4. Can you see a difference between the two images?

   ____

   ____

5. What do you conclude about covering the photocell from this activity?

   ____

   ____

   ____

ACTIVITY 18.C

LAB ASSIGNMENT—CENTERING THE BODY PART OVER THE PHOTOCELL

MATERIALS

A radiographic phantom that can be exposed using the Bucky (abdomen, chest, pelvis)
Two loaded cassettes big enough to fit an image of the phantom you are using
A radiographic room equipped with automatic exposure control (phototiming)
A processor
A densitometer

PROCEDURE

For all the exposures, place the phantom on the center of the x-ray tabletop. Detent the x-ray tube or center the x-ray tube to the Bucky tray. Use a 40-inch SID and position the x-ray tube so that it is centered over the phantom. Do not angle the x-ray tube. Place the cassette in the Bucky tray and center the cassette to the x-ray tube and phantom. Adjust the collimation size to the size of the cassette or use automatic collimation. Activate the automatic exposure control on the control panel. Use a high mA station, the optimum kVp for the type of phantom, and set the backup time to .5 second. Set the phototimer density to the normal setting. Activate the center photocell.

Exposure 1. Make the first exposure with the phantom centered as directed above. This should place the spine portion of the phantom directly over the center photocell. Label this image exposure 1.

Exposure 2. Make the second exposure with the phantom off-centered laterally so that the central ray is directed 3 inches to one side of the spine. Label this image exposure 2.

Answer the lab analysis questions.

NAME ______________________

DATE ______________________

ACTIVITY 18.C

LAB ANALYSIS—CENTERING THE BODY PART OVER THE PHOTOCELL

1. What type of phantom did you use for your experiment?

   ____

2. Using the densitometer measure 5 spots within the image from both exposures. Measure one spot in the center of the image, and one spot on each of the 4 edges. Measure the same spots on each of the images. Record the readings.

Exposure 1		**Exposure 2**	
Edges	Center	Edges	Center
1. ____________	____________	1. ____________	____________
2. ____________		2. ____________	
3. ____________		3. ____________	
4. ____________		4. ____________	

3. Did the measurements from the two images differ? Explain.

   ____

   ____

   ____

4. Can you see a difference between the two images?

   ____

   ____

5. What do you conclude about centering the body part over the photocell from this activity?

   ____

   ____

   ____

NAME ______________________

DATE ______________________

ACTIVITY 18.D

CHAPTER REVIEW

MULTIPLE CHOICE

_____ 1. The device used to measure the exit radiation with automatic exposure control is a/an:
   a. exposure meter
   b. voltmeter
   c. ammeter
   d. photocell

_____ 2. When using automatic exposure control with the center photocell activated, if the centering point for an AP lumbar spine is over the liver instead of over the spine:
   a. the radiograph will be too light
   b. the radiograph will be too dark
   c. the radiograph should be good

_____ 3. The backup time should be set:
   a. above the expected exposure time
   b. below the expected exposure time
   c. equal to the expected exposure time
   d. at 1 second for all exposures

_____ 4. When using automatic exposure control with the center photocell activated, if the centering point for a lateral chest is at the level of T-11 instead of at T-6:
   a. the radiograph will be too light
   b. the radiograph will be too dark
   c. the radiograph should be good

_____ 5. If the center photocell is used instead of the two outside photocells for a PA chest exposure:
   a. the radiograph will be too light
   b. the radiograph will show motion
   c. the radiograph will have too much contrast
   d. the radiograph will be too dark

_____ 6. If a low mA is selected the automatic exposure control will:
   a. produce a radiograph with less density
   b. use a long exposure time
   c. increase the kVp
   d. produce a radiograph with more density

_____ 7. The kVp used for automatic exposure control should be:
   a. high
   b. low
   c. optimum
   d. set at 80 kVp for all exposures

_____ 8. Which one of these would be the best for a radiographer to do to control motion when using automatic exposure control?
a. decrease the back up time
b. increase the kVp
c. use a high mA
d. use a density setting lower than normal

_____ 9. When using automatic exposure control, the timer on the control panel:
a. determines the length of the exposure
b. is a backup time
c. doesn't serve any function
d. measures exit radiation

_____ 10. When using automatic exposure control, if the centering point for a lateral knee is at the patella and the center photocell is used:
a. the radiograph will be too light
b. the radiograph will be too dark
c. the radiograph should be good

_____ 11. Which one of these changes will produce a radiograph with higher contrast when using automatic exposure control?
a. decrease the mA
b. increase the back up time
c. decrease the kVp
d. decrease the density setting below normal

_____ 12. If the minimum reaction time is .01 second, what will happen to the radiograph if the required exposure time is .03 second
a. the radiograph will be too light
b. the radiograph will be too dark
c. the radiograph should be good

_____ 13. Which one of these changes will make the radiograph more dense when using automatic exposure control?
a. increase the mA
b. increase the back up time
c. increase the kVp
d. increase the density setting above normal

_____ 14. If the minimum reaction time is .01 second what should the radiographer do if the required exposure time on a very small patient is .005 second:
a. increase the back up time
b. increase the kVp
c. decrease the mA
d. decrease the density setting below normal

For questions 15–20, place an A if the center photocell should be used and a B if the two outside photocells should be used.

_____ 15. lateral chest

_____ 16. KUB

_____ 17. lateral thoracic spine

_____ 18. PA chest

_____ 19. lateral skull

_____ 20. AP left hip

Index